The importance of the ~~relation~~ processes and health has been increasingly recognised over recent years. The development of the field is reflected in the growth of disciplines such as health psychology, psychosocial epidemiology and behavioural medicine. Understanding the links between the social environment, emotion, behaviour and illness is a growing theme in medical and health education. The basic literature is, however, widely dispersed across medical and social science journals.

This book makes available within a single volume some of the most important articles that have been published over the past 30 years. The 31 articles are grouped round six themes: *Life stress, social support and health*; *Psychophysiological processes in disease*; *Personality, behaviour patterns and health*; *Health practices and the modification of health risk behaviour*; *Coping with illness and disability*; and *Behavioural interventions in medicine*. Each is prefaced by a state-of-the-art review of the theme by the editors. These readings will be a most valuable resource for medical, psychology and health sciences teachers, students and clinicians.

1

Psychosocial Processes and Health:
A Reader

Compiled and edited by

ANDREW STEPTOE

Department of Psychology,
St George's Hospital Medical School,
University of London

JANE WARDLE

Imperial Cancer Research Fund Health Behaviour Unit,
Institute of Psychiatry,
University of London

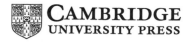
CAMBRIDGE
UNIVERSITY PRESS

Published by the Press Syndicate of the University of Cambridge
The Pitt Building, Trumpington Street, Cambridge CB2 1RP
40 West 20th Street, New York, NY 10011-4211, USA
10 Stamford Road, Oakleigh, Melbourne 3166, Australia

First published 1994

Printed in Great Britain at the University Press, Cambridge

A catalogue record for this book is available from the British Library

Library of Congress cataloguing in publication data

Steptoe, Andrew.
    Psychosocial processes and health: a reader / compiled and edited
by Andrew Steptoe, Jane Wardle.
        p.   cm.
    Includes bibliographical references and index.
    ISBN 0 521 41610 8 (hardback). – ISBN 0 521 42618 9 (pbk.)
    1. Clinical health psychology.   2. Social psychology.   I. Wardle,
Jane.   II. Title
    [DNLM: 1. Psychology, Social – collected works.   2. Health –
collected works.   3. Psychophysiology – collected works.   HM 251
S837p 1994]
    R726.7.S75   1994
    155.9′2 – dc20
    DNLM/DLC
    for Library of Congress   93-49004 CIP

ISBN 0 521 41610 8   hardback
ISBN 0 521 42618 9   paperback

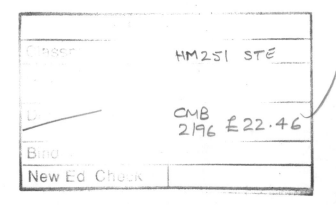

Contents

Preface

The interrelationships between psychosocial processes, behaviour and health have become the subject of increasing interest to clinicians and biomedical and social scientists over recent years. The development of disciplines such as behavioural medicine, psychosocial epidemiology, medical sociology and health psychology reflects the attention that is now being paid to this field. Material on the links between the social environment, emotion, behaviour and illness is being incorporated into the training of medical students and health professionals. Teaching on these topics has also been introduced into the graduate medical curriculum, and undergraduate and clinical psychology courses.

This growth of activity has been accompanied by the publication of specialist journals such as *Health Psychology, Annals of Behavioral Medicine, Journal of Behavioral Medicine, Stress Medicine, International Journal of Behavioral Medicine*, and *Psychology and Health*. Textbooks for medical students and health psychologists have been introduced, while numerous edited volumes attest to the fertility of this field. However, it is our experience that access to important source material on psychosocial processes and health is limited. Students working within medical institutions may not have access to the relevant social science journals and *vice versa*. Key papers are published across a wide range of journals from general medical periodicals such as the *Lancet* and the *New England Journal of Medicine*, through specialist epidemiology and social science journals, to discipline-specific publications such as the *American Heart Journal* and the *Journal of the National Cancer Institute*.

This set of readings has therefore been devised with the specific purpose of making available within a single book a series of important papers that have been published over the past 30 years in the area of psychosocial processes and health. Some of these papers are classics in the field, in that they were instrumental in bringing particular theoretical orientations into a wider scientific consciousness, or in establishing important empirical findings with significant clinical implications. Other papers illustrate themes in research or important research findings that we have found to be of value in kindling the interest of students at many stages of their education. We have chosen to orientate the readings around six broad areas that have proved useful for teaching, namely: *Life stress, social support and health* (Section 1); *Psychophysiological processes in disease* (Section 2); *Personality, behaviour patterns, and health* (Section 3); *Health practices and the modification of health risk behaviour* (Section 4); *Coping with illness and disability* (Section 5); and *Behavioural interventions in medicine* (Section 6). Each set of readings is preceded by an introduction in which we have attempted to place papers in their clinical and scientific context. (Discussion of the readings is indicated by italicizing the names of authors.) The subsequent impact of these papers and more recent relevant scientific research is also discussed. The papers have been reproduced as written, and only their appearance has been altered.

Inevitably, our choice is a personal one, and other compilers might have arrived at a different selection. We are conscious of many omissions, including papers concerned with child health, doctor–patient communication, pain management, the problems surrounding AIDS, social inequalities in health, and many other topics. Nevertheless, we hope that the readings we have chosen will provide useful material for teachers and students alike, and act as a starting point for clinicians and scientists who want to find out about the links between psychosocial processes and health.

A.S.
J.W.

Section 1

Life stress, social support and health

Readings

Unemployment and mortality in the OPCS Longitudinal Study.
  K. A. Moser, A. J. Fox and D. R. Jones. *Lancet*, **ii**, 1324–9, 1984.

Job strain, work place social support, and cardiovascular disease: a cross-sectional study of a random sample of the Swedish working population.
  J. V. Johnson and E. M. Hall. *American Journal of Public Health*, **78**, 1336–42, 1988.

Social networks, host resistance, and mortality: a nine-year follow-up study of Alameda County residents.
  L. F. Berkman and S. L. Syme. *American Journal of Epidemiology*, **109**, 186–204, 1979.

Goal frustration and life events in the aetiology of painful gastrointestinal disorder.
  T. K. J. Craig and G. W. Brown. *Journal of Psychosomatic Research*, **28**, 411–21, 1984.

Psychosocial assets, life crisis and the prognosis of pregnancy.
  K. B. Nuckolls, J. Cassel and B. H. Kaplan. *American Journal of Epidemiology*, **95**, 431–41, 1972.

Introduction

Section 1 is concerned with the role of life stress in the development of illness. A variety of health problems are addressed, ranging from symptoms of cardiovascular and gastrointestinal disorders to mortality. The readings have been selected to illustrate a number of important themes.

The first theme is the operationalisation of adverse life experience. One of the major difficulties that bedevilled early work in psychosomatic medicine and stress research was that life experience was poorly characterised, and was assessed primarily through respondents' retrospective reports. The fact that people with illnesses say that they were under stress before onset, contributes little to our understanding, since these reports may be biased by the person's health status, and by *post hoc* interpretations of their experience. The readings in Section 1 have taken various approaches to assessing life experience in a more objective way, involving the measurement of specific life events (*Craig and Brown; Nuckolls et al.*), chronic adverse circumstances such as job strain (*Johnson and Hall*), and the condition of unemployment (*Moser et al.*). They illustrate various strategies for deriving information about peoples' experience of life that can be quantified and related to health outcome in a systematic fashion.

The second theme is that life stress is not simply a product of unpleasant occurrences, but also depends on the person's social and personal resources. Personality and behaviour patterns are discussed further in Section 3, so in this section the focus is on the social environment. The impact of social networks and supports on health has been acknowledged increasingly over recent years (Cohen and Syme, 1985; Shumaker and Czajkowski, 1993). What is also becoming apparent is that social support is not a unitary concept. The extent of the social network is conceptually distinct from the degree of emotional and material support that is provided in times of crisis. Some social contacts may have negative rather than positive consequences, and social conflict is a potent source of psychological distress. It cannot be assumed that a person reporting close contact with family and friends will necessarily have access to effective support in times of crisis. Support itself has many dimensions, including emotional support, tangible or material assistance, and support in terms of information and advice. The relative impact of these will vary in different circumstances. These distinctions may account for some of the discrepant results in the debate concerning whether social support has a 'main effect' on health, or whether it acts as a 'buffer' to life stress. The readings illustrate both effects, with results from the Alameda County study showing that networks are directly associated with mortality (*Berkman and Syme*), while studies of job strain (*Johnson and Hall*) and the stressors encountered by pregnant women (*Nuckolls et al.*) demonstrate that social support protects people who are under particular pressure.

The third major theme is the design of studies relating life stress with health. The fundamental issue concerns the analysis of causation. The most convincing test of causation used in science is the experimental design, in which exposure to the putative causal factor is evaluated in a randomised prospective study. Such a procedure cannot reasonably be used in studies of life stress and health, so investigators are reliant on a range of observational study designs in which conditions are not manipulated experimentally. Three general approaches are illustrated in Section 1: the cross-sectional survey in which putative causal factors and health outcomes are assessed simultaneously (*Johnson and Hall*); the case–control study, in which the experiences of people with a particular disorder are contrasted with those of comparison subjects (*Craig and Brown*); and the longitudinal cohort study, in which populations with different levels of exposure to the putative causal factor are followed up, and differential health consequences are measured (*Moser et al*; *Berkman and Syme*; *Nuckolls et al.*). Each of these designs has different strengths in terms of such factors as the representativeness of samples, their abilities to uncover the sequence of events as they unfold, and the speed with which results can be obtained. They also have different limitations such as the number of participants required, openness to bias, and competing explanations of results. These properties have been lucidly compared by Elwood (1988). The reader may also identify an important tension between population-based studies which involve large representative samples (*Moser et al*; *Johnson and Hall*; *Berkman and Syme*), and clinically based studies that explore in detail the experience of individuals suffering from particular problems (*Craig and Brown*; *Nuckolls et al.*). This contrast between the individual and population level is one that runs through much of the literature on psychosocial processes and health, and will reemerge in later sections of the volume, particularly in relation to disease prevention through population-based programmes (Section 4) as against intensive interventions with individual people at risk (Section 6).

Unemployment and mortality

The paper by *Moser, Fox and Jones* uses longitudinal data from a national register to evaluate the association between unemployment and mortality. Unemployment has important political and social ramifications, and there is little doubt that it may have adverse effects on well-being. Health consequences have been investigated extensively over recent years, with studies of mental health (Warr, 1987), suicide (Brenner, 1985), and physiological function (Kasl *et al.*, 1968; Mattiasson *et al.*, 1990). The strength of the study by Moser et al. lies in their imaginitive use of routine census data to investigate the relationship of unemployment to the most convincing health endpoint of all – mortality. Data were derived from a large representative sample of the population, and show that mortality among men aged 15–64 years who were seeking work in the week prior to the 1971 census was significantly elevated over the subsequent 10 years. This effect has been replicated using 1981 census data, where similar results emerge despite the overall level of unemployment being much higher than a decade earlier (Moser *et al.*, 1987). Rates of deaths through violence or suicide were especially high among unemployed men, although raised risk of death from cardiovascular disease and cancer was evident as well. Comparable observations have been made in Denmark, Finland and other countries (Iversen *et al.*, 1987; Martikainen, 1990).

A particular feature of this reading is that *Moser et al.* were able to use their data to explore alternative explanations of the results. One obvious possibility is that men were unemployed because of poor health, and that excess mortality might be the result of preselecting a 'sick' group. If this were the explanation, one would expect the elevated mortality rate to diminish over time, as the proportion of unhealthy subjects in the unemployed category was reduced. In fact, there is little evidence for such an effect. It is also interesting that the impact of unemployment was experienced by the wives of men in the study, and that they too showed excess mortality. Again, this argues against a selection factor being responsible for the mortality among the unemployed. The explanation favoured by the authors is that the stress of unemployment has an effect on the family and not solely on the index subjects.

The results of this analysis illustrate another important association between psychosocial factors and mortality, namely the socioeconomic status mortality gradient. *Moser et al.* used conventional measures of social class to classify subjects, but similar patterns are seen in *Berkman and Syme*'s results using different indices of social status. There are many competing explanations of social inequalities of health, and these have been clearly discussed by Blane (1985). While selection processes and population drift may account for some of the effects, the major responsibility probably lies in the different social and personal experiences of people with differing social status (Marmot *et al.*, 1991). Social gradients in mortality and morbidity appear to increase as people move from early adulthood to late middle-age, so are particularly worrying in the context of demographic trends in the population (House *et al.*, 1992).

One benefit of the research strategy described by *Moser et al.* is that, through studying a large, representative sample, it was possible to establish strong relationships between life stress and health. The limitation of this approach is that little is known about the individuals involved. It is possible, for example, that many of those designated as unemployed found work soon afterwards, while others lost their jobs over the 10-year follow-up. Some men will have been able to cope with unemployment more effectively than others. Such effects would be likely to dilute the impact of unemployment as defined in the study.

Job stress and social support

The second reading pursues the theme of life stress and health by evaluating dimensions of work-related strain in relation to cardiovascular symptoms. People who are employed spend a substantial portion of their waking lives at work, so it is not surprising that a large literature has investigated the impact of job stress on health and well-being. A particularly influential approach to occupational stress is the demand–control model developed by Robert Karasek (1979). This model proposes that job strain will arise when high levels of job demand are coupled with low levels of control over decision making and job content. Thus, a demanding job will not in itself lead to ill-effects, since the worker may be able to exert considerable discretion over how the job is done. This approach has not gone uncriticised (see Ganster, 1989); nevertheless, a body of evidence has emerged suggesting that the demand–control approach may be particularly relevant to cardiovascular disease (Karasek and Theorell, 1990).

Johnson and Hall's study illustrates this association with cardiovascular disease, while also adding the element of social support. They find that symptoms of cardiovascular disease are particularly prevalent among high job strain workers who report little work-related social support. This illustrates a buffering effect of social support, in that the impact of social relationships was more pronounced among workers who experienced high job strain. The study investigated a large random sample of the working population, and sophisticated statistical procedures were used to show that the impact of high job strain coupled with low support is not a marker of some other potential causal factor such as socioeconomic status, gender or cigarette smoking. The study also introduces the concept of domain-specific social support, suggesting that the measurement of social relationships in the work setting may be particularly useful when evaluating job-related experience. Another intriguing observation is that high levels of job control may not always be beneficial, since the prevalence of cardiovascular symptoms among subjects reporting high control coupled with high demands and low support was substantial. High control over a job may bring with it heavy responsibility, and when this is experienced in social isolation, the result may be negative.

The limitations of the study design, acknowledged by *Johnson and Hall*, are also illuminating. The cross-sectional approach limits causal interpretation. It is possible that some aspect of cardiovascular disease or its symptoms leads workers to become socially isolated, and to perceive their work as being excessively demanding. The reliance on self-report of health status may lead to misclassification and bias. However, longitudinal analyses have confirmed the impact of these factors on mortality, so bias in symptom reporting is unlikely to be responsible (Johnson *et al.*, 1989). The study has therefore helped to establish the three-way interaction between demands, perceptions of control, and social support as being important to the investigation of life stress and health.

Social networks and mortality

It has been believed since the seminal work of Emil Durkheim that social ties and social networks protect people against ill-health. *Berkman and Syme*'s paper was perhaps the first convincingly to show an association between mortality and the extent of social networks. They had the advantage of being able to utilise data from the Alameda County study, a systematic survey of nearly 7000 randomly selected adults that was first assessed in 1965. The sample has been investigated from a number of aspects, and is notable for the high response rate and minimal attrition. Both these features add to the confidence that can be placed on the longitudinal cohort design. A further reading using the Alameda County data is included in Section 4 (*Wingard et al.*).

Berkman and Syme demonstrate that mortality in men and women is associated with social relationships, assessed both at the most individual level (marriage) and in terms of broader networks. Mortality was more frequent during the follow-up period in those with few social connections, and this was apparent in men and women from early to late adult life. As in the study by *Moser et al.*, it was possible to tease out competing explanations of this pattern by carrying out subsidiary analyses. Thus, it can be seen that the results were not simply due to people with few social connections being more unhealthy from the start of the survey, or using health services less effectively. The degree to which people follow a healthy lifestyle (regular exercise, moderate alcohol consumption, not smoking, etc.) may play a part in the social network difference, but only goes a small way towards accounting for mortality effects. Similarly, the strong association between socioeconomic status and mortality contributes to the link between networks and death, without being entirely responsible.

It is therefore argued by *Berkman and Syme* that social isolation may reduce peoples' resistance to sources of ill-health through failures of psychological coping and through stress-related physiological processes. These possibilities are elaborated further through readings in

Sections 2 and 3. It is suggested that social networks contribute to the individual's resistance in a general fashion, rather than affecting vulnerability to specific disorders. This non-specificity hypothesis has been elaborated in detail by Cassel (1976). The associations between social support and mortality described in this reading have been confirmed in other surveys (House *et al.*, 1988).

It should be noted that although social networks are often associated with a protective effect, this is not invariably the case. Having an extensive social network may have negative as well as positive consequences. The more contacts the person has, the greater the opportunities for adverse emotional experiences such as bereavement, separation and loss of friendship. Moreover, people with wide networks may be called upon to provide support to many others, and this can also be emotionally demanding (Buunk and Hoorens, 1992). The summary measures of social networks obtained in the Alameda County study do not provide information about the way in which social connections operated, or how they were mobilised in times of difficulty.

Life events and gastrointestinal disorder

The next reading illustrates a very different approach to the investigation of psychosocial factors and health. The notion that life stress could be quantified through the measurement of discrete objective 'life events' was first systematically introduced by Holmes and Rahe (1967). Their original instrument, the Schedule of Recent Experiences, was a list of 43 events, and this has been elaborated subsequently and used extensively in many different health settings. The Schedule of Recent Experiences and its successors have been severely criticised on many counts (Brown, 1974). These arguments are well summarised by Paykel (1983), and concern the accuracy and reliability of event recording, and the evaluation of the significance of events for the individual under investigation.

The paper by *Craig and Brown* illustrates a powerful alternative strategy for assessing life events and chronic life difficulties. This is the Life Events and Difficulties Schedule developed by Brown and his associates. It is an interview method which not only provides accurate information about events through probing and cross-checking, but also includes an independent method of assessing the threat associated with each incident. This technique has been applied principally to psychiatric disorders, although research on physical complaints has been gathering momentum (Brown and Harris, 1978, 1989).

The study applies the life event method to patients with gastrointestinal disorders. *Craig and Brown* found that severe life events or chronic difficulties over the previous nine months were significantly more common among patients with functional gastrointestinal disorders (such as irritable bowel syndrome and dyspepsia) than in healthy controls or patients with organic disorders. In contrast, experiences involving the frustration of desired goals following a period of sustained striving were more frequent in the organic disorder group. The result is important as a demonstration of the way in which associations can be found at the clinical level between stressful experiences and ill-health, and also as an example of the operationalisation of subtle concepts such as goal frustration within a framework of objective assessment. Interestingly, the basic pattern of results has been confirmed in an independent study in which a specific association between duodenal ulcer and goal frustration was identified (Ellard *et al.*, 1990). The data run counter to the theory that life stress has a non-specific generalised impact on health status, since different types of experience were found to be related to different outcomes. Results from psychophysiological experiments likewise challenge the notion of non-specificity in stress processes (Steptoe, 1983).

Studies like the one described by *Craig and Brown* involve intensive assessments on the individual participants, so are inevitably smaller in scale than surveys. This means that some of the numbers are extremely small in the various subsidiary comparisons, so their representativeness is unknown. The information on life events and difficulties is collected retrospectively, although the interviewer is not aware of the diagnostic status of participants. This approach therefore has both strengths and limitations, and can be seen as complementary to the larger-scale cohort studies.

Pregnancy complications and life events

The last reading of Section 1 focuses on another set of health problems (complications of pregnancy) and another aspect of the association between life stress and health, namely the protective influence of psychosocial assets. *Nuckolls, Cassel and Kaplan* studied a cohort of women bearing their first child, and recorded life events before and during pregnancy, together with the women's social and personal resources and assets. They found an interaction between life stress and assets, so that high levels of pregnancy complications were observed among women with poor resources who experienced severe life change both before and during pregnancy. In this way, the study documented an interaction between stressful life experience and support, for neither events nor assets proved to be significant in isolation.

Some features of this study can be criticised on methodological grounds, although the general pattern of results has been confirmed at least in part by other researchers (Norbeck and Tilden, 1983; Newton and Hunt, 1984). *Nuckolls et al.* used the type of life schedule that was criticised by *Craig and Brown*. The participants had a difficult rating task, being required on a single occasion to recall life events both during pregnancy and during the year prior to pregnancy. The pregnancy complication rate was surprisingly high (47% of the sample), so different patterns of results might emerge from a present-day obstetric unit. Nevertheless, the study has a number of strengths that make it an important illustration of links between life stress and health. The authors were able to conduct a prospective study on a rather homogeneous cohort, with psychosocial measures being obtained before the medical events occurred. Such a design was possible because complications were frequent in the population. Much larger cohorts are required to investigate relatively rare events like premature mortality. A careful analysis was performed on those who did not complete the study, strengthening the confidence that could be placed on results. It is also notable that the psychosocial assets found in this study to buffer severe life events include personal as well as social resources. Factors such as self-esteem and attitudes to pregnancy were incorporated into the assets measure, suggesting that a broad conceptualisation may be helpful. The relevance of personal factors of this kind to stress resistance and vulnerability to adverse life events is a thread that is taken up again in Section 3. Finally, it should be noted that the beneficial effects of social support during pregnancy, labour and postpartum have been amply confirmed by other investigations, with emotional, tangible and informational support all having a positive influence on women's health (Gjerdingen *et al.*, 1991).

References

Blane, D. (1985). An assessment of the Black Report's explanations of health inequalities. *Sociology of Health and Illness*, **7**, 423–45.

Brenner, M. H. (1985). Economic change and the suicide rate: a population model including loss, separation, illness and alcohol consumption. In: *Stress in Health and Disease*, pp. 160–85. M. R. Zales (ed.). New York: Brunner/Mazel.

Brown, G. W. (1974). Meaning, measurement and stress of life events. In: *Stressful Life Events: Their Nature and Effects*, pp. 217–43. B. S. Dohrenwend and B. P. Dohrenwend (eds.). New York: John Wiley.

Brown, G. W. and Harris, T. O. (1978). *Social Origins of Depression*. London: Tavistock.

Brown, G. W. and Harris, T. O. (eds.) (1989). *Life Events and Illness*. London: Unwin Hyman.

Buunk, A. P. and Hoorens, V. (1992). Social support and stress: the role of social comparison and social exchange processes. *British Journal of Clinical Psychology*, **31**, 445–57.

Cassel, J. (1976). The contribution of the social environment to host resistance. *American Journal of Epidemiology*, **104**, 107–23.

Cohen, S. and Syme, L. S. (eds.) (1985). *Social Support and Health*. New York: Academic Press.

Ellard, K., Beaurepaire, J., Jones, M., Piper, D. and Tennant, C. (1990). Acute and chronic stress in duodenal ulcer disease. *Gastroenterology*, **99**, 1628–32.

Elwood, J. M. (1988). *Causal Relationships in Medicine*. Oxford: Oxford University Press.

Ganster, D. C. (1989). Worker control and well-being: a review of research in the workplace. In: *Job Control and Worker Health*, pp. 3–23. S. L. Sauter, J. J. Hurrell and C. L. Cooper (eds.). Chichester: John Wiley.

Gjerdingen, D. K., Froberg, D. G. and Fontaine, P. (1991). The effects of social support on women's health during pregnancy, labour and delivery, and the post-partum period. *Family Medicine*, **23**, 370–5.

Holmes, T. H. and Rahe, R. H. (1967). The social readjustment rating scale. *Journal of Psychosomatic Research*, **11**, 213–18.

House, J. S., Landis, K. R. and Umberson, D. (1988). Social relationships and health. *Science*, **241**, 540–4.

House, J. S., Kessler, R. C., Herzog, A. R., Mero, R. P., Kinney, A. M. and Breslow, M. J. (1992). Social stratification, age, and health. In: *Aging, Health Behaviors, and Health Outcomes*, pp. 1–32. K. W. Schaie, D. Blazer and J. S. House (eds.). Hillsdale: LEA.

Iversen, A., Andersen, O., Andersen, P. K., Christoffersen, K. and Keiding, N. (1987). Unemployment and mortality in Denmark, 1970–80. *British Medical Journal*, **295**, 879–84.

Johnson, J. V., Hall, E. M. and Theorell, T. (1989). Combined effects of job strain and social isolation on cardiovascular disease morbidity and mortality in a random sample of the Swedish male working population. *Scandinavian Journal of Work and Environmental Health*, **15**, 271–9.

Karasek, R. (1979). Job demands, job decision latitude, and mental strain: implications for job redesign. *Administrative Science Quarterly*, **24**, 285–308.

Karasek, R. and Theorell, T. (1990). *Healthy Work*. New York: Basic Books.

Kasl, S. B., Cobb, S. and Brooks, G. W. (1968). Changes in serum uric acid and cholesterol levels in men undergoing job loss. *Journal of the American Medical Association*, **206**, 1500–7.

Marmot, M. G., Davey-Smith, G., Stansfeld, S., Patel, C., North, F., Head, J., White, I., Brunner, E. and Feeney, A. (1991). Health inequalities among British civil servants: the Whitehall II Study. *Lancet*, **337**, 1387–93.

Martikainen, P. T. (1990). Unemployment and mortality among Finnish men, 1981–5. *British Medical Journal*, **301**, 407–11.

Mattiasson, I., Lindgärde, F., Nilsson, J. A. and Theorell, T. (1990). Threat of unemployment and cardiovascular risk factors: longitudinal study of quality of sleep and serum cholesterol concentrations in men threatened with redundancy. *British Medical Journal*, **301**, 461–6.

Moser, K. A., Goldblatt, P. O., Fox, H. A. and Jones, D. R. (1987).

Unemployment and mortality: a comparison of the 1971 and 1981 longitudinal census samples. *British Medical Journal*, **294**, 86–90.

Newton, R. W. and Hunt, L. P. (1984). Psychosocial stress in pregnancy and its relationship to low birth weight. *British Medical Journal*, **288**, 1191–4.

Norbeck, J. S. and Tilden, B. P. (1983). Life stress, social support, and emotional disequilibrium in complications of pregnancy: a prospective, multivariate study. *Journal of Health and Social Behavior*, **24**, 30–46.

Paykel, E. S. (1983). Methodological aspects of life events research. *Journal of Psychosomatic Research*, **27**, 341–52.

Shumaker, S. and Czajkowski, S. M. (eds.) (1993). *Social Support and Cardiovascular Disease*. New York: Plenum.

Steptoe, A. (1983). Stress, helplessness and control: the implications of laboratory studies. *Journal of Psychosomatic Research*, **27**, 361–7.

Warr, P. (1987). *Work, Unemployment and Mental Health*. Oxford: Oxford University Press.

Unemployment and mortality in the OPCS Longitudinal Study

K. A. Moser, A. J. Fox and D. R. Jones

Social Statistics Research Unit, City University, London EC1V 0HB, UK

Summary

The mortality of men aged 15–64 who were seeking work in the week before the 1971 census was investigated by means of the OPCS Longitudinal Study, which follows up a 1% sample of the population of England and Wales. In contrast to the current position, only 4% of men of working age in 1971 fell into this category. The mortality of these unemployed men in the period 1971–81 was higher (standardised mortality ratio 136) than would be expected from death rates in all men in the Longitudinal Study. The socioeconomic distribution of the unemployed accounts for some of the raised mortality, but, after allowance for this, a 20–30% excess remains; this excess was apparent both in 1971–75 and in 1976–81. The data offer only limited support for the suggestion that some of this excess resulted from men becoming unemployed because of their ill-health; the trend in overall mortality over time and the pattern by cause of death were not those usually associated with ill-health selection. Previous studies have suggested that stress accompanying unemployment could be associated with raised suicide rates, as were again found here. Moreover, the mortality of women whose husbands were unemployed was higher than that of all married women (standardised mortality ratio 120), and this excess also persisted after allowance for their socioeconomic distribution. The results support findings by others that unemployment is associated with adverse effects on health.

Introduction

Perhaps because of the steep rises in the late 1970s in the proportion of the working populations of western countries who were unemployed, several groups have been trying to assess the impact of unemployment on health. The published work, ranging from aggregated, national data to detailed case-reports, has lately been reviewed by Brenner and Mooney,[1] Warr,[2] and Cook and Shaper.[3] Although Brenner's econometric

Reprinted from Unemployment and mortality in the OPCS Longitudinal Study. Moser, K. A., Fox, A. J. and Jones D. R. *Lancet*, ii, 1324–9. © Crown copyright (1984).

studies,[4,5] which seek to explain variations in annual UK mortality rates in terms of the unemployment rate and various other measures of economic growth, have received wide attention, investigation of the impact of unemployment on the health of an individual (and his/her family) requires a disaggregated study design. Few results from epidemiological studies of adequate power, specifically designed to measure the mortality consequences of unemployment, have been reported. Small investigations of groups of men being made redundant have been inconclusive. In larger studies, such as the Regional Heart Study,[6] the Department of Health and Social Security cohort study,[7,8] and the Office of Population Censuses and Surveys (OPCS) Longitudinal Study reported on here,[9] the relation between unemployment and mortality has not been the primary interest. As a result, weaknesses of study size, outcome and explanatory variables, control-group selection, and response and follow-up rates have reduced the weight to be attached to the results. Although there is some evidence from these studies of raised morbidity and mortality among the unemployed, potential confounding factors remain unmeasured, and inevitably the causal mechanism remains unestablished. Some light has been shed on the morbidity consequences (in particular the psychological consequences) of unemployment in case studies and other research entailing detailed interviewing of small, but high-risk, groups (see Warr[2]). Whilst these investigations are likewise subject to methodological limitations, they suggest that, at least in some population subgroups, being, and in particular, *becoming* unemployed is associated with increased morbidity, including depression, anxiety, and stress-related behaviour such as smoking and alcohol consumption. Age, sex, occupational group, and length of unemployment are among the effect-modifying factors suggested.

In this paper we use data from the OPCS Longitudinal Study (LS) to examine further the relation between unemployment and mortality. Unemployed men in the LS sample have already been shown to have high mortality in 1971–75 and several possible explanations have been offered.[9] Firstly, men's health may suffer *as a result of* unemployment, perhaps owing to a fall in income and social status, increased stress, and consequent behaviour. Secondly, men in poor health may be more likely to *become* unemployed, and the raised mortality of unemployed men may simply reflect their health status *before* unemployment. Thirdly, the high mortality may reflect the social distribution of unemployed men *before* unemployment and the strong relation between mortality and measures of socioeconomic status.

In this paper we examine the importance that can be attached to these three explanations by (i) using mortality data for the ten years 1971–81; (ii) controlling for the socioeconomic distribution of the unemployed men; and (iii) looking at the mortality of women married to unemployed men. The interpretation of our analysis is limited because our indicator of unemployment relates to one week in April, 1971, and we have no information on how long these men had been or were subsequently, unemployed.

Subjects and methods

Source of data

The LS is based on a 1% sample of individuals enumerated in England and Wales in the 1971 census. Census records for sample members have been linked with information on subsequent events about which details are routinely collected, principally births, deaths, and cancer registrations. This analysis focuses on deaths in the period 1971–81. Some census information on other persons in any household containing an LS member is also linked to the information about the sample member.

In this analysis the unemployed group comprises those men who indicated, in response to the 1971 census question on economic position, that they were seeking work or waiting to take up a job in the week before the census; we shall refer to them either as "seeking work" or as unemployed. This excludes other categories of economic position such as in employment, temporarily or permanently sick, and retired or otherwise inactive. Perception of economic position is dependent on many factors— primarily age, sex, and (especially for women) marital status and prevailing socioeconomic climate. Women reporting themselves as "seeking work" were a select group; 38% of women aged 15–59 in our sample were placed in the inactive category to which housewives were allocated. Consequently, we have limited ourselves here to an investigation of *male* unemployment and, principally, to mortality of men in the working age range 15–64. Of the quarter of a million men in the sample in 1971, 161 699 were aged 15–64 and, of these, 5861 (3·6%) were "seeking work".

The 1971 census provided some sociodemographic information on respondents. We were able to classify men "seeking work" into social classes from details of their most recent jobs. The LS also contains information on the household and other household members, and we have used this to investigate the mortality of women married to men "seeking work".

Methods

Throughout the analysis the standardised mortality ratio (SMR, the ratio of observed [O] to expected [E] deaths × 100) is used as a summary index

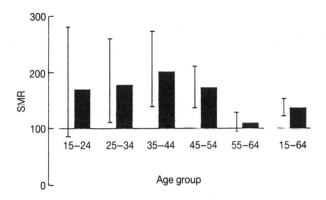

Fig. 1. Mortality 1971–81 of men seeking work in 1971 by age at death.

of mortality. Expected deaths are obtained by applying the death rates by 5-year age groups in the standard group to the person-years-at-risk in the study group.[10] In most of the analyses the standard group comprises all men in the LS aged 15 and over at census. Where a different standard group is used this is indicated in the text. Approximate 95% confidence limits for the ratio of observed to expected deaths are also presented.[11]

Results

The SMR for 1971–81 for men aged 15–64 years at death, seeking work in 1971, was 136 with approximate 95% confidence limits 122–152. It rose from 129 for 1971–75 to 144 for 1976–81. Although the mortality of these men was raised at all ages, the excess seems greater at younger ages (fig 1). In age groups 25–34, 35–44 and 45–54 the SMR exceeded 170.

Effects of socioeconomic distribution

How much of the excess mortality among the unemployed men can be explained by their socioeconomic distribution? The difference between the social class distribution of unemployed men and all men in the LS is shown in fig 2. Unemployed men were concentrated in the lower social classes. For example, social class V contained 16% of all unemployed men but only 7% of all men. For one-fifth of the unemployed it was not possible to allocate them to a social class on the basis of their most recent job; this is the case for less than 2% of all men. Those allocated to this "inadequately described" group mainly comprised men whose failure to complete the census question on most recent occupation reflected either the fact that they were out of work or that they were enumerated in institutions such as hospitals.

Table I. *Mortality 1971–81 of all men and men seeking work in 1971, by social class*

| | | Men "seeking work" in 1971 aged 15–64 at death | |
Social class	All men aged 15–64 at death SMR	SMR	SMRs standardised for social class
I	73 (263)	79 (3)	103
II	78 (1224)	109 (28)	139
IIIN	98 (828)	113 (20)	116
IIIM	94 (2693)	123 (90)	132
IV	103 (1468)	155 (67)	150
V	120 (727)	150 (61)	124
Armed forces	84 (31)	—	—
Inadequately described	183 (176)	165 (59)	87
Unoccupied	264 (651)	—	—
Total	100 (8061)	136 (328)	121

Figures in parentheses are numbers of observed deaths.

There was a strong mortality gradient with social class among all men (with a social class I SMR of 73 and a social class V SMR of 120), which was also present, indeed wider, among men "seeking work" (table I). Within each social class the SMR for men "seeking work" was higher than that for all men, indicating that the raised mortality of the unemployed was maintained through all the classes. As would be expected, this is not so for the residual group, the "inadequately described"; many of this group were in hospitals and other institutions, so those among them who were "seeking work" would have been a comparatively healthy subset.

To take account of the social class distribution of the unemployed, new values for the expected deaths were calculated, with standardisation for age and class. The SMR for all unemployed men, standardised for age and class, was 121 with approximate 95% confidence limits 108–135; this suggests that some but not all of the excess mortality among unemployed men may be explained by their class distribution.

Standardisation for the distribution of unemployed men by social class but with exclusion of men with "inadequately described" occupations suggests that the component of the raised mortality of men "seeking work" which could be explained by their social class composition was somewhat less than indicated above.[12] Standardisation for housing

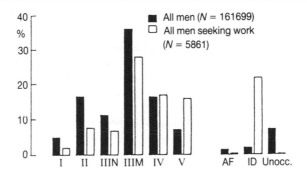

Fig. 2. Percentage distribution of all men seeking work aged 15–64 by social class in 1971. I–V = social class; AF = armed forces; ID = inadequately described occupations; Unocc = unoccupied.

tenure—an alternative measure of socioeconomic status[9]—reduced the SMR of men "seeking work" from 136 to 127 (table II).

The increase in SMR in unemployed men, from 129 in 1971–75 to 144 in 1976–81, seemed to be accounted for by the social class distribution; SMRs standardised for age and social class were 122 and 123 for the two time-periods. The effect of standardising the SMRs for social class was greater in 1976–81 than in 1971–75 because there was a steeper social class gradient in mortality in 1976–81 than in 1971–75. This results largely from dissipation of the effects of selective health-related mobility out of employment which affected mortality differentials in the earlier period.[13]

Mortality seems to have been particularly high for malignant neoplasms and for accidents, poisonings, and violence (table III). Raised mortality from malignant neoplasms (O=94, E=66·5) appears to have been attributable in the main to deaths from lung cancer (O=48, E=27·4). A clear excess from this cause remained after allowance for social class.

High mortality from accidents, poisonings, and violence (O=46, E=22·8) was only partly explained by the very high mortality from suicide (O=20, E=8·3). Although SMRs for both these causes were reduced by social class standardisation, substantial excesses remained.

Effects of health-related selection in the unemployed group

We now examine evidence for the suggestion that the men who were unemployed in 1971 became unemployed *because* of poor health.[14] If ill-health were a major influence on the selection of this group we would expect the health, and the relative mortality, of the group to improve over time. Such a change would be expected because of the high initial mortality of those selected on the basis of ill-health; the proportion of sick men in this category would decline over time. This and other

Table II. *Mortality 1971–81 of men seeking work in 1971, aged 15–64 at death, standardised for age and social class, and age and housing tenure*

Expected deaths based on:	SMR	Approx 95% confidence interval
Age specific rates	136	122–152
Age and *social class* specific rates	121	108–135
Age and *housing tenure* specific rates	127	113–141

Table III. *Mortality 1971–81 of men seeking work in 1971, aged 15–64 at death, by cause of death*

Cause of death	SMR	Approx 95% CI	SMR standardised for social class	Approx 95% CI
All causes	136 (328)	122–152	121	108–135
Malignant neoplasms	141 (94)	114–172	128	103–155
Lung cancer	175 (48)	128–229	154	113–202
Circulatory diseases	116 (132)	97–138	109	90–128
Ischaemic heart disease	111 (93)	89–135	107	86–130
Respiratory diseases	146 (27)	95–208	132	86–187
Bronchitis, emphysema and asthma	119 (12)	60–197	117	59–193
Accidents, poisonings and violence	202 (46)	147–266	149	108–196
Suicide &c*	241 (20)	145–361	169	102–254
Other accidents, poisonings, & violence	179 (26)	116–257	140	90–200

Figures in parentheses are numbers of observed deaths.
*ICD 8th revision 850–877, 942, 950–959, 980–989.

mechanisms would lead to a reduction in mortality over time, as has been observed in other areas of our work.[13,15] On the other hand, if this group were selected on the basis of positive health, we would expect the health of the group to worsen, and their relative mortality to rise with time. A further component of the analysis involves examination of patterns of cause-specific mortality over time, since the time scales for changes in mortality for acute causes would be shorter than those for chronic causes if the selection mechanism were valid.

Although we have 10 years' mortality data, this is a short time-span over which to observe trends in cause-specific mortality for such a small

Table IV. *Mortality 1971–75 and 1976–81 of men seeking work in 1971, aged 15–64 at death, by cause of death*

Cause of death	SMR	Approx 95% CI	SMRs standardised for social class	Approx 95% CI
All causes				
1971–75	129 (167)	110–150	122	104–142
1976–81	144 (161)	122–168	123	105–143
Lung cancer				
1971–75	208 (31)	140–290	189	127–263
1976–81	137 (17)	79–212	118	68–182
Ischaemic heath disease				
1971–75	108 (48)	79–142	114	84–150
1976–81	114 (45)	82–150	100	73–133
Bronchitis, emphysema, and asthma				
1971–75	30 (2)	3–87	33	3–97
1976–81	278 (10)	130–481	250	117–433
Suicide &c				
1971–75	250 (9)	111–444	148	66–262
1976–81	244 (11)	119–414	186	91–316
Other accidents, poisonings, and violence (excluding suicide)				
1971–75	203 (16)	114–316	147	83–229
1976–81	147 (10)	69–255	156	73–271

Figures in parentheses are numbers of observed deaths.

subgroup of the population. The lack of power of this analysis of short-term trends by cause of death is apparent from the wide confidence intervals around the SMRs in table IV. As we have said, the SMRs for all causes of death standardised for social class showed no trend between the two time periods.

The fall in SMRs (standardised for social class) for lung cancer and ischaemic heart disease might be construed as evidence of ill-health selection, but they were not based on sufficient numbers of deaths for firm conclusions to be drawn about their trends with time. Interpretation of the pattern of deaths from bronchitis is even more problematical.

Although these data provide no strong evidence for a selection effect, we cannot rule out the possibility that there is one operating. The complexity of the hypothesis and the large sampling variation make conclusive interpretation of the data difficult.

Table V. *Mortality 1971–81 of women whose husbands were seeking work in 1971,*
by cause of death

Cause of death	SMR	Approx 95% CI
All causes	120 (173)	102–139
Malignant neoplasms	112 (59)	85–143
Lung cancer	88 (7)	34–166
Circulatory diseases	129 (76)	101–161
Ischaemic heart disease	157 (47)	115–206
Respiratory diseases	127 (14)	68–204
Bronchitis, emphysema and asthma	93 (4)	23–209
Accidents, poisonings, and violence	86 (5)	26–181
Suicide &c	160 (4)	40–360

Figures in parentheses are numbers of observed deaths. The standard population
used in calculating the expected deaths was all married women resident in private
households.

Effects of unemployment on the health of other household members

Any adverse effects of unemployment—through, for example, a fall in
income, or an increase in stress—may be expected to have repercussions
on all members of the unemployed person's family or household. By
examining mortality among people other than the unemployed man
himself we partly eliminate any health-selection effect, unless the
ill-health of others in the household was associated with his being less
available for work. Any adverse health experience among these family
members could therefore be interpreted as more directly attributable to
the effects of unemployment.

Table V shows the mortality in 1971–81 of the 2906 married women in
private households whose husbands were unemployed at the 1971 census.
The standard population used in calculating the expected deaths was all
married women resident in private households. The overall SMR for
1971–81 was 120 (approximate 95% confidence intervals 102–139), which
suggests that mortality among this group of women was higher than
would have been expected. The SMR rose from 108 in 1971–75 to 129 in
1976–81; the approximate 95% confidence intervals were 83–138 and
105–154, respectively.

Although some cause-specific SMRs were raised, the numbers of
deaths from specific causes were in the main too small to make any clear
interpretations of the results. However, for ischaemic heart disease the
SMR was 157 with approximate 95% confidence intervals 115–206. There

was no apparent trend over time for this cause; the SMR for 1971–75 was 155 and that for 1976–81 was 159.

As with the excess mortality for unemployed men, part of the excess mortality among women whose husbands were unemployed may have been due to the socioeconomic composition of this group. The data on tenure suggest that a high proportion of these women lived in local-authority housing; 45% lived in council housing and 34% owned their houses as compared with 27% and 56%, respectively, among married women whose husbands were *in* employment.

The tenure mortality gradient was far steeper among women with unemployed husbands (owner occupiers had an SMR of 101 while council tenants had an SMR of 144) than among women with husbands in employment (corresponding SMRs 90 and 114). Within each tenure group the women with unemployed husbands had considerably higher mortality; the overall SMR of these women was 124, compared with 100 for women whose husbands were in employment. However, standardisation for tenure distribution reduced the SMR only from 124 to 121. This suggests that housing tenure explained little of the excess mortality among women with unemployed husbands.

Discussion

Limitations and strengths of the analysis

This paper has been concerned with *male* unemployment and its relation with the mortality of unemployed men and that of women married to unemployed men. Unfortunately we have not been able to consider female unemployment and its effect on health, mainly because of difficulties in interpreting responses to the question on economic position in the 1971 census.

Although we have followed about 6000 men unemployed in 1971 for up to 10 years, the 328 deaths which occurred amongst this group were too few in number to enable us to test specific relations satisfactorily—for example, for selected causes of death and by year of death. In particular, the assessment of evidence for a health-related selection effect was severely hampered.

Our indicator of unemployment relates to one week in April, 1971, and we have no information on how long these men had been, or were subsequently, unemployed.

The principal strength of the investigation is that it is a *prospective* study of individuals who were unemployed in 1971, rather than a study of histories collected retrospectively, or an analysis of aggregate data. In this extension of the earlier analysis[9] we have examined the social class composition of unemployed men to establish the extent to which the raised mortality of these men is explained by social class differentials in mortality. As well as looking at the mortality among unemployed men, we have now started to investigate the mortality experienced by other members of households containing an unemployed man. This is useful not only because it enables us to assess the wider health effects of unemployment but also for the light it sheds on the role of health-related selection, the weakest element of our analysis of mortality among the unemployed themselves. These issues are discussed more fully in a working paper.[12]

Findings

Among men who were "seeking work" in 1971, our data indicate high mortality (SMR 136) over the next 10 years. The analysis suggests that some of this excess mortality may be explained by the fact that unemployed men were more concentrated in social classes IV and V; nonetheless, a 20–30% excess remained unexplained. However, it should be noted that, without details of the timing of unemployment in relation to social mobility, it is difficult to establish the direction of the causal relation.

The evidence in support of some health-related selection of unemployed men remains very unclear, although it seems probable that men "seeking work" were partly selected for *good* health since the least healthy men, who were not in employment, would have been recorded either as "out of work, sick" or "permanently sick". Two causes of death, lung cancer and suicide, stand out as having significantly raised levels of mortality among men "seeking work" after allowance for social class. Both causes have been linked elsewhere to stress and stress-related activity.[16,17] However, to explain an excess of lung cancer mortality in 1971–81, one must probably invoke exposure to a risk factor *before* 1971.

Women whose husbands were "seeking work" had raised mortality (SMR 120 compared with all married women resident in private households), most of which remained after controlling for tenure distribution. As any health-related selection effect is expected to be small among women whose husbands were unemployed—indeed the SMR rose with increased follow-up—it is reasonable to suggest that their high mortality was largely attributable to other factors, such as a direct effect of their spouses' unemployment. The excess mortality from ischaemic heart disease may support this hypothesis since this disease has been linked with stress.[18] Further work now in progress on the mortality of *other* members of the households where there was an unemployed man in 1971 should therefore be of particular interest.

Between 1971 and 1981 unemployment became a more common experience among men in the working age range and durations of unemployment increased. These changes make it difficult to extrapolate from our findings to estimate the impact of unemployment on health today. Once we have access to mortality data for the 1980s and information from the 1981 census on the employment status and socioeconomic circumstances of the LS sample members at this second point in time, we should be able to assess the changing health effects of unemployment.

To summarise, although effects of other factors remain to be investigated, the results of this investigation do provide evidence suggesting that *some* of the excess mortality among unemployed men may be explained by their socioeconomic circumstances before unemployment. However, this alone does not account for all of the high mortality in unemployed men and in women married to unemployed men.

Acknowledgements

The analyses are part of a review by the Social Statistics Research Unit at City University of mortality data available from the OPCS Longitudinal Study. (Crown copyright is reserved.) This programme is supported by a grant from the Medical Research Council. The views expressed are those of the authors.

References

1. Brenner, MH, Mooney, A. Unemployment and health in the context of economic change. *Soc Sci Med* 1983; **17**: 1125–38.
2. Warr P. Twelve questions about unemployment and health. In: Roberts B, Finnegan R, Gallie D, eds. New approaches to economic life: Manchester: University Press (in press).
3. Cook D, Shaper AG. Unemployment and health. In: Harrington M, ed. Recent advances in occupational health, vol. 2. Edinburgh: Churchill Livingstone (in press).
4. Brenner MH. Mortality and the national economy: a review, and the experience of England and Wales, 1936–1976. *Lancet* 1979; **ii**: 568–73.
5. Brenner MH. Unemployment and health. *Lancet* 1979; **ii**: 874–75.
6. Cook DG, Cummins RO, Bartley MJ, Shaper AG. Health of unemployed middle-aged men in Great Britain. *Lancet* 1982; **i**: 1290–94.
7. Wood D. The DHSS cohort study of unemployed men (working paper no 1). London: Department of Health and Social Security, 1982.
8. Ramsden S, Smee C. The health of unemployed men: DHSS cohort study. *Employment Gazette* September, 1981, 397–401.
9. Fox AJ, Goldblatt PO. Socio-demographic mortality differentials: longitudinal study 1971–75, series LS no 1. London: HM Stationery Office, 1982.
10. Berry G. The analysis of mortality by the subject-years method. *Biometrics* 1983; **39**: 173–84.

11. Vandenbroucke JP. A shortcut method for calculating the 95 per cent confidence interval of the standardised mortality ratio. *Am J Epidemiol* 1982; **115**: 303–04.

12. Moser KA, Fox AJ, Jones DR, Goldblatt PO. Unemployment and mortality in the OPCS longitudinal study. London: SSRU, City University. Working paper no 18, 1984.

13. Fox AJ, Goldblatt PO, Jones DR. Social class mortality differentials: artefact, selection or life curcumstances? *J Epidemiol Commun Health* (in press).

14. Stern J. The relationship between unemployment, morbidity and mortality in Britain. *Population Studies* 1983; **37**: 61–74.

15. Fox AJ, Goldblatt PO, Adelstein AM. Selection and mortality differentials. *J Epidemiol Commun Health* 1982; **36**: 69–79.

16. Cooper CL. Psychosocial stress and cancer. *Bull Br Psychol Soc* 1982; **35**: 456–59.

17. Platt S. Unemployment and suicidal behaviour: a review of the literature. *Soc Sci Med* 1984; **19**: 93–115.

18. Jenkins CD. Recent evidence supporting psychologic and social risk factors for coronary disease. *N Engl J Med* 1976; **294**: 987–94, 1033–38.

Job strain, work place social support, and cardiovascular disease: a cross-sectional study of a random sample of the Swedish working population

Jeffrey V. Johnson, PhD, and Ellen M. Hall, MA

Jeffrey V. Johnson, PhD, Assistant Professor, Division of Occupational Medicine, Department of Environmental Health Sciences, School of Hygiene and Public Health, Johns Hopkins University, 615 North Wolfe Street, Baltimore, MD 21205, USA. Ms. Hall is Project Coordinator for this research project.

Abstract

This cross-sectional study investigates the relationship betwen the psychosocial work environment and cardiovascular disease (CVD) prevalence in a randomly selected, representative sample of 13,779 Swedish male and female workers. It was found that self-reported psychological job demands, work control, and co-worder social support combined greater than multiplicatively in relation to CVD prevalence. An age-adjusted prevalence ratio (PR) of 2.17 (95% CI–1.32, 3.56) was observed among workers with high demands, low control, and low social support compared to a low demand, high control, and high social support reference group. PRs of approximately 2.00 were observed in this group after consecutively controlling for the effects of age together with 11 other potential confounding factors. The magnitude of the age-adjusted PRs was greatest for blue collar males. Due to the cross-sectional nature of the study design, causal inferences cannot be made. The limitations of design and measurement are discussed in the context of the methodological weaknesses of the work stress field. (*Am J Public Health* 1988; 78:1336–1342.)

Introduction

The role of a stressful work environment in the development of cardiovascular disease (CVD) is a matter of current interest.[1-6] A model

Reprinted from Job strain, work place social support, and cardiovascular disease: a cross-sectional study of a random sample of the Swedish working population. Johnson, J. V. and Hall, E. M. *American Journal of Public Health*, **78**, 1336–42, 1988. © American Public Health Association.

of job stress—the demand control model—has been proposed by Karasek.[7] The model predicts that biologically aversive strain will occur when the psychological demands of the job exceed the resources for control over task content. The research of Karasek, Theorell and colleagues suggests that it is this combination of high demands and low control that produces job strain.[7-12] Workers in high strain jobs have been shown to have greater risk of developing CVD.[7-9,11]

However, important methodological challenges to etiological inference remain in the occupational stress field[13,14] despite 20 years of research. These include: an over-reliance on cross-sectional as opposed to prospective designs; lack of generalizability due to the frequent restriction of samples to healthy, employed males; lack of valid and reliable measures of chronic disease outcomes; lack of exposure data with stress being evaluated on the basis of only a single measure in time; and incomplete models of the stress process. Investigations using the demand–control model have addressed a number of these problems.[15] However, the model itself has been criticized for not including other, equally important, psychosocial work characteristics.[9]

Although the cross-sectional design of the present study does not permit causal inferences, it does address two of the difficulties mentioned above: restricted samples and incomplete modeling. Our study group consists of a random sample of both men and women which is representative of the entire working population of Sweden. Also, the demand–control model has been redefined by the addition of work related social support. Previous research has suggested that social support may serve to modify the impact of psychological demands both on and off the job.[2,6] A number of prospective studies have found an association between general social network interaction and total mortality incidence.[16-21] Inadequate work place social support and social isolation has been shown to be associated with a higher incidence of angina pectoris among male workers in Israel;[22] a greater incidence of coronary heart disease among female clerks;[23] psychological problems among air traffic controllers;[24] higher cholesterol values among those whose work mates were constantly changing;[25] higher levels of illness among the unemployed;[26,27] a greater physical health impact from perceived stress among male petrochemical workers[28,29] and increased job stress and psychological strain among men in 23 occupations.[30] Studies which have looked at the moderating or so-called "buffering" effect of social support have found that it ameliorates the impact of perceived stress and job strain on physical and mental health.[30-32]

None of the research on social support and CVD to date has been linked with the demand–control formulation. This was an impetus to the present study and to the development of the model shown in Figure 1.

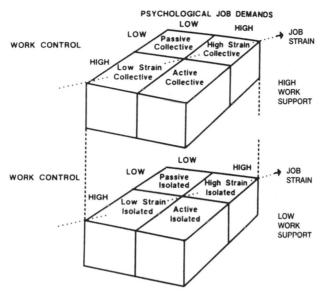

Figure 1. Demand–Control–Support Model.

In the Demand–Control–Support model work-related social support has been dichotomized into isolated or collective conditions, thereby redefining the process of job strain (indicated by the diagonal arrows in Figure 1). This model permits us to examine whether the lack of social support combines with job strain to further increase the likelihood of CVD prevalence.

Methods

Study sample

The data used were the Swedish Central Bureau of Statistics (SCB) Survey of Living Conditions ("ULF" in Swedish). This ongoing survey was mandated in the early 1970s by the Swedish Parliament as the major social accounting system to investigate the distribution of health status, income, education, and various aspects of the social and work environment. Over the past 14 years, considerable effort has been devoted to constructing reliable and valid indicators which, according to the survey's director, "are not colored by the respondent's ambitions, and reference frames. Among other matters this means that wishes, demands, opinions, etc. are not in principle surveyed."*

*Vogel J: The Swedish annual Level of Living Survey: Social indicators and social reporting as an official statistics program. Paper presented at the Tenth World Congress of Sociology, Mexico City, August 16, 1982, p. 30.

The Living Conditions Survey is conducted annually. A systematic random sample of individuals born on the 15th of each month was obtained from the National Registry of Births. Spouses were also interviewed. The present study combined two annual samples. In 1976, the sample consisted of 14,000 subjects and in 1977 of 14,500. Response rates were 79 per cent in 1976 and 81 per cent in 1977. Later studies on the effects of non-response on variables concerning illness were found to be minimal.[33,34]

The survey data were collected in a one-hour personal or telephone interview performed by a trained SCB interviewer. The present investigation used a sub-sample of 13,779 subjects consisting of employed persons from the ages of 16 to 65 (mean age 39); 52 per cent were males, 48 per cent females.

Measurement of job characteristics

The psychological job demands indicator was constructed from two items:

- Is your job hectic?
- your job psychologically demanding?

A Guttman scale was constructed using the combined responses to these questions. The proportions reporting low, medium, and high demands were: 34.7, 36.7 and 28.6 per cent, respectively. The Guttman coefficient of reproducibility for the scale was .92 and the coefficient of scalability was .79.

This measure can be criticized as providing an overly simplistic assessment of actual levels and types of demands, and for measuring subjective appraisals as opposed to objective psychosocial conditions. However, it correlates highly with other known occupational stressors such as lack of rest breaks, anticipation of job loss, and piece rate work,[10] and it has been used in earlier prospective studies of the relation between job strain and coronary heart disease.[7]

The work control scale is a linear composite which measures decision-making authority, task variety, and personal freedom on the job. The following items were scored according to whether the subject had never (0), sometimes (1), or often (2) any of the following:

- Influence over the planning of work
- Influence over the setting of the work pace
- Influence over how time is used in work
- The planning of work breaks
- The planning of vacations
- Flexible working hours
- Freedom to receive a phone call during working hours

- Freedom to receive a private visitor at work
- Varied task content
- Varied work procedures
- Possibilities for on-going education as part of the job

Scores range from 0 to 22 with a mean of 12. The standard deviation was 4.4; scores were normally distributed. The Cronbach's alpha for the scale was .70; the average item to total scale correlation was .52. This measure is similar to indicators used by Swedish and American investigators to measure comparable aspects of job content.[7,10,12]

Work-related social support was measured using a scale consisting of five dichotomous items. Respondents were asked whether they:

- Could talk to co-workers during breaks
- Could leave their job to talk with co-workers
- Could interact with co-workers as part of their work
- Met with co-workers, outside of the work place
- Had met with a co-worker during the last six months

The total scale was constructed by adding the responses, across items. The scores ranged from 0–5, with a mean of 3, and a standard deviation of 1.5. The Cronbach's alpha was .75; the average item-to-total correlation being .70. This scale measures two aspects of support: opportunity to interact at work and if co-worker interaction is carried over into non-work life. It measures the basic prerequisites for social support but does not evaluate whether social contact at work is positive or negative and therefore may tend to overestimate the degree of social support found in Swedish work places. However, in a separate analysis we found that it correlated highly with more sensitive measures of social support available in the 1976 ULF, which included instrumental aid from co-workers, free time activities performed with co-workers, and supportive discussions between co-workers.[35]

The three psychological work environmental scales are weakly associated with each other. The Pearson correlation coefficients between the measures are: demands and control = .01, demands and support = .09, control and support = .12; indicating that these are relatively independent characteristics.

Cardiovascular disease indicator

The measure of CVD prevalence was based on the SCB's health classification system. As part of the larger SCB effort information on all types of long-term illness and disability was obtained in a personal interview. The respondent was asked a general question concerning health status: "Do you suffer any longstanding illness, effects of an injury, any disability or weakness?" Given an affirmative response, the interviewer probes: "Could you explain that a little more?", "What did the doctor say it was?". "What part of the body or organ system is affected?" The respondents were also questioned concerning use of regular medication, in order to include symptom free conditions, not covered by the previous questions. The description of any illness was coded by a central unit of the SCB, using a coding system developed and tested by two Swedish physicians, who worked as consultants to the SCB. They matched symptoms with the International Classification of Disease, 8th revision. Based on the total set of responses, SCB coders classified 804 subjects with ICD codes 3900–4589 as having CVD. The prevalence rate for the entire study group was 5.83 per cent, 395 females with CVD with a prevalence rate of 6.03 per cent and 409 males with a prevalence rate of 5.66 per cent. These differences in sex-specific rates are similar to those reported in other studies of cardiovascular prevalence in Sweden and Britain.** Karasek found that the CVD prevalence rate in Swedish employed males was 5.9 per cent, as measured by having two or more self-reported symptoms on the Karasek–Theorell CVD indicator.[7] The difference in prevalence estimations between the SCB and the Karasek–Theorell indicators may be due to the much larger sample size of the present study, and/or to the divergence in diagnostic methods.

The predictive validity of the CVD indicator was examined by observing whether or not individuals who report symptoms were later at risk for CVD mortality. The survey group was linked to the National Mortality Registry using the individual person number assigned to all Swedish residents. Incidence of cardiovascular related mortality was identified by combining all deaths for arteriosclerotic heart disease, cerebrovascular and peripheral vascular disease (ICD codes, 8th Revision, 400–404, 410–414, 427, 430–436, 440–445). During the six-year follow-up period, individuals classified as having CVD had an age- and sex-adjusted relative risk ratio of 3.32 (95% CI–3:00, 3.64) for cardiovascular-related mortality, as compared to persons who were classified as not having CVD. In order to test the discriminant validity of the CVD prevalence measure, an indicator of all noncardiovascular mortality was constructed. CVD prevalence cases had a much lower, and age- and sex-adjusted relative risk ratio of 1.15 (95% CI–.71, 1.59) for noncardiovascular-related mortality.

**Lundberg O: Social class and inequalities in morbidity—Some recent Swedish findings. Paper presented at the Fourth Nordic Social Policy Research Seminar, Hasselby Slott, Sweden, October 1984.

Potential confounding factors and effect modifiers

Twelve variables were examined to see if they confounded or otherwise modified the relationship between work environment characteristics and CVD. These factors are displayed in Appendix I and are described in more detail elsewhere.[21,35]

Statistical analysis

The data were analyzed using a series of epidemiologic programs developed by Rothman and Boice.[36] The most frequent measure of association was the relative prevalence ratio. The Mantel–Haenszel Chi was used for hypothesis testing[37] and confidence limits were constructed from the point estimates of the PR and the Mantel–Haenszel test statistic, using test-based interval estimation.[38–40]

When controlling for confounding factors the data were first stratified into categories of the confounding factor, and a weighted average of the stratum specific rate ratios was obtained using Mantel–Haenszel procedures.[36,37] Hypothesis testing and confidence interval estimation in the stratified analysis were performed using Mantel-Haenszel[36] and Miettinen's techniques.[40]

To analyze for interactions, an index of synergy—the Rothman Interaction Ratio—was used to evaluate whether two or more factors combine greater than additively in relation to risk.[41,42] This expression is the ratio of the observed effect of combined exposure to two or more risk factors, divided by that effect which would be expected if the factors were acting independently. If the interaction ratio exceeds 1, it is an index of synergism and if the value of the ratio is less than 1, it is an index of antagonism. A slight modification of Rothman's approach has been used in the study in that the independent contribution of each risk factor is arrived at by simultaneously controlling for the other factors following the modeling procedure proposed by Breslow and Day.[43]

Results

The combined effects of psychological job demands, work control, and work-related social support on CVD are shown for prevalence rates in Table 1 and for age-adjusted PRs in Table 2. The demand-control model is reproduced in each of these tables for high, medium, and low levels of social support. The reference category used for the age adjustment calculations is the low demand, high control, and high support group. These workers were identified as the low exposure group based on the

Table 1. *Prevalence rates for cardiovascular disease in the Demand–Control–Support Model*

	Psychological Job Demands		
	Low Demand	Medium Demand	High Demand
High Work Support			
% Low Work Control (n)	[1] 5.48 (675)	[2] 7.26 (822)	[3] 6.36 (566)
% Medium Work Control (n)	[4] 4.95 (808)	[5] 4.33 (876)	[6] 5.66 (672)
% High work Control (n)	[7] 2.88 (729)	[8] 3.25 (862)	[9] 5.11 (880)
Medium Work Support			
% Low Work Control (n)	[10] 4.46 (493)	[11] 7.39 (555)	[12] 7.44 (363)
% Medium Work Control (n)	[13] 7.51 (506)	[14] 6.50 (523)	[15] 7.25 (331)
% High Work Control (n)	[16] 3.99 (376)	[17] 5.84 (411)	[18] 5.34 (393)
Low Work Support			
% Low Work Control (n)	[19] 8.22 (426)	[20] 8.33 (492)	[21] 9.25 (400)
% Medium Work Control (n)	[22] 5.59 (420)	[23] 8.53 (305)	[24] 6.81 (191)
% High Work Control (n)	[25] 6.25 (352)	[26] 6.94 (216)	[27] 11.03 (136)

Note: Numbers 1 through 27 in brackets correspond to "cells" referred to in text.

theoretical criteria of the model which distinguishes this as having the fewest demands combined with the maximum psychosocial resources.

We can first examine the impact of the introduction of social support on the demand–control model by comparing the overall magnitude of the prevalence rates and ratios at each level of social support. With few exceptions for each demand–control combination prevalence rates and ratios increase with decreasing levels of social support. Within the high social support category, PRs relative to the reference category are highest in high strain combinations where the level of job demands exceed that of work control (i.e., cells 2, 3, and 6 in Table 2). Moreover, the job combinations predicted by the model to be the highest strain groups (high demands and low control) demonstrate an increase in the magnitude of the PRs with decreasing levels of social support.

The demand–control model hypothesizes that a pattern of increasing strain will occur along a strain diagonal, shown for high and low levels of social support in Figure 1. The results for CVD prevalence along this diagonal are shown in Table 1 and 2. As the job combinations change from low demand and high control (cells 7, 16, 25) to medium demands and medium control (cells 5, 14, 23) to high demands and low control (cells 3, 12, 21) the prevalence rates and ratios increase. However, as the level of social support decreases, CVD prevalence rates and PRs increase at each point along the strain diagonal.

Table 2. *Age-adjusted prevalence ratios for cardiovascular disease in the Demand–Control–Support Model*

	Psychological Job Demands		
	Low Demand	Medium Demand	High Demand
High Work Support			
% Low Work Control	[1] 1.44	[2] 1.69	[3] 1.82
95% CI	(.87, 2.39)	(1.05, 2.73)	(1.10, 3.01)
% Medium Work Control	[4] 1.59	[5] 1.34	[6] 1.74
95% CI	(.96, 2.62)	(.80, 2.25)	(1.06, 2.87)
% High Work Control	[7] 1.00	[8] 1.11	[9] 1.58
95% CI	(Reference Category)	(.64, 1.92)	(.97, 2.58)
Medium Work Support			
% Low Work Control	[10] 1.69	[11] 1.88	[12] 1.94
95% CI	(1.00, 2.85)	(1.14, 3.09)	(1.14, 3.31)
% Medium Work Control	[13] 1.85	[14] 1.70	[15] 1.86
95% CI	(1.12, 3.06)	(1.02, 2.84)	(1.07, 3.22)
% High Work Control	[16] 1.14	[17] 1.80	[18] 1.30
95% CI	(.60, 2.17)	(1.04, 3.12)	(.72, 2.29)
Low Work Support			
% Low Work Control	[19] 1.95	[20] 2.10	[21] 2.17
95% CI	(1.18, 3.23)	(1.30, 3.38)	(1.32, 3.56)
% Medium Work Control	[22] 1.49	[23] 2.08	[24] 1.57
95% CI	(.85, 2.60)	(1.22, 3.56)	(.81, 3.06)
% High Work Control	[25] 1.43	[26] 1.77	[27] 2.55
95% CI	(.81, 2.53)	(.94, 3.30)	(1.38, 4.71)

Note: Numbers 1 through 27 in brackets correspond to "cells" referred to in text.

The potential modifying effect of work control on the relation between job demands and cardiovascular prevalence is also evident in the low social support condition of the high demand–high control group (cell 27). The PR for this group is the highest observed. It was not predicted by the model. These results suggest that the modifying effect of work control on the job demand and CVD relationship is evident only under a particular contingency: when social support from co-workers is present. If workers have few social interaction opportunities, there is an elevation in cardiovascular prevalence in the high demand–high control combination.

Other job combinations exhibit elevated prevalence rates and ratios relative to the reference category, not predicted by the basic demand–

Table 3. *Rothman's interaction analysis for cardiovascular disease*

Excess Prevalence Risk Analysis:

Job Variable or Combination	Controlling For:	Prevalence Ratio (95% CI)	% Excess Prevalence Risk
Job Demands	Age	1.24	
	Control Support	(1.06, 1.47)	24
Work Control	Age	1.25	
	Demands Support	(1.06, 1.47)	25
Work Support	Age	1.29	
	Demands Control	(1.10, 1.52)	29
High Demand, Low Control Combination	Age Support	1.69 (1.25, 2.28)	19
High Demand, Low Support Combination	Age Control	1.56 (1.15, 2.10)	3
Low Control, Low Support Combination	Age Demands	1.71 (1.33, 2.25)	17

Interaction Analysis:
Additive Expected Excess Prevalence Risk: 78%
Observed Combined Excess Prevalence Risk: 117% (From Table 4, cell 21)
Rothman's Interaction Ratio (observed/expected): 1.50
Multiplicative Expected Prevalence Ratio: 2.00
Multiplicative Interaction Ratio: 1.09.

control formulation. The low demand–low control cells characterized in Figure 1 as passive work situations (cells 1, 10, 19) show substantially elevated PRs when social support is medium (PR = 1.69) or low (PR = 1.95).

The statistical interactions of the three job characteristics were examined using Rothman's technique.[42,43]

Each factor, taken individually, contributed about the same amount of excess prevalence for CVD with PRs ranging from 1.24 to 1.29 (Table 3). The additive expected excess prevalence risk was 78 per cent and the observed combined excess prevalence risk was 117 per cent. By dividing the observed excess prevalence risk by the expected prevalence risk the Rothman's interaction ratio of 1.50 was obtained. This finding indicates that demands, control, and support combine 50 per cent more than additively. Indeed, as the multiplicative interaction ratio of 1.09 indicates, the three-factor interaction is 9 per cent more than multiplicative.

The influence of potential confounding factors such as health behaviors, other types of job demands, and sociodemographic factors was

Table 4. *Controlling for potential confounding factors and effect modifiers in the Demand–Control–Support and cardiovascular disease (CVD) relationship*[a]

Confounding Factor or Effect Modifier	Prevalence Ratio for CVD	95% CI
Crude	3.12	1.96–5.26
Age	2.17	1.32–3.56
(All subsequent analyses are age-adjusted)		
Sex	1.87	1.13–3.11
Physical Exercise[b]	1.96	1.04–3.70
Intergenerational Class Mobility	1.97	1.12–3.46
Marital Status	2.00	1.21–3.29
Non-work Social Support	2.16	1.32–3.53
Immigrant Status	2.16	1.30–3.56
Occupational Class Level	2.17	1.12–4.19
Rural vs Urban	2.19	1.33–3.56
Smoking[b]	2.31	1.20–4.48
Household Disposable Income	2.35	1.40–3.95
Physical Job Demands	3.41	1.59–7.36

[a]High demand, low control, low support workers are compared with low demand, high control, and high support workers.
[b]Information on smoking and exercise available only in 1977 survey group.

considered. In this series of analyses, the theoretically lowest exposure group (low demands–high control–high social support) was compared to the theoretically highest exposure category (high demands, low control, low social support) within each level or strata of the potential confounding factor. After testing for age and finding that this decreased the crude relative risk from 3.21 to 2.17, age was included in all subsequent analysis.

In Table 4, it can be seen that after controlling for the various potential confounding factors the PR remains elevated above 1.00; the potential confounding factors have been ordered along a continuum according to whether they decrease, have no effect on, or increase the PR. Controlling for sex and physical exercise reduces the PR to some degree. Adjusting for occupational mobility, marital status, social class level, etc. did not alter the PR. When controlling for the smoking, income, and physical job demand variables the association between the adverse work combination and CVD increased. This was particularly pronounced when controlling for physical job demands.

The individual and combined effects of demands, control and support were examined within four sex-class groups: blue collar males (n = 4,242), blue collar females (n = 3,661), white collar males

Table 5. *Individual and combined cardiovascular disease (CVD) prevalence ratios of job demands, work control, and work social support for sex and class groups*

Job Variable or Combination	Blue Collar Males	White Collar Males	Blue Collar Females	White Collar Females
High Job Demands[a]	1.36	1.32	1.21	1.14
95% CI	(.99, 1.86)	(.93, 1.86)	(.88, 1.66)	(.76, 1.70)
Low Work Control[b]	1.42	1.03	1.12	1.07
95% CI	(.96, 2.09)	(.60, 1.75)	(.77, 1.62)	(.70, 1.66)
Low Social Support[c]	1.13	1.16	1.27	1.33
95% CI	(.82, 1.57)	(.77, 1.74)	(.97, 1.67)	(.89, 2.01)
High Job Demands, Low Work Control[d]	3.55	1.03	1.43	1.13
95% CI	(1.64, 7.69)	(.36, 2.91)	(.88, 2.30)	(.36, 2.91)
High Job Demands, Low Social Support[e]	1.82	1.81	1.68	2.06
95% CI	(1.06, 3.15)	(1.02, 3.22)	(1.07, 2.63)	(1.05, 4.01)
Low Work Control, Low Social Support[f]	1.97	1.86	1.86	1.44
95% CI	(1.04, 3.73)	(.98, 3.51)	(.93, 3.71)	(.75, 2.77)
High Job Demands, Low Work Control, Low Social Support[g]	7.22	2.44	2.19	1.95
95% CI	(1.60, 37.39)	(.95, 6.28)	(.77, 6.23)	(.74, 5.12)

[a]Compared to low demand group, controlling for age, control, support.
[b]Compared to high control group, controlling for age, demand, support.
[c]Compared to high support group, controlling for age, demand, control.
[d]Compared to low demand, high control group, controlling for age, support.
[e]Compared to low demand, high support group, controlling for age, control.
[f]Compared to high control, high support group, controlling for age, demand.
[g]Compared to low demand, high control, high support group, controlling for age.

(n = 2,987), and white collar females (n = 2,889). These results are shown in Table 5.

In all four sex-class groups the three work factors taken individually were only slightly associated with cardiovascular prevalence, while the combinations of work characteristics show the highest PRs.

There is a differential pattern of association among the various sex-class groups. The blue collar male group is most affected by the combination of the three job characteristics, particularly in the high demand–low control combination, with a PR 3.55 (95% CI–1.64, 7.69); and in the high demand–low control–low support combination with a PR 7.72 (95% CI-1.60, 37.39).

The combined effects are less evident in white collar males, although the basic hypothesized relations are still discernible.

For females the combined effects can also be seen but are less pronounced than among blue collar males and there is no obvious difference between blue and white collar workers.

Discussion

We are able to corroborate some of the basic predictions of the demand–control formulation in this study. As Karasek and others have previously reported, increasing levels of job strain are associated with increasing rates of cardiovascular prevalence. Work-related social support appears to accentuate the impact of job strain, in that workers with the lowest levels of social support had higher prevalence rates and ratios at each level of job strain. What was not predicted by the earlier demand–control model, however, was the elevated PRs found among active-isolated workers. Although we can only speculate as to the explanation for this finding, it is possible that in some working situations, high levels of control may accentuate rather than reduce the impact of demands. Our indicator of control may actually be measuring responsibility pressure, which in some occupations might constitute another component of job demands. This suggests the need to further refine our measurement of work control in order to at least distinguish control as a resource from responsibility as a demand.

Low social support in combination with low control was also associated with increased PRs, even in the absence of psychological job demands. This suggests that earlier insights concerning the negative impact of understimulation and qualitative underload on the cardiovascular system may still be relevant.[44]

The findings for the various sex and class groups clearly demonstrate that blue collar male workers have the strongest associations between adverse work combinations and CVD. However, it should be noted that one effect of reproducing the analysis performed in the total population for subgroups is to restrict the overall variance of work characteristics. This probably had the greatest effect on restricting the subgroup variation of work control, most strongly associated with sex and class, thereby diminishing its association with CVD.

Many of the work stress studies to date have been restricted to males.[45] It is often assumed that job characteristics that are important predictors for males are important for females as well. The findings reported here indicate that there may be sex as well as class differences. The sex-class analysis suggests that among women social support may be a more important predictor for CVD prevalence than work control. However, these findings can only be interpreted as suggestive and as an indication of the need to focus more attention on the specific differences between the various sex and class groups in the working population.

While this investigation supports the other research linking psychosocial work organization and CVD, it shares certain methodological weaknesses common to the field as a whole. As noted, because of the cross-sectional design, it is not possible to discern causal relationships. Since we cannot temporally separate work exposure from the manifestation of the disease, it is impossible to rule out alternative explanations to the observed associations. Although we have adjusted for a variety of individual characteristics, including class mobility, differential selection factors could provide alternative explanations to the observed findings. Although, as Theorell and his colleagues point out,[15] it is unlikely that individuals with CVD would select themselves into high strain occupations, it is plausible that individuals previously employed in high strain jobs who have experienced cardiovascular symptoms could move into passive isolated jobs.

Due to lack of information in the ULF data, it was not possible to examine the potential confounding effects of diet. It is unlikely, however, that diet would explain the associations observed in this study, for dietary practices observed in Sweden are markedly homogenous. Although men in lower level occupations may tend to have a higher relative weight than those in upper level occupations,[15] since we have controlled for occupational class level in our analysis, the effects of class differences in diet and weight would at least be partly accounted for.

Another threat to causal interpretation arises from the fact that the presence of cardiovascular illness might affect the way in which individuals perceive their working situation, leading them to report it as being more psychologically demanding.

Although there is evidence of the predictive and discriminant validity of the CVD prevalence indicators, a more objective measure would be preferable. The measures of demand, control, and support used in this study also could be further refined. In the present study the evaluation of psychological job demands, in particular, is determined by the subjective perception of employees. Also, it is not clear that the social support measure reflects more than the frequency and opportunity for interaction. In general, research into the effects of the psychosocial environment would be strengthened if there were more objective exposure data.

In a recent review discussing many of the problems in research methodology which retard the development of the occupational stress field, Kasl notes a dilemma faced by many researchers: "better research designs are more a function of the resources available to the investigator and less a reflection of his/her level of methodological sophistication."[14]

Large data sets, such as the one used in this study, are resources, but within these extensive samples, one must make use of the information as it exists. Certain strengths, i.e., a large, representative sample, a good response rate, and the ability to identify and control for a variety of confounding factors are important advantages; relying on survey questions which were not specifically formulated to meet the requirements of stress research has distinct disadvantages.

In conclusion, the addition of social support expands the demand–control formulation from an emphasis on the individual connection between a person and their job into the domain of collective relationships between people. Although recent reviews have pointed out that the findings concerning work place social support have been weak and confusing,[46] our results can only suggest that social support may have to be linked to influence processes such as work control to have any substantial effect on cardiovascular health.

Acknowledgements

Much of this research was performed in Sweden at the Research Unit for the Social Psychology of Work, University of Stockholm. The authors wish to acknowledge the many theoretical and practical contributions of the director of this unit, the late Bertil Gardell, PhD, Professor of Work Psychology. We also would like to thank Robert Karasek, PhD, and Tores Theorell, MD, PhD, for their thoughtful suggestions during each stage of this research effort. In addition, we thank Anders Ahlbom, PhD, for his valuable suggestions on statistical procedures; and Per-Olof Fredericksson, Gudrun Lindberg, and Joachim Vogel, PhD, for their advice and practical support with the data analyses.

The study was financially supported by the Swedish Work Environment Fund. Dr. Johnson was also supported during the study period by National Heart Lung and Blood Institute Cardiovascular Risk Reduction Training Grant 5T32HL07180 and Public Health Service Biomedical Research Support Grant S07RR05445.

References

1. Levi L, Frankenhaeuser M, Gardell B: Work stress related to social structures and processes: *In:* Elliott G, Eisdorfer C (eds): Stress and Human Health. New York: Springer, 1982; 119–146.
2. House J, Cottington E: Health and the workplace. *In:* Aiken L, Mechanic D (eds): Applications of Social Science to Clinical Medicine and Health Policy. New Brunswick: Rutgers University Press, 1986; 392–416.
3. Kasl S: The challenge of studying the disease effects of stressful work conditions. Am J Public Health 1981; 71:628–630.
4. Kasl S: Epidemiological contributions to the study of work stress. *In:* Cooper C, Payne R (eds): Stress at Work. New York: Wiley, 1977; 3–48.

5. Frankenhaeuser M: Psychoneuroendocrine approaches to the study of stressful person-environment transactions. *In:* Selye H (ed): Selye's Guide to Stress Research. New York: Van Nostrand Reinhold, 1980; 46–70.

6. House J, Jackson M: Occupational stress and health. *In:* Ahmed P, Coelho C (eds): Towards a New Definition of Health. New York: Plenum, 1979.

7. Karasek R, Baker D, Marxer F, Ahlbom A, Theorell T: Job decision latitude, job demands, and cardiovascular disease: A prospective study of Swedish men. Am J Public Health 1981; 71:694–705.

8. Alfredsson L, Karasek R, Theorell T: Myocardial infarction risk and psychosocial work environment characteristics: An analysis of the male Swedish work force. Soc Sci Med 1982; 16:463–467.

9. Baker D: The study of stress at work. Annu Rev Public Health 1985; 6:367–381.

10. Karasek R: Job demands, job decision latitude, and mental strain: Implications for job redesign. Admin Sci Q 1979; 24:285–308.

11. Karasek R, Theorell T, Schwartz J, Pieper C, Alfredsson A: Job psychological factors and coronary heart disease. Adv Cardiol 1982; 29:62–76.

12. Karasek R: Job socialization and job strain: Implications of two related psychosocial mechanisms for job design. *In:* Gardell B, Johansson G (eds): Working Life. Chichester, England: John Wiley and Sons, 1981.

13. House J, Strecher V, Metzner H, *et al:* Occupational stress and health among men and women in the Tecumseh Community Health Study. J Health Soc Behav 1986; 27:62–77.

14. Kasl SV: Methodologies in stress and health: Past difficulties, present dilemmas, future directions. *In:* Kasl S, Cooper C (eds): Stress and Health Issues in Research Methodology. Chichester, England: John Wiley and Sons, 1987

15. Theorell T, Alfredsson L, Knox S, Perski A, Svensson J, Waller D: On the interplay between socioeconomic factors, personality and work environment in the pathogenesis of cardiovascular disease. Scan J Work Environ Health 1984; 10:373–380.

16. Berkman L: The relationship of social networks and social support to morbidity and mortality. *In:* Cohen S, Syme SL (eds): Social Support and Health. New York: Academic Press, 1985; 240–259.

17. Berkman L, Syme SL: Social networks, host resistance and mortality: A nine year study of Alameda county residents. Am J Epidemiol 1979; 109:186–204.

18. House J, Robbins C, Metzner H: The association of social relationships and activities with mortality. Prospective evidence from Tecumseh community health study. Am J Epidemiol 1982; 116:123–140.

19. Blazer D: Social support and mortality in an elderly community population. Am J Epidemiol 1982; 115:684–694.

20. Schoenbach V, Kaplan BH, Fredman L, Kleinbaum D: Social ties and mortality in Evans County, Georgia. Am J Epidemiol 1986; 123:577–591.

21. Orth-Gomer K, Johnson JV: Social network interaction and mortality: A six year follow-up of a random sample of the Swedish Population. J Chronic Dis 1987; 40:949–957.

22. Medalie J, Kahn HA, Neufeld H, Rise R, Goldbourt U: Five year myocardial infarction incidence: 2. Association of single variables to age and birthplace. J Chronic Dis 1973; 26:329–349.

23. Haynes S, Feinleib M: Women, work and coronary heart disease: Prospective findings from the Framingham Heart Study. Am J Public Health 1980; 70:133–141.
24. Rose R, Hurst M, Herd A: Cardiovascular and endocrine responses to work and the risk of psychiatric symptoms among air traffic controllers. *In:* Barrett J (ed); Stress and Mental Disorder. New York: Raven Press, 1979.
25. Cassel J: The use of medical records: Opportunities for epidemiological studies. JOM 1963; 5:185–190.
26. Cobb S, Kasl S: Termination: The consequences of job loss. NIOSH Pub. No. 77–224. Cincinnati, Ohio: National Institute for Occupational Safety and Health, 1977.
27. Jahoda M: Employment and Unemployment: A Socio-Psychological Analysis. Cambridge: Cambridge University Press, 1982.
28. House J: Work Stress and Social Support. Reading, Mass: Addison, Wesley, 1981.
29. House J, McMichael A, Wells J, Kaplan B, Landerman L: Occupational stress and health among factory workers. J Health Soc Behav 1979; 20:139–160.
30. Pinneau S: Effect of social support on psychological and physiological strain. Doctoral dissertation, University of Michigan, 1975.
31. LaRocco J, House J, French J: Social support, occupational stress and health. J Health Soc Behav 1980; 21:202–218.
32. Karasek R, Triantis K, Chaudhry S: Co-worker and supervisor support as moderators of associations between task characteristics and mental strain. J Occ Behav 1982; 3:147–160.
33. Bergman L, Hanve R, Rappe R: Why do some people refuse to participate in interview surveys? Stat Rev 1978; 5:286–301.
34. Lindstrom H: Non-response estimates due to illness: S.C.B. Report No. 24. Stockholm: Swedish Statistical Bureau, 1981.
35. Johnson J: The impact of workplace social support, job demands and work control. Environmental and Organizational Psychology Research Reports, 1, Stockholm: University of Stockholm, 1986.
36. Rothman K, Boice J: Epidemiologic Analysis with a Programmable Calculator. Boston: Epidemiology Resources, 1982.
37. Mantel N, Haenszel W: Statistical aspects of the analysis of data from retrospective studies of disease. JNCI 1959; 22:719–748.
38. Miettinen O: Confounding and effect modification. Am J Epidemiol 1974; 100:350–353.
39. Miettinen O: Simple interval estimation of risk ratio. Am J Epidemiol 1974, 100:515–516.
40. Miettinen O: Estimability and estimation in case-referent studies. Am J Epidemiol 1976; 103:226–235.
41. Rothman K: Synergy and antagonism in cause-effect relationships. Am J Epidemiol 1974; 99:385–388.
42. Rothman K: The estimation of synergy or antagonism. Am J Epidemiol 1976; 103:506–511.
43. Breslow N, Day N: Statistical methods in cancer research. Lyon International Agency for Research on Cancer, 1980.
44. Frankenhaeuser M, Gardell B: Overload and underload in working life:

Outline of a multidisciplinary approach. J Human Stress 1976; 2:35–46.

45. Haw M: Women, work and stress: A review and agenda for the future. J Hlth Soc Behav 1982; 123:132–144.

46. Kasl S, Wells J: Social support and health in the middle years. *In:* Cohen S, Syme SL (eds): Social Support and Health. New York: Academic Press 1985; 143–165.

Appendix I. *Potential confounding factors and effect modifiers*

Factor	Categories	Percentage
1. Age	16–44	66
	45–65	34
2. Sex	Female	48
	Male	52
3. Marital Status	Married	64
	Single	36
4. Income	Low	33
	Medium	34
	High	32
5. Intergenerational Class Mobility	Upwardly mobile	35
	Downwardly mobile	35
	No change in class	30
6. Occupational Class Level	Lower level manual	39
	Upper level manual	18
	Lower level office	18
	Upper level office	25
7. Immigrant Status	Native Swedish	87
	Immigrant	13
8. Region	Urban	65
	Rural	35
9. Smoking	Nonsmoker	61
	Smoker	39
10. Physical Exercise	Sedentary	60
	Active	40
11. Physical Job Demands	Low	29
	Medium	32
	High	39
12. Non-work Related Social Support	Low	33
	Medium	32
	High	34

Social networks, host resistance, and mortality: a nine-year follow-up study of Alameda County residents

Lisa F. Berkman and S. Leonard Syme

Department of Epidemiology and Public Health and Institution for Social and Policy Studies, Yale University, New Haven, CT 06520, USA
Program in Epidemiology, School of Public Health, University of California, Berkeley, CA, USA

Abstract

Berkman, L. F. (Dept. of Epidemiology and Public Health, Yale U., New Haven, CT 06520), and S. L. Syme. Social networks, host resistance, and mortality: A nine-year follow-up study of Alameda County residents. *Am J Epidemiol* 109:186–204, 1979.

The relationship between social and community ties and mortality was assessed using the 1965 Human Population Laboratory survey of a random sample of 6928 adults in Alameda County, California and a subsequent nine-year mortality follow-up. The findings show that people who lacked social and community ties were more likely to die in the follow-up period than those with more extensive contacts. The age-adjusted relative risks for those most isolated when compared to those with the most social contacts were 2.3 for men and 2.8 for women. The association between social ties and mortality was found to be independent of self-reported physical health status at the time of the 1965 survey, year of death, socioeconomic status, and health practices such as smoking, alcoholic beverage consumption, obesity, physical activity, and utilization of preventive health services as well as a cumulative index of health practices.

health surveys; marriage; mortality; smoking; social class; social isolation

Previous research has suggested that social ties and relationships may play a critical role in the determination of health status. Individuals undergoing rapid social and cultural changes (1–5) as well as those living in situations characterized by social disorganization (6–8), and poverty

Reprinted from Berkman, L. F. and Syme, S. L. Social networks, host resistance, and mortality: a nine-year follow-up study of Alameda County residents. *American Journal of Epidemiology*, **109**, 186–204, 1979.

(9–12) appear to be at increased risk of acquiring many diseases. These situations have frequently been described in terms of the absence of stable social ties and resources available to individuals living in such circumstances. Other studies of army wives (13) and men undergoing job loss (14) suggest that social supports may be protective against the harmful health consequences associated with stressful life events.

Furthermore, it repeatedly has been observed that people who are married have lower mortality rates than those who are single, widowed, or divorced (15–17). The relationship between widowhood and increased morbidity and mortality is particularly striking. The results of several investigations (18–21) indicate that widows, especially in the first year following bereavement, have many more complaints about their health, have more mental and physical symptoms, believe they have sustained a lasting deterioration to their health, and have increased mortality rates. Recent evidence reveals that these differences do not appear to be totally attributable to some primary selection process in marriage (22), homogamy (23), or differences in such risk factors as serum cholesterol, blood pressure, or obesity (24).

The literature cited above provides some preliminary evidence that social and community ties may play some role in the etiology of disease. However, in most of these studies, investigators have not directly measured social contacts. Further, most of these findings have been derived from observations of special population groups such as widowers, army wives, or particular occupational groups. In this paper, results are reported of a study in which the impact of a range of social ties and networks was directly examined in relation to mortality from all causes in a large sample of a general population.

Methods

Study population

The data utilized in this report are based on information collected by the Human Population Laboratory (HPL), part of the California State Department of Health. In 1965, a survey was conducted based on a stratified systematic sample of Alameda County housing units. Institutionalized populations were not included. The sampling procedure, explained in greater detail elsewhere (25), resulted in the selection of 4452 occupied housing units. Each of these units was visited by an enumerator who gathered demographic data on all household members of all ages and left a questionnaire for all persons aged 20 or over, or for younger people who were married. Of the households, 8023 adults were identified as eligible for the study. Of these, 6928, or 86 per cent, finally

Table 1. *Age-specific mortality rates per 100 (all causes) men and women, ages 30–69. Human Population Laboratory Study of Alameda County, 1965–1974*

Age	No. of respondents	No. of deaths	% died
	Men		
30–39	673	16	2.4
40–49	729	36	4.9
50–59	501	68	13.6
60–69	326	91	27.9
Total	2229	211	9.5 (crude rate)
	Women		
30–39	728	16	2.2
40–49	807	32	4.0
50–59	574	45	7.8
60–69	387	67	17.3
Total	2496	160	6.4 (crude rate)

returned questionnaires. When compared to respondents, the small group of non-respondents included proportionately more older people, males, whites, and single or widowed persons (26). However, the differences between respondents and non-respondents have a negligible effect on population estimates, and respondents have been judged to be a representative sample of adults in the county. The present analysis is restricted to 2229 men and 2496 women between the ages of 30–69.

Mortality follow-up

Mortality data were collected for the nine-year period from 1965 to 1974, when a follow-up survey was conducted. A computer matching file was created with the California Death Registry to obtain the records of those people who died within the state. The exact description of the matching process is given elsewhere (27). Additional out-of-state death clearance information was obtained for those respondents believed to have moved out of state between the two survey periods. Through these methods, death certificates were located for 682 people. Through extensive follow-up in 1974, all but 302 respondents, or 4 per cent, of the original sample were located. Those lost to follow-up were not found to differ markedly on the health measures in the 1965 survey. The collection of mortality data therefore seems to be fairly complete and unbiased.

Statistical analysis

The chi square statistics presented in this paper are based on a modification of the Mantel–Haenszel chi square (28) developed by Brand and Sholtz (29). The Mantel–Haenszel statistic has been modified to include more than two comparison groups. In this paper, the statistic is adjusted for both age and a second covariable of interest, e.g., health practices or socioeconomic status. All age-adjusted mortality rates presented were adjusted by the indirect method (30, 31).

Results

Age-specific mortality rates from all causes for men and women between the ages of 30 and 69 are shown in table 1. As expected, women have lower mortality rates than men, and mortality rates increase sharply with age. The age- and sex-specific mortality rates in the Human Population Laboratory sample are similar to mortality rates for Alameda County.

Four sources of social contact

Table 2 shows the age- and sex-specific mortality rates for each of four sources of social contact examined: 1) marriage; 2) contacts with close friends and relatives; 3) church membership; and 4) informal and formal group associations. With few exceptions, respondents with each type of social tie had lower mortality rates than respondents lacking such connections.

In each age and sex group, people who are married have lower mortality rates than the non-married, i.e., separated, widowed, single, and divorced. The relative risks for non-married women compared to married women are approximately 1.4 for each age group. For men, the relative risks in the two younger groups are much larger: 2.9 and 2.1, respectively, for 30–49-year-old men and 50–59-year-old men. The age-adjusted chi square value for the differences in mortality rates among men of different marital status is highly significant; for women, the same chi square value fails to reach statistical significance.

Three questions on the Human Population Laboratory survey comprise an Index of contacts with friends and relatives: 1) "How many close friends do you have?"; 2) "How many relatives do you have that you feel close to?"; 3) "How often do you see these people each month?" Considered individually, none of these questions were important predictors of mortality; however, when combined, they are associated with signficant increases in risk. As seen in table 2, in every age and sex category, people who report having few friends and relatives and/or who

Table 2. *Age and sex-specific mortality rates per 100 (all causes) by source of social contact, Human Population Laboratory Study of Alameda County, 1965–1974*

	30–49		50–59		60–69		p^*
	No.	% died	No.	% died	No.	% died	
Men							
Marital status							
Married	1227	3.0	446	12.1	268	26.9	$p \leqslant 0.001$
Non-married	175	8.6	55	25.5	98	33.7	
Contacts with friends and relatives							
High	276	2.9	127	11.0	81	22.2	
Medium	865	3.4	303	14.2	173	24.9	$p \leqslant .001$
Low	236	5.1	62	14.5	59	40.7	
Church member							
Member	391	2.8	168	11.3	88	21.6	$p \leqslant .05$
Non-member	1011	4.1	333	14.7	238	30.3	
Group member							
Member	1066	3.6	394	11.9	223	28.2	ns†
Non-member	336	3.9	107	19.6	103	27.2	
Women							
Marital status							
Married	1249	3.0	407	7.1	208	14.4	ns
Non-married	286	3.8	167	9.6	179	20.7	
Contacts with friends and relatives							
High	266	1.9	166	6.6	105	11.4	
Medium	1007	2.9	340	7.6	223	17.0	$p \leqslant .001$
Low	239	5.4	57	12.3	42	31.0	
Church member							
Member	484	1.4	217	6.9	152	15.8	$p \leqslant .05$
Non-member	1051	3.9	357	8.4	235	18.3	
Group member							
Member	1005	2.4	347	7.2	173	15.0	$p \leqslant .05$
Non-member	535	4.5	227	8.8	214	19.2	

*Chi square values were calculated for differences in age-adjusted mortality rates among categories.
†Not significant.

see them infrequently have higher mortality rates than those people who have many friends and relatives and see them frequently. The age-adjusted chi square values for both men and women are highly significant ($p \leqslant .001$).

It is interesting to note that these differences in mortality rates between people who score high and low on the combined measure of contacts are greater for women than for men. The relative risks for men are 1.8 for men between 30–49 years of age; 1.3 for 50–59-year-old men; and 1.8 for men 60–69 years old. For women in these age groups, the relative risks are 2.8, 1.9 and 2.7, respectively.

As shown in table 2, individuals who belong to a church or temple have lower mortality rates than those who do not. These differences are not as large as those observed for other kinds of contacts, i.e., marital status, friends and relatives, although they are consistent. The age-adjusted chi square values are significant for differences in mortality rates among church members and non-members for both men and women ($p \leqslant .05$).

Analysis of mortality by membership in all other groups yields similar findings, as shown in table 2. With the exception of older men, both men and women who belong to one or more formal and informal groups have lower mortality rates than individuals who do not belong to any groups. The differences for men are not significant, although they are significant for women.

In a separate multivariate analysis not shown here, each of the four sources of social contacts shown in table 2 was found to predict mortality independently of the other three. However, the more intimate ties of marriage and contact with friends and relatives were stronger predictors than were ties of church and group membership.

The Social Network Index

To summarize the effects on mortality of increasing social isolation, a Social Network Index was constructed. Briefly, the Social Network Index considers not only the number of social ties but also their relative importance. Thus, intimate contacts are weighted more heavily than church affiliations and group memberships. Four network categories were developed to reflect differences in type and extent of social contact. The procedure by which this Index was developed and the precise description of methods used to score it are available elsewhere (22).

The age- and sex-specific mortality rates from all causes for the Social Network Index are shown in figure 1. The figure reveals a consistent pattern of increased mortality rates associated with each decrease in social connection. The only exception to this pattern is found among women aged 50–59 where those moderately connected had lower rates than those who had the most social ties. The relative risks of those most isolated compared to those with most connections are shown at the base of the figure. For men in the 30–49-year age group, the relative risk is 2.5; for men 50–59 it is 3.2; and for those aged 60–69 it is 1.8. For women, the relative risks are 4.6, 2.1 and 3.0, from the youngest to the oldest age

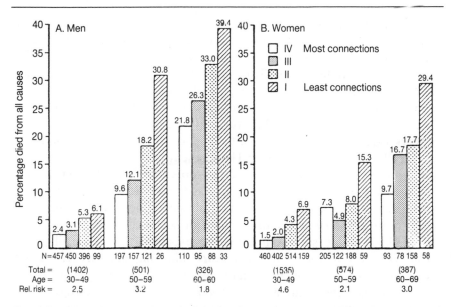

Figure 1. Age- and sex-specific mortality rates from all causes per 100 for Social Network Index, Human Population Laboratory Study of Alameda County, 1965–1974.

groups, respectively. Age-adjusted relative risks are 2.3 for men and 2.8 for women. The chi square value for the age-adjusted differences in mortality among the four network categories is highly significant ($p \le .001$).

The relative risks associated with low rank on the Social Network Index are greater than those of any single network measure or of a combined measure of marital status and contacts with friends and relatives.

The impact of sickness on social networks

While it is apparent that social networks are associated with mortality rates, the reasons for this association are unclear. A commonly expressed hypothesis is that people with few connections are probably sick and physically unable to maintain many ties. This is a difficult problem to assess, but two separate attempts were made to describe the direction of causality.

In the first attempt, the relationship between social networks and mortality was examined while controlling for physical health status at the time of the survey in 1965. Baseline physical health status was assessed by an index developed as a global measure of general physical health (32). This index measures physical health along a spectrum ranging from disability to chronic conditions to symptoms to no health problems.

Age-adjusted mortality rates from all causes, calculated by the indirect method, are shown in table 3 for each category of the Social Network Index and physical health status. From the table it can be seen that the Social Network Index is associated with mortality rates independently of baseline health status. In every category of health status for both men and women, those with the most social contacts have lower mortality rates than those most isolated. The gradient from high to low in the four network categories is consistent with only an occasional deviation and is statistically significant ($p \leqslant .001$). The gradient is least clear, however, for women who reported having no health problem or few symptoms.

A second approach to this problem was to examine the distribution of network responses by year of death. If physical illness at the time of the survey were responsible for the amount of social diconnection reported during the baseline survey, it would be expected that those ill people would be likely to die in the first years following the survey. Table 4 shows the distribution of the social network responses by year of death. As seen in the table, only a small proportion of the isolates died in the first two years following the survey. Furthermore, among both men and women the percentage of people with few connections who died in the first two years following the survey is similar to the percentage of people with many social contacts who died in that same time period. The figures in this table are not age-adjusted; however it has previously been shown that the Social Network Index is associated with mortality independently of age (see table 3 and figure 1). Though not conclusive, these findings suggest that physical illness alone does not appear capable of accounting for the association between social disconnection and increased mortality rates.

Socioeconomic status

A second potentially confounding factor which might be responsible for the observed association between social connections and mortality is socioeconomic status. In order to explore this issue, the Social Network Index was reduced from four categories to two because of the small number of deaths in some cells. By combining the "connected" and "moderately connected" categories into one category, and the two more isolated categories into another, five categories of socioeconomic status could be maintained.

Measures of income and educational level were used to develop an index of socioeconomic status. Occupation was not used because this resulted in inappropriate coding for women in some instances. Each of the measures, i.e., income and education level, were divided into five categories approximating a normal curve so that the middle category

Table 3. *Age-adjusted mortality rates from all causes per 100 for men and women, ages 30–69, for Social Network Index and Physical Health Spectrum, Human Population Laboratory Study of Alameda County, 1965–1974*

Social Network Index	Physical Health Spectrum									
	Disability	(n)	Chronic condition	(n)	Symptoms	(n)	No health problems	(n)	Total	(n)
Men										
I (fewest connections)		(23)*	13.9	(62)		(29)*	8.1	(44)	15.6	(158)
II	28.2	(54)	9.7	(189)	14.3	(152)	8.6	(210)	12.2	(605)
III	18.0	(40)	8.8	(270)	6.0	(181)	5.6	(211)	8.6	(702)
IV (most connections)	18.5	(45)	6.3	(258)	4.8	(183)	5.4	(278)	6.4	(764)
Total (n)	22.7	(162)	8.6	(779)	8.1	(545)	6.5	(743)	9.5	(2229)
Women										
I (fewest connections)	23.0	(53)	8.3	(81)	7.0	(74)	7.7	(68)	12.1	(276)
II	12.2	(112)	8.3	(312)	2.7	(247)	4.5	(189)	7.2	(860)
III	12.8	(55)	4.2	(209)	3.1	(201)	2.8	(137)	4.9	(602)
IV (most connections)	6.6	(72)	2.7	(263)	4.3	(226)	5.1	(197)	4.3	(758)
Total (n)	14.1	(292)	5.8	(865)	3.8	(748)	4.5	(591)	6.4	(2496)

*Rates not calculated for cells with 30 or fewer individuals.

Table 4. Distribution of Social Network Index responses by year of death for men and women, ages 30–69, Human Population Laboratory Study of Alameda County 1965–1974

Social Network Index	Year of death											
	1965–66		1967–68		1969–70		1971–72		1973–74		Total deaths	
	%	(n)	%	(n)	%	(n)	%	(n)	%	(n)	%	(n)
Men												
I (fewest connections)	15	(4)	26	(7)	26	(7)	18	(5)	15	(4)	100	(27)
II	19	(14)	18	(13)	21	(15)	21	(15)	21	(15)	100	(72)
III	16	(9)	19	(11)	17	(10)	32	(19)	16	(9)	100	(58)
IV (most connections)	15	(8)	19	(10)	19	(10)	27	(15)	20	(11)	100	(54)
Women												
I (fewest connections)	16	(6)	14	(5)	32	(12)	22	(8)	16	(6)	100	(37)
II	9	(6)	22	(14)	14	(9)	26	(17)	29	(19)	100	(65)
III	4	(1)	22	(6)	19	(5)	22	(6)	33	(9)	100	(27)
IV (most connections)	16	(5)	16	(5)	39	(12)	16	(5)	13	(4)	100	(31)

contained approximately a third of the sample, the two surrounding groups included about 20 per cent of the sample in each group, and the two extreme categories included the remaining 15 per cent of the sample in each of those categories. Five new groups were then constructed from the combination of the measures of income and education.

Table 5 shows age-adjusted mortality rates in relation to the Social Network and Socioeconomic Indices. In all five social class categories for both men and women, without exception, those with few social contacts had higher mortality rates than those with many contacts. The chi square values for the differences in mortality rates between the two network risk groups (after adjusting for age and socioeconomic status) were highly significant for both men and women ($p \leq .001$). These data support the conclusion that the Social Network Index predicts mortality independently of socioeconomic status.

Health practices

A third set of factors which might account for the observed association between networks and mortality are health practices. Thus, people who are socially isolated might have engaged in health practices known to be associated with poor health outcomes:

Smoking

Smoking was assessed by smoking status in 1965, i.e., current smoker, past smoker, and never smoked. Table 6 shows the age-adjusted mortality rates within social network and cigarette smoking categories. While there is an association between smoking and the Social Network Index, it can be seen that the mortality gradient among different network groupings persists and is statistically significant ($p \leq .001$) while controlling for smoking status and age.

Obesity

Obesity was measured by the Quetelet Index. This Index adjusts weight for height so that people of comparable proportions are classified together. This Index is calculated as: weight in pounds/(height in inches)^2. Three categories were devised for this index (33): 1) those 10 per cent or more underweight; 2) those between 9.99 per cent underweight and 29.9 per cent overweight; and 3) those 30.00 per cent or more overweight. Age-adjusted mortality rates for the Social Network and Quetelet Indices are shown in table 7. Although there were too few numbers in most cells to calculate adjusted mortality rates among those respondents 10 per cent

Table 5. *Age-adjusted mortality rates from all causes per 100 for men and women, ages 30–69, by Social Network Index and socioeconomic status, Alameda County, 1965–1974*

Social Network Index	Socioeconomic status												
	Lower	(n)	Lower-Middle	(n)	Middle	(n)	Upper-Middle	(n)	Upper	(n)	Total	(n)
Men												
I and II (fewest connections)	11.8	(86)	12.7	(110)	16.6	(243)	11.7	(242)	7.3	(67)	13.1	(748)
III and IV (most connections)	8.0	(89)	11.1	(168)	6.3	(501)	8.1	(498)	4.2	(192)	7.5	(1448)
Total (n)	9.9	(175)	11.7	(278)	9.5	(744)	9.1	(740)	5.2	(259)	9.4	(2196)
Women												
I and II (fewest connections)	9.9	(121)	7.3	(209)	8.2	(431)	6.8	(302)	5.7	(40)	8.0	(1103)
III and IV (most connections)	7.3	(69)	1.1	(151)	4.9	(487)	4.1	(514)	5.2	(123)	4.4	(1344)
Total (n)	8.8	(190)	4.6	(360)	6.6	(918)	5.2	(816)	5.4	(163)	6.1	(2447)

Table 6. *Age-adjusted mortality rates from all causes per 100 for men and women,*
ages 30–69, by Social Network Index and smoking history, Alameda County,
1965–1974

Social Network Index	Smoking history							
	Present	(n)	Past	(n)	Never	(n)	Total	(n)
Men								
I (fewest connections)	17.2	(91)		(29)*	14.7	(36)	15.8	(156)
II	16.8	(315)	10.1	(139)	5.7	(149)	12.1	(603)
III	10.5	(371)	5.9	(162)	7.2	(165)	8.5	(698)
IV (most connections)	10.2	(348)	6.6	(196)	2.5	(214)	6.8	(758)
Total (n)	12.8	(1125)	7.5	(526)	5.5	(564)	9.4	(2215)
Women								
I (fewest connections)	14.9	(136)	19.8	(31)	7.2	(107)	12.2	(274)
II	7.4	(379)	12.1	(102)	5.8	(365)	7.2	(846)
III	5.1	(276)	2.4	(54)	5.2	(256)	4.9	(586)
IV (most connections)	5.4	(254)	6.5	(83)	3.1	(412)	4.2	(749)
Total (n)	7.5	(1045)	9.9	(270)	4.9	(1140)	6.4	(2455)

*Rates not calculated for cells with 30 or fewer individuals.

or more underweight, a clear gradient among network categories is observable in the other two weight/height groups. Thus, the Social Network Index predicts mortality independently of obesity ($p \leq .001$).

Alcohol consumption

In table 8 age-adjusted mortality rates are shown for the Social Network Index in relation to alcoholic beverage ingestion. Alcohol ingestion was divided into three categories: 1) those drinking 46 or more drinks a month; 2) those drinking between 17 and 45 drinks a month; and 3) those abstaining or drinking up to 16 drinks a month. Drinks of wine, beer, or liquor were counted equally in this analysis. Among both men and women, the social network-mortality association exists independently of alcoholic beverage consumption. The chi square value for differences in mortality rates among network categories while adjusting for both age and level of alcohol consumption is statistically significant ($p \leq .001$).

Table 7. *Age-adjusted mortality rates from all causes per 100 for men and women, ages 30–69, by Social Network Index and obesity (Quetelet Index), Alameda County, 1965–1974*

Social Network Index		Quetelet Index							
	≥10% underweight	(n)	9.9% underweight–29.9% overweight	(n)	≥30% overweight	(n)	Total	(n)	
Men									
I (fewest connections)		(12)*	15.5	(117)		(28)*	15.5	(157)	
II		(23)*	11.5	(516)	15.1	(60)	12.5	(599)	
III		(18)*	7.8	(609)	11.3	(71)	8.5	(698)	
IV (most connections)		(10)*	6.9	(670)	5.9	(79)	6.9	(759)	
Total (n)	19.1	(63)	9.2	(1912)	10.0	(238)	9.5	(2213)	
Women									
I (fewest connections)		(16)*	10.4	(193)	15.9	(67)	12.1	(276)	
II	10.7	(57)	6.6	(629)	8.1	(174)	7.3	(860)	
III	9.5	(39)	4.0	(464)	5.9	(99)	4.9	(602)	
IV (most connections)		(24)*	4.0	(589)	4.6	(145)	4.3	(758)	
Total (n)	10.8	(136)	5.7	(1875)	7.7	(485)	6.4	(2496)	

*Rates not calculated for cells with 30 or fewer individuals.

Table 8. *Age-adjusted mortality rates from all causes per 100 for men and women, ages 30–69, by Social Network Index and alcohol consumption, Alameda County, 1965–1974*

Social Network Index	46+	(n)	17–45	(n)	0–16	(n)	Total	(n)
	Drinks per month							
	Men							
I (fewest connections)	17.6	(40)	17.9	(38)	13.8	(80)	15.6	(158)
II	20.0	(146)	7.9	(185)	11.5	(274)	12.2	(605)
III	6.4	(164)	5.2	(256)	12.4	(282)	8.6	(702)
IV (most connections)	13.3	(131)	5.1	(242)	6.2	(391)	6.9	(764)
Total (n)	13.2	(481)	6.5	(721)	9.9	(1027)	9.5	(2229)
	Women							
I (fewest connections)	15.9	(31)	9.6	(43)	12.3	(202)	12.1	(276)
II	8.4	(72)	7.0	(176)	7.0	(612)	7.2	(860)
III	6.6	(67)	5.0	(155)	4.6	(380)	4.9	(602)
IV (most connections)	5.8	(49)	4.5	(157)	4.1	(552)	4.3	(758)
Total (n)	8.5	(219)	6.0	(531)	6.4	(1746)	6.4	(2496)

Physical activity

Physical activity was assessed by responses to four questions involving how often respondents participated in 1) active sports; 2) swimming or taking long walks; 3) physical exercises; 4) gardening, hunting, or fishing. An index was created based on the degree to which respondents participated in any of these activities. In the Index, the first three activities were given equal weight; and the final item was given half the weight of the first three. Table 9 shows that the differences in mortality risk among network categories do not appear attributable to different levels of physical activity among respondents in network groups. The chi square value for differences in mortality rates among network categories while adjusting for both age and level of physical activity is statistically significant ($p \leqslant .005$).

A cumulative index of health practices

While these health behaviors, considered one at a time, may not account for the association between social networks and mortality, it is possible that a combination of health practices might be responsible for such an association. A cumulative index of seven health practices developed by

Table 9. *Age-adjusted mortality rates from all causes per 100 for men and women ages 30–69, by Social Network Index and physical activity, Alameda County, 1965–1974*

Social Network Index	Physical activity							
	Least activity	(n)	Moderate activity	(n)	Most activity	(n)	Total	(n)
			Men					
I (fewest connections)	18.2	(57)	17.1	(71)		(30)*	15.6	(158)
II	14.4	(150)	12.4	(314)	8.9	(141)	12.2	(605)
III	9.9	(129)	8.8	(377)	6.6	(196)	8.6	(702)
IV (most connections)	9.2	(109)	7.6	(368)	4.4	(287)	6.9	(764)
Total (n)	12.4	(445)	9.8	(1130)	5.9	(654)	9.5	(2229)
			Women					
I (fewest connections)	14.8	(137)	8.1	(115)		(24)*	12.1	(276)
II	8.8	(289)	6.3	(444)	5.8	(127)	7.2	(860)
III	7.4	(190)	3.5	(286)	2.3	(126)	4.9	(602)
IV (most connections)	6.0	(173)	4.6	(412)	0.8	(173)	4.3	(758)
Total (n)	9.0	(789)	5.2	(1257)	2.9	(450)	6.4	(2496)

*Rates not calculated for cells with 30 or fewer individuals.

Belloc and Breslow was used to assess this possibility. A detailed description of the Index and its relationship to physical health has been previously reported (34, 35).

Respondents received a score on this index indicating their number of "good" health practices. One point was received for each of the following practices: 1) does not smoke cigarettes; 2) drinks "moderately" (no more than four drinks per sitting); 3) eats breakfast regularly; 4) does not eat between meals regularly; 5) sleeps seven or eight hours per night; 6) engages in regular physical activity; and 7) is within a certain range of weight for height.

Table 10 shows age-adjusted mortality rates for the Social Network Index and the Index of Health Practices. Examination of the column and row totals shows that both social networks and health practices are strongly associated with mortality. Further, these two variables are associated with one another. At each health practice level, however, the mortality gradient persists among social network level categories although the magnitude of the association is somewhat diminished when health practices are taken into consideration. Differences in mortality rates among the social network groups remain highly significant for both men

Table 10. Age-adjusted mortality rates from all causes per 100 for men and women, ages 30–69, by Social Network Index and Health Practices Index, Alameda County, 1965–1974

Social Network Index	Health practices							
	0–4 positive*	(n)	5 positive	(n)	6–7 positive	(n)	Total	(n)
	Men							
I (fewest connections)	21.5	(73)	9.9	(48)	10.5	(37)	15.6	(158)
II	14.6	(251)	11.7	(162)	9.9	(192)	12.2	(605)
III	10.3	(229)	9.9	(215)	6.6	(258)	8.6	(702)
IV (most connections)	7.8	(230)	9.5	(239)	4.2	(295)	6.2	(764)
Total (n)	12.3	(783)	10.2	(664)	6.7	(782)	9.5	(2229)
	Women							
I (fewest connections)	15.2	(123)	8.5	(83)	10.0	(70)	12.1	(276)
II	10.4	(323)	7.5	(272)	4.0	(265)	7.2	(860)
III	5.8	(202)	4.7	(189)	4.3	(211)	4.9	(602)
IV (most connections)	6.5	(191)	2.4	(234)	4.4	(333)	4.3	(758)
Total (n)	9.3	(839)	5.6	(778)	4.7	(879)	6.4	(2496)

*Good health practices.

and women when adjusting simultaneously for age and health practice score ($p \leqslant .001$).

Health services

Finally, the possibility was explored that the relationship between social networks and mortality, while not due to any health practices, could be due to differential use of medical services by people with few social resources. An index of preventive utilization of health services was developed based on three questions: 1) "Do you have health insurance?"; 2) "Have you had a dental check-up in the past year, even though you felt well?"; 3) "Have you had a medical check-up in the past year, even though you felt well?" Respondents who had both dental and medical check-ups in the past year were classified as high scorers. Low scorers were respondents who had neither a dental nor a medical check-up although they may have had health insurance; moderate scorers included all other respondents.

Age-adjusted mortality rates for the Social Network Index and an index of preventive utilization of health services are shown for men and women in table 11. This table reveals that people who use preventive health services have slightly lower mortality rates than those who make little or moderate use of such services. People with few social contacts are less likely to use such preventive services. The social network gradient in mortality, however, is still seen in each health care category, with some deviation in pattern. While this measure of health services may not be a sensitive measure of use of preventive health care, variations in mortality observed among people with different kinds of social contacts are not accounted for by the more obvious differences in use of preventive health services ($p \leqslant .005$).

Discussion

The preceding analyses have shown that social and community ties are associated with risk of mortality. Four sources of social relationships were examined: 1) marriage; 2) contacts with close friends and relatives; 3) church membership and 4) informal and formal group associations. In each instance, people with social ties and relationships had lower mortality rates than people without such ties. Each of the four sources was found to predict mortality independently of the other three; the more intimate ties of marriage and contact with friends and relatives were stronger predictors than were the ties of church and group membership.

To assess the cumulative effects of these ties and relationships, a Social Network Index was created based on these four sources of contact. When

Table 11. *Age-adjusted mortality rates from all causes per 100 for men and women, ages 30–69, by Social Network Index and level of preventive care, Alameda County, 1965–1974*

Social Network Index	Level of preventive health care							
	Low	(n)	Medium	(n)	High	(n)	Total	(n)
Men								
I (fewest connections)	15.4	(49)	9.7	(48)		(29)*	14.2	(126)
II	11.4	(162)	9.8	(203)	9.2	(118)	10.2	(483)
III	7.8	(180)	6.5	(236)	4.5	(170)	6.1	(586)
IV (most connections)	5.8	(181)	5.6	(241)	6.1	(197)	5.8	(619)
Total (n)	8.6	(572)	7.8	(728)	6.9	(514)	7.7	(1814)
Women								
I (fewest connections)	6.8	(66)	11.4	(78)	8.4	(50)	8.8	(194)
II	8.4	(171)	5.4	(241)	5.4	(236)	6.1	(648)
III	2.7	(115)	6.7	(199)	4.0	(184)	4.7	(498)
IV (most connections)	3.6	(117)	3.5	(238)	3.6	(253)	3.6	(608)
Total (n)	5.6	(469)	5.6	(756)	4.6	(723)	5.2	(1948)

*Rates not calculated for cells with 30 or fewer individuals.

the sample was stratified according to the level of social contact and source of affiliation, the most isolated group of men was found to have an age-adjusted mortality rate 2.3 times higher than men with the most connections; for women who were isolated, the rate was 2.8 times higher than the rate for women with the most social connections. For every age group examined, and for both sexes, people with many social contacts had the lowest mortality rates and people with the fewest contacts had the highest rates. The relative risks between these groups range from just under 2 to over 4.5.

The association between the Social Network Index and mortality was found to be independent of self-reported physical health status at the time of the survey, year of death, socioeconomic status, and such health behaviors as smoking, alcohol ingestion, physical inactivity, obesity, and low utilization of preventive health services, and a cumulative index of health practices.

On the basis of the findings in this study, future research might focus on more sophisticated network models tapping many more dimensions of social and community ties. Of particular interest is the number of possible relationships that place an individual in a particular risk category. For instance, people who were not married but who had many friends and relatives were found to have mortality rates equal to those who were married but who had fewer contacts with friends and relatives. Similarly, it did not seem important whether contacts were among friends or relatives; it was only in the absence of either of these sources of contacts that there was a significant increase in the risk of death during the follow-up period. Trade-offs and substitutions such as this assured that about 60 per cent of the sample, through one kind of contact or another, managed to maintain reasonably low mortality risk. It was only in the presence of mounting social disconnection, when individuals failed to have links in several different spheres of interaction, that mortality rates rose sharply.

Limitation of mortality data

Two limitations involved with the use of mortality data have implications for the conclusions which can be drawn from these results. First, there is the continuing thought that people who died during the nine-year follow-up period were ill at the time of the initial survey. The association between physical health status as determined at the baseline survey and subsequent mortality supports this suspicion. It is therefore possible that the relationship between networks and mortality is due to the fact that isolated people were ill at the time of the survey and were unable physically to maintain extended contacts. This is a serious issue and one which was explored in some depth. The results presented do not support this possible explanation. While controlling for health status at the time of the baseline survey, the Social Network Index continued to predict mortality. In an analysis of year of death, it was shown that the percentage of isolated people who died in the first years following the survey is similar to the percentage of people with many social contacts who died in that same period. If these two analyses involved valid and accurate indicators of illness status at the time of the survey, it does not appear likely that the relationship between networks and mortality is merely a reflection of underlying poor health. On the other hand, if these measures are not valid and accurate indices of health status in 1965, this issue remains unresolved.

The second limitation of mortality data is also related to the association between mortality and morbidity. Throughout this research, the implication has been that social factors influence susceptibility to disease, i.e., disease incidence. In fact, from studies involving mortality data, it is unknown whether the risk factors influence disease incidence or "survival time" between the incidence or diagnosis of disease and death. It should be noted that in either case, host resistance may be the involved mechanism. Previous work on social supports and incidence of pregnancy complications (13) and on cultural and social mobility and coronary heart disease (4) suggests that social factors are capable of influencing disease incidence; however, from the data in this study, it cannot be concluded which end of the disease spectrum is most influenced by social networks.

Mechanisms

Although the hypothesis has been supported that social and community ties may be protective against a wide variety of disease outcomes, the mechanisms by which networks influence health status remain unclear. A critical issue is how social isolation might affect health status. It is interesting to note that the Network Index was found to be associated not only with overall mortality but with four separate causes of death: ischemic heart disease, cancer, cerebrovascular and circulatory diseases, and a category including all other causes of death, e.g., diseases of the digestive and respiratory system, accidents, and suicide. Since social isolation is associated with so many causes of death, it is possible that there are several pathways that might lead from social isolation to illness. One pathway might be through the use of health practices which may lead to poor health consequences. The association between isolation and such practices suggests that this is likely. However, since health practices do not seem capable of explaining more than a small part of the social network/mortality association, other pathways must also be involved.

A second pathway may be through psychological responses to isolation such as depression or changed coping and appraisal processes. Such psychological responses might predispose an individual to suicide or to risk-taking behavior which could result in accidents. It has been suggested that the critical role psychosocial factors play in the causation of disease is not due to stressful objective circumstances, but to the way in which these circumstances are more subjectively perceived and mediated by the individual. In an analysis of psychological factors, social networks, and mortality to be presented in another paper, it was found that none of the psychological factors developed from items from the 1965 Human Population Laboratory survey mediated between social networks and risk of mortality. The correlations between the psychological factors and networks were only moderate, and in all cases the Network Index continued to predict mortality independently of psychological status. It should be noted, however, that the Human Population Laboratory psychological items were not originally created as mediating variables between social circumstances and health outcomes and may therefore not tap the crucial dimensions of such psychological factors.

Another pathway might lead directly from social isolation to physiologic changes in the body which increase general susceptibility to disease. Previous research on the impact of the social environment on a wide range of health outcomes suggests that many social "risk factors," e.g., poverty, migration, may not be etiologically specific for any single disease (36). Kaplan et al. (37), Cobb (38) and Antonovsky (39, 40) recently have proposed that social and community ties may serve as important factors in promoting host resistance to disease. These investigators have proposed that stressful social circumstances such as lack of social ties and resources may alter host susceptibility and consequently would be expected to be associated with a wide range of disease outcomes and with increased morbidity and mortality rates. Nervous, hormonal, and immunologic control systems have frequently been invoked as potential pathways by which stressful circumstances might cause disease. Evidence is clear from animal experiments that stressful social circumstances may modify control systems leading to changes in health status (41–44). Adequate tests of the hypothesis that social circumstances alter general susceptibility to disease in humans will not be possible, however, until data are available on physiologic mechanisms capable of mediating the relationship between social events and disease outcomes.

The role which stressful social circumstances play in the causation of disease may be dependent upon their absolute strength and their strength relative to other causal agents. Thus, when agents are particularly pathogenic and exposure is widespread, the effects of social factors may be small. However, when disease agents are less obviously pathogenic or virulent, social factors may play a significant role in determining variations in health status. The findings from this study suggest that social circumstances such as social isolation may have pervasive health consequences; and they support the hypothesis that social factors may influence host resistance and affect vulnerability to disease in general.

Acknowledgements

Supported by a National Instutute of Mental Health Grant No. T01 MH 13561 and a National Center for Health Services Research Grant No. HS 00368.

The authors gratefully acknowledge the staff of the Human Population Laboratory, California State Department of Health Services (where Dr. Berkman was employed from 1977–1978) for their assistance and support in the preparation of this manuscript. They also thank Dr. Richard Brand, School of Public Health, University of California, Berkeley, for his help with parts of the statistical analyses.

References

1. Marmot MG, Syme SL: Acculturation and coronary heart disease. Am J Epidemiol 104:225–247, 1976
2. Cassel J, Tyroler HA: Epidemiological studies of culture change: I. Health status and recency of industrialization. Arch Environ Health 3:25–33, 1961
3. Tyroler HA, Cassel J: Health consequences of cultural change: II. The effect of urbanization on coronary heart mortality among rural residents. J Chronic Dis 17:167–177, 1964
4. Syme SL, Hyman MM, Enterline PE: Some social and cultural factors associated with the occurrence of coronary heart disease. J Chronic Dis 17:277–289, 1964
5. Mancuso TF, Sterling TD: Relation of place of birth and migration in cancer mortality in the U.S. J Chronic Dis 27:459–474, 1974
6. Nesser WB, Tyroler HA, Cassel JC: Social disorganization and stroke mortality in the black populations of North Carolina. Am J Epidemiol 93:166–175, 1971
7. James S, Kleinbaum DG: Socioecologic stress and hypertension related mortality rates in North Carolina. Am J Public Health 66:354–358, 1976
8. Harburg E, Erfurt JC, Chape C, et al: Socioecologic stressor areas in black–white blood pressure: Detroit. J Chronic Dis 26:595–611, 1973
9. Antonovsky A: Social class, life expectancy and overall mortality. Milbank Mem Fund Q 45:31–73, 1967
10. Kitagawa EM, Hauser PM: Differential Mortality in the United States. Cambridge, Harvard University Press, 1973
11. Nagi MH, Stockwell EG: Socioeconomic differentials in mortality by cause of death. Health Serv Rep 88:449–465, 1973
12. Syme SL, Berkman LF: Social class, susceptibility, and sickness. Am J Epidemiol 104:1–8, 1976
13. Nuckolls KB, Cassel J, Kaplan BH: Psychosocial assets, life crisis, and the prognosis of pregnancy. Am J Epidemiol 95:431–441, 1972
14. Gore S: The influence of social support and related variables in ameliorating the consequences of job loss. Doctoral dissertation. University of Pennsylvania, 1973
15. Ortmeyer CF: Variations in mortality, morbidity, and health care by marital status. Edited by CE Erhardt, JE Berlin. In Mortality and Morbidity in the United States. Cambridge, Harvard University Press, 1974, pp 159–588
16. Durkheim E: Suicide. New York, The Free Press, 1951
17. Price JS, Slater E, Hare EH: Marital status of first admissions to psychiatric beds in England and Wales in 1965 and 1966. Social Biology 18:574–594, 1971
18. Maddison D, Viola A: The health of widows in the year following bereavement. J Psychosom Res 12:297–306, 1968
19. Marris R: Widows and Their Families. London, Routledge and Kegan Paul, 1958
20. Parkes CM: The effects of bereavement on physical and mental health—a study of the medical records of widows. Br Med J 2:274–279, 1964
21. Rees WP, Lutkins SG: Mortality of bereavement. Br Med J 4:13–16, 1967
22. Berkman LF: Social networks, host resistance, and mortality: A follow-up

study of Alameda County residents. Doctoral dissertation. University of California, Berkeley, 1977

23. Parkes CM, Benjamin B, Fitzgerald RG: Broken heart: A statistical study of increased mortality among widowers. Br Med J: 1:740–743, 1969

24. Weiss NS: Marital status and risk factors for coronary heart disease. Br J Prev Soc Med 27:41–43, 1973

25. California State Department of Public Health: Alameda County Population 1965. April 1966

26. Hochstim JR: Health and ways of living—the Alameda County Population Laboratory. Edited by II Kessler, ML Levin. *In* The Community as an Epidemiological Laboratory. Baltimore, Johns Hopkins University Press, 1970, pp 149–176

27. Belloc N, Arellano M: Computer record linkage on a survey population. Health Serv Rep 88:344–350, 1973

28. Mantel N, Haenszel W: Statistical aspects of the anlysis of data from retrospective studies of disease. J Natl Cancer Inst 22:719–748, 1959

29. Brand RJ, Sholtz RI: A multiple adjustment method for combining $J \times 2$ contingency tables for prospective and survival study analysis. Presented at Biometrics Society Meeting, March, 1976

30. Lilienfeld AM, Pedersen E, Dowd JE: Cancer Epidemiology: Methods of Study. Baltimore, Johns Hopkins University Press, 1967

31. Fleiss J: Statistical Methods for Rates and Proportions. New York, Wiley and Sons, 1973

32. Breslow L: A quantitative approach to the World Health Organization definition of health: Physical, mental and social well-being. Int J Epidemiol 1:347–355, 1972

33. Metropolitan Life Insurance Company: Overweight: Its Significance and Prevention, 1960

34. Belloc N, Breslow L: Relationship of physical health status and health practices. Prev Med 1:409–421, 1972

35. Belloc N: Relationship of health practices and mortality. Prev Med 2:67–81, 1973

36. Cassel J: The contribution of the social environment to host resistance. Am J Epidemiol 104:107–123, 1976

37. Kaplan BH, Cassel JC, Gore S: Social support and health. Medical Care (supplement) 15(5):47–58, 1977

38. Cobb S: Social support as a moderator of life stress. J Psychosom Med 38:300–314, 1976

39. Antonovsky A: Breakdown: A needed fourth step in the conceptual armamentarium of modern medicine. Soc Sci Med 6:537–544, 1972

40. Antonovsky A: Conceptual and methodological problems in the study of resistance resources and stressful life events. Edited by BS Dohrenwend, BP Dohrenwend. *In* Stressful Life Events: Their nature and effects. New York, Wiley and Sons, 1974, pp 245–259

41. Calhoun JB: Population density and social pathology. Sci Am 206:139–148, 1962

42. Ader R, Kreutner A, Jacobs HL: Social environment, emotionality and alloxan diabetes in the rat. Psychosom Med 25:60–68, 1963

43. Ratcliffe HL, Cronin MIT: Changing frequency of arteriosclerosis in mammals and birds at the Philadelphia Zoological Garden. Circulation 18:41–52, 1958
44. Gross WB: Effects of social stress on occurrence of Marek's Disease in chickens. Am J Vet Res 33:2275–2279, 1972

Goal frustration and life events in the aetiology of painful gastrointestinal disorder

T. K. J. Craig and G. W. Brown

Department of Social Policy and Social Science, Bedford College,
11 Bedford Square, London WC1B 3RA, UK

Abstract

Life events and difficulties were recorded for the year preceding onset of abdominal pain in 135 consecutive referrals to three gastrointestinal clinics, and for the equivalent time period in a matched, healthy community comparison series. Fifty-six patients were found to have an organic gastrointestinal disorder. Severely threatening events and major difficulties known to play a critical aetiological role in clinical depression, occurred with much the same frequency during the 38 weeks before onset of non-organic ('functional') gastrointestinal disorder. There was no such relationship between the severity of threat and organic disorder. A measure of 'goal frustration' reflecting the degree to which the subjects' aims and ambitions were insurmountably obstructed by the occurrence of the event, was significantly associated with organic disorder. This finding may explain the often reported association between life stress and organic gastrointestinal disorder.

Introduction

Impressive arguments have been developed stating that stress research has been led astray by its emphasis on *particular* social stresses leading to specific diseases, rather than seeing stressors raising susceptibility to disease in general [1]. Although we do not wish to deny the cogency of the argument, the fact is that our own experience within psychiatry points to the value of studying particular conditions and their link with particular kinds of stress. There is now clear evidence that the stressors for

Reprinted from *Journal of Psychosomatic Research*, **28**, Craig, T. K. J. and Brown, G. W. Goal frustration and life events in the aetiology of painful gastrointestinal disorder, 411–21. Copyright (1984), with kind permission from Pergamon Press Ltd, Headington Hill Hall, Oxford OX3 0BW, UK.

depression [2–4], differ in important ways from those for anxiety [3], and for schizophrenia [2, 5], and see no reason why a similar approach should not pay off in the area of physical disease.

In the case of gastrointestinal disorder, speculation about the role of life stress can be traced to virtually the first clinical descriptions [6–8].

But until recently work has been based on a small number of patients and although these early studies provided important insights they were unable to demonstrate convincing causal links even when supported by direct observation of the physiologic reactions of the gut to a variety of noxious stimuli [9–11]. In the last 20 years the development of the Bedford College Life Events and Difficulties Schedule (LEDS) has met many of the problems of low reliability and low validity that have plagued life stress research [12–14]; the instrument has been used largely with psychiatric conditions [2, 3, 5, 15, 16]; it has, however, also been employed in a few studies of physical disorder [17–20], one of which has a direct bearing on this report. In this study of those undergoing appendectomy, Creed demonstrated that severely threatening events played an important aetiological role but only in patients whose appendix turned out to be normal histologically. Patients with clear evidence of inflammation had no higher rate of such events than a normal comparison series but did have a somewhat raised rate of less severely threatening events [20]. The present investigation was partly conceived to explore this latter association.

Subjects and method

Patients between the ages of 18 and 60 were selected from a continuous series of attenders at three gastrointestinal clinics. Each had presented for the first time at the clinic with an onset of abdominal pain which had occurred within the previous twelve months. Patients suffering from a recurrence of symptoms were included only where first ever onset was within the previous three years, and the patient had been symptom free in the absence of medication for the last twelve months before the current episode. All were interviewed before the completion of any physical investigative procedures, usually at the first out-patient appointment or within a few days of that. In all instances the interview was prior to their second visit to the hospital.

A non-hospitalised comparison group, that had been free of gastrointestinal illness for at least two years, was selected from a random sample of persons registered with five general practices in the catchment area of the hospitals. This provided the basis of pairwise match for each patient on the basis of age, sex, marital state, social class, country of birth and life-stage (an index reflecting age and the presence of children in the respondents' household and known to be related to the frequency of certain life events in the general population).

The LEDS has been described extensively elsewhere [2]. It is an interview-based instrument and unlike many other life-event instruments it is concerned with ongoing difficulties as well as with discrete events. Each category of event or difficulty is extensively defined and in the interview itself this list is explored in detail with each subject, searching for the occurrence and precise dating of each potential event or difficulty. It is known to have high reliability [2, 21, 22]. As an additional check on accuracy, we confirmed dates of events and difficulties where possible by examining official records, travel documents, business letters, personal diaries and the like. Once the presence of an event or difficulty was established, further questions were asked in order to be able to rate a number of qualitative dimensions. These were rated by members of the wider research team involved on other life stress projects in the unit; raters were kept unaware as to whether the subject was a patient or belonged to the comparison group, and were similarly kept ignorant about the presence of psychiatric symptoms. Although the interviewer was present at these rating meetings he deferred in all instances to the decision of the rating team so as to avoid possible bias arising from information relating to the mental or physical state of the subject. Two of these qualitative dimensions are to be described in detail.

Long-term threat

In essence, this rating provides a measure of how distressing or unpleasant the average person would find such an event or difficulty given similar biography and current circumstances. For events this long-term aspect reflects the likely consequences and implications of the event some 7–10 days after its occurrence. The rating was *contextual* in the sense that raters were not told of the subject's account of his or her responses to the event or difficulty; they made judgements only in terms of how the average person in similar biographical and environmental circumstances would be likely to respond, basing these judgements on precedents describing these 'average' responses which have been collected over the past 15 yr of research with this method. So for example in rating a birth, raters would be told of the ease of delivery and any complications, the financial circumstances of the family, the current state of the marital relationship, and whether the pregnancy had been planned or was the result of a contraceptive failure.

In studies of depression, what have been termed *severe events* (the top two points of a four-point scale of severity of long-term threat and focused on the subject alone or jointly with another) and *major difficulties* (of a similar order of threat and of two or more years duration) were found to be of aetiological significance [2]. The term *provoking agent* was developed in research on depression to refer to any experience of either severe events or major difficulties (or both), since, although they formed a minority of the events and difficulties in the general population, it was just those that played an aetiological role in depression.

Goal frustration

This measure was developed specifically for the present study with the aim of exploring one aspect of early theoretical formulations of psycho-somatic disease—that the experience of the frustration of ambition is of direct causal significance in organic gastrointestinal disease. Like other contextual measures in the LEDS the rating is made by team workers other than the interviewer, on a four-point scale of severity, the top two points being taken to indicate marked, irrevocable goal frustration. The requirement for making such a rating was that there should be evidence that the subject had made consistent and sustained efforts to obtain his or her goal. An example rating and case history is given in the section reporting results.

Physical diagnosis

Only after all interviews were complete and events and difficulties had been rated for both patient and community samples were details of the physical diagnosis of the patients obtained. These were provided by the patient's consultant physician on the basis of all available investigative diagnostic tests. Subjects were classed as *definitely organic* where there was confirmatory laboratory evidence of disease (such as endoscopically visualised active peptic ulceration) or as having a *functional* disorder where there was no such confirmatory diagnosis.

All statistical analyses have used the chi-squared test except where otherwise indicated.

Results

One hundred and forty-five patients were approached as meeting our basic criteria for entry to the study. Of these, two refused to participate, and three failed to complete the interview.

Physical diagnosis

Fifty-six of the patients had definite organic gastrointestinal disorder, supported by at least one major confirmatory diagnostic investigation (usually direct visualisation on endoscopy). In addition to these 56 there were five patients with other systemic disease which accounted for their gastrointestinal symptoms and these have been excluded from this analysis. The remaining 79 had a 'functional' disorder. Twenty-one of the latter had the characteristic clinical picture of the irritable bowel syndrome; 14 gave convincing clinical descriptions of dyspepsia in the absence of structural change and 35 had abdominal pain in the absence of dyspeptic or typical bowel symptoms. The remaining eight had histories highly suggestive of organic disease, but the confirmatory tests were inconclusive and they were classed as functional. Twenty-eight of the 135 patients included in the study were recurrences of an old gastrointestinal disorder (15 organic and 13 functional).

Demographic characteristics

Patients with functional disorder were on the whole more likely to be female (73% functional disorder and 48% organic, $p < 0.01$), single (40 and 22%, $p < 0.02$), and slightly younger (mean 34.6 and 38.3 yr). There were no differences in social class or country of birth. Since the comparison group were pairwise matched for these characteristics they showed a closely similar distribution.

Smoking

Patients with organic disorder were more likely to be heavy smokers, 41% (23/56) smoked 20 or more cigarettes (or equivalent) daily compared with 27% (21.79) of the functionally ill and 22% (30/135) of the healthy comparison group ($p < .01$). There were also non-signficant tendencies for patients with organic disorder to consume more alcohol and eat irregularly.

Life events and difficulties

Severe events and provoking agents

For the study of provoking agents we included events or difficulties occurring in a 38-week period before onset: most recent studies using the LEDS have used this period which was first utilised in the study of depressed patients. Fifty-seven per cent of patients with a functional diagnosis experience a severely threatening event focused on the subject prior to onset compared with 23% of those with an organic diagnosis and 15% of the comparison group (Table I). The high rate of severe events among the functionally ill, is closely comparable to that among the

Table I. *Proportion experiencing at least one event or difficulty of the specified type in a 38-week period before onset/interview*

Type of gastrointestinal disorder	Severe event (%)	Provoking agent (severe event or major difficulty) (%)	Goal frustration (%)
Functional	57 (45/79)	67 (53/79)	24 (19/79)
Organic	23 (14/56)	23 (14/56)	54 (30/56)
Healthy comparison	15 (20/135)	23 (31/135)	9 (12/135)
	Row 1 vs 2, $p < 0.001$.	Row 1 vs 2, $p < 0.001$.	Row 1 vs 2, $p < 0.001$.
	Row 1 vs 3, $p < 0.001$.	Row 1 vs 3, $p < 0.001$.	Row 1 vs 3, $p < 0.01$.
			Row 2 vs 3, $p < 0.001$.

non-inflamed appendix group studied by Creed [20], as well as that found for depressed patients [2], and there is good reason to believe that severe events play a similarly important aetiological role in all three conditions. The majority of severe events in the functional group involve losses and disappointments and do not appear to differ in content from those known to produce depression [2].

The findings remain unaltered when the combined category of provoking agent (i.e. severe event or major difficulty) is considered (Table I, column 2), and analysis by sex does not affect these findings.

Goal frustration events and difficulties

Goal frustration, in complete contrast to severe threat, was far more common among those with organic disorder: 54% experienced such an event or difficulty in the 38 weeks before onset compared with 24% of those with functional disorder, and 9% of the comparison subjects (Table I, column 3). While both groups of patients have more experience of goal frustration than healthy subjects, the organic has double the rate of functional. Interpretation is complicated by the fact that goal frustration is correlated with severity of threat (gamma = 0.66), and its high rate among the functional patients might be explained simply by their much higher rate of provoking agents. This indeed proved to be the case: controlling for the presence of a provoking agent shows that for those with *functional disorder* there are no events or difficulties characterised by marked goal frustration which are not also provoking agents, while 43%

Table II. *Proportion experiencing a goal frustration event or difficulty in 38 weeks before onset of gastrointestinal disorder by presence of a provoking agent*

Type of gastrointestinal disorder	No provoking agent (%)	Provoking agent (%)
Functional	0 (0/26)	36 (19/53)
Organic	43 (18/42)	86 (12/14)
Healthy comparison	3 (3/104)	29 (9/31)

of those with organic disorder had experienced goal frustration in the absence of a provoking agent (Table II). Furthermore, when those with and without a provoking agent are considered the functional and comparison groups do not differ in their experience of goal frustration (Table II). This suggests that goal frustration as such plays no aetiological role in functional disorder.

For the organic patients for which there is evidence of a powerful causal effect the mean time between the goal frustration and the onset of symptoms was 4.8 weeks.

Goal frustration, demographic characteristics and diagnosis

It is perhaps not surprising that almost three times more men in the *general population* experienced a goal frustrating event or difficulty (16 vs 5%, $p = 0.05$). One possible explanation is that men are more likely to have greater competitive investment in work or career, and are possibly thereby more often exposed to frustration of their ambitions. Indeed for men in the general population occupational ambitions were involved in 70% of the goal frustration events and difficulties, while for women three-quarters concerned failure to achieve a desired outcome in personal relationships. Among patients by contrast, there is no such sex difference, and while work or career ambitions accounted for two-thirds of the reported goal frustration events and difficulties for men, they were almost as common for women where over half involved work or career plans. The female patients in our series would therefore seem to be more ambitious, at least in work terms, than their healthy counterparts.

There was no relationship between goal frustration and age, cultural background, marital status, or social class, and the results remain unaltered if subjects with a relapse of an old gastrointestinal disorder are excluded from the analysis. Similarly there was more goal frustration among the organically ill for all degrees of tobacco or alcohol consumption. There is a tendency for goal frustration to be associated with

Table III. *Proportion of patients experiencing goal frustration by diagnosis*

Type of gastrointestinal disorder	Diagnosis	Goal frustration (%)
Organic	Oesophageal ulceration	75 (3/4)
	Gastric ulcer/gastritis	64 (7/11)
	Duodenal ulcer/duodenitis	67 (8/12)
	Ulcerative colitis	54 (7/13)
	Regional enteritis	50 (1/2)
	Pancreatitis	100 (2/2)
	Cholecystitis	0 (0/4)
	Other GI	25 (2/8)
Functional	Dyspepsia	29 (4/14)
	Irritable bowel	14 (3/21)
	Other	27 (12/44)

Grouped brackets: Oesophageal ulceration, Gastric ulcer/gastritis, Duodenal ulcer/duodenitis → 67 (18/27); Ulcerative colitis, Regional enteritis → 53 (8/15); Pancreatitis, Cholecystitis, Other GI → 29 (4/14); combined 53 (8/15) and 29 (4/14) → 41 (12/29).

acid-peptic disorders—67% (18/27) vs 41% (12/29) though this fails to reach statistical significance. There is no such trend amongst diagnostic groups in the functionally ill (Table III).

Goal frustration and striving

Severity of goal frustration, as we have conceived it, depends a great deal on the degree of effort that has been made to attain a goal. Of course effort is itself likely to be closely related to the desirability of the goal and to the presence of obstacles to its acquisition. In every instance where there was a goal frustration such efforts involved some long-term movement toward a valued goal. However, there was at least one shorter period of intense and sustained striving aimed at overcoming a particular obstacle. The length of the period of *general* goal directed actively did not differ between patients and comparison subjects, ranging between 3 months and 3 yr with a mean length of 25 weeks. The short periods of *intense* striving lasted for only a few weeks at a time and always began with some obstructing incident, which, in most instances, was an event in terms of our definition. For example, a building contractor received a bill demanding payment for work that had been incomplete. Feeling that this demand was unreasonable, he refused to pay and was eventually threatened with court action 6 months later. During this initial period of general goal directed activity (the goal being to avoid paying for unfinished work), he wrote letters pointing out that the work had been incomplete and that he was only prepared to pay for what he felt had been completed. His solicitor advised against going to court but, in spite of this, he remained determined to defend his refusal to settle the account. The first goal frustration event occurred when he lost his case. Rather than stop at this point, he decided to take the matter before an appeal court, and in so doing alienated his solicitor to the extent that he refused to act for him. In the weeks leading up to the appeal he strove to perfect his defence, working long hours over what he saw as the critical points in his favour. This period of intense striving ended when he lost his appeal and this time was ordered to pay both his and the claimants' costs, as well as the sum owing. Onset of his organic gastrointestinal disorder occurred within a week of this final event. (See Fig. 1 for a schematic representation.)

This example illustrates that periods of striving could be responses to an indication that the goal might be in jeopardy. Forty-one per cent of all marked goal frustration events in patients were preceded by an incident which could be conceived as giving a *specific warning* of the subsequent goal frustration preceding onset. In the example there were two such specific warnings—the first occurring when he was summoned to appear in court, and the second at the point where he lost the first case and decided to appeal. (Receiving a summons, for instance, *specifically* forecasts the appearance in court.) Such warnings were particularly common among patients: of those with goal frustration 41% (20/49) had at least one compared with only 8% (1/12) in the comparison population ($p < 0.05$). The 'final' goal frustration occurred in all instances within three months of this specific warning. When faced with this first warning that something might well go wrong the patients did not abandon their course of action, even when, as in most instances, it was quite clear that success was most unlikely and an alternative approach might be more appropriate. Furthermore in most instances where there was a warning, the patients striving, as in the example, clearly made the situation worse than it might otherwise have been. This was evident in nine of the fourteen organic patients and three of the six functional patients whose goal frustration was preceded by a specific warning.

About a quarter of those with goal frustration (13/49) had difficulties only. However in every instance, there proved to be at least one incident before onset which, although not meeting the formal criteria for an event in terms of the LEDS, was clearly a significant marker of goal frustration. For example, the discovery by a business man that a company was withdrawing the offer of a contract to him *before formal agreement had been reached*, while not included as an LEDS-defined event, was clearly a significant incident in the context of his company's long-term financial difficulties. Of course, searching *post hoc* for such explanatory incidents only in those that have experienced a goal frustration difficulty must be treated with caution given the frequency of incidents not rateable as

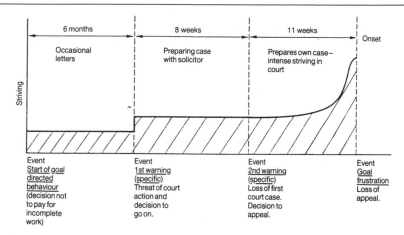

Fig. 1.

events under the existing LEDS. Nevertheless it is sufficient to suggest that there is no reason to believe any different aetiological principle is involved among these 13 patients.

Discussion

The association we have documented between severely threatening events and difficulties (provoking agents) and functional gastrointestinal disease is perhaps hardly surprising given the frequency with which stressful experience has been previously linked with functional disorders. For example, Chaudry and Truelove in their study of antecedent factors in the aetiology of the irritable bowel syndrome reported that threequarters of their patients had a psychological factor which could be related to onset or exacerbation of symptoms. Among women the most common stressors were difficulties in marriage, in family relationships and with their children and among men worries about work [23], see also [24, 25]. More important is the direct confirmation of Creed's finding (using the same life event instrument) concerning abdominal pain mimicking appendicitis, and the fact that both studies are an almost exact replication of work with depression where the same type of severely threatening events are of critical aetiological importance [20, 2].

For organic disease, on the other hand, evidence for stressful experience has been less consistent and impressive. Early studies using unstandardised instruments suggested some kind of link with stressful events but with the introduction of more systematic measurement of both physical disorder and life stress there has been increasing doubt about the validity of these earlier reports. Piper and his colleagues found no relationship between the mean frequencies of life events, their undesirability and subsequent onset or relapse of gastric or duodenal ulcer disease [26–28]. Similarly negative relationships have been reported in studies of ulcerative colitis [29, 30]. These together with the study of appendicitis [20] and our own suggest that the bulk of evidence is against *severe longterm threat*, being of significance in gastrointestinal organic disease. If stress does play a role it is likely to be of a different order from that involved in affective psychiatric disorder or functional states. We believe that it is possible and that this is a good part of the reason why many of the earlier, more impressionistic studies, concluded that there was a link between stress and organic illness. Indeed we decided to explore the possible importance of goal frustration because of our belief that this was the common thread running through so many of the case histories dealing with life stress in the early psychosomatic literature [31–37].

In one of these earlier less systematic studies, Davies and Wilson noted the aetiological significance of life-event stress among 205 cases of peptic ulcer, arguing that in 84% the symptoms had first begun after an event affecting the subject's finances, work or the health of his family [36–37]. On the basis of personality measures they argued that ulcer patients were more liable to rebuff and failure because "through their keenness they expose themselves to affronts, failures and disappointments more frequently than their placid neighbours." Although these conclusions were based on rather idiosyncratic measures of personality, the order of difference between the ulcer patients and comparison subjects was high: 58% of the ulcer patients demonstrated such personality traits and 14% of the comparison series. There are some similarities between the implications of a personality influence and our finding that the ultimate severity of the goal frustration experience appeared often to be the result of the subject's own actions. Early reports often emphasised attributes of the ulcer personality, notably that sufferers were ambitious, efficient and striving [38–40], but for the most part they concentrated on patient populations and overlooked the possibility that such attributes were common in healthy individuals. However other studies, early and late, failed to confirm that patients were unusually ambitious [41–42] and it seems likely that having ambition or working industriously toward desired goals is insufficient in itself to bring about organic illness. Our findings by contrast suggest that it is the *frustration* of these plans and ambitions that is of prime importance. In short, it may well be that there are many who strive earnestly, but that relatively few experience severe goal frustration as reported by us, and it is only these few who are at risk of becoming ill.

Effective theory will also need to concern itself with the emotional response provoked by the goal frustration event as a key component in the final pathway to organic change. This emotional response is likely to be different from the depression which follows the experience of loss and the anxiety which follows a danger event. The obvious candidate is anger and this has been suggested on a number of occasions in the past [9, 10]. The emotion of sadness, and the associated cognition of giving-up in the face of a loss, or the apprehension and vigilance associated with danger events, can be contrasted with the tenacity shown by our subjects in striving to achieve their goals. Both the hopelessness of the giving-up response to loss and the vigilance in danger situations are more passive responses than the striving posture adopted by those experiencing obstacles to ambitions. Here it is an active, assertive process involving fight rather than flight or withdrawal. This contrast will be the focus of further analysis of our material on psychiatric symptoms intervening between the events and the two types of gastrointestinal disorder and of data on cognitive sets.

The analysis so far has highlighted the need for aetiological studies of gastrointestinal disorder to integrate many different types of factors simultaneously into their causal models; for by pinpointing the importance of the goal frustration experience it has raised further hypotheses about the cognitive, emotional, psychiatric and somatic processes which mediate between the environment and physical illness.

Acknowledgements

The project was supported by the Medical Research Council. We thank Drs. R. Pounder of the Royal Free Hospital and R. Vicary of the Whittington and Royal Northern Hospitals for allowing us to study their patients; the general practitioners of the five surgeries in North London who allowed us access to their registers when drawing our comparison sample; Miss J. Duffell for her invaluable assistance in data collection and administration of the project; Tirril Harris for her helpful guidance; Prof. A. Wakeling of the Royal Free for his support, and the administrative staff of hospitals and surgeries for their friendly assistance in tracing records. A special note of gratitude to Miss Fee for her patient secretarial assistance. Finally we thank the many patients and population subjects who agreed to participate in the study and gave so much of their time.

References

1. CASSEL J. Psychological processes and 'stress': theoretical formulation. *Int J Hlth Serv* 1974; **4**:471–482.
2. BROWN GW, HARRIS TH. *The Social Origins of Depression: A Study of Psychiatric Disorder in Women.* London: Tavistock Publications. New York: Free Press, 1978.
3. FINLAY-JONES RA, BROWN GW. Types of stressful life event and the onset of anxiety and depressive disorders. *Psychol Med* 1981; **11**: 803–815.
4. PAYKEL ES, MYERS JK, DIENELT MN, KLERMAN GL, LINDENTHAL JJ, PEPPER MP. Life events and depression: a controlled study, *Arch Gen Psychiat* 1969; **21**: 753–760.

5. LEFF J, KUIPERS L, BERKOWITZ R, VAUGHN C, STURGEON D. Life events, relatives expressed emotion and maintenance neuroleptics in schizophrenic relapse. *Psychol Med* 1983; **13**: 799–806.

6. BRINTON W. *On the Pathology, Symptoms and Treatment of Ulcer of the Stomach.* London: John Churchill 1857.

7. MURREY CD. Psychological factors in the etiology of ulcerative colitis and bloody diarrhoea. *Am J Med Sci* 1930; **180**: 239–245.

8. STEWART W. Psychosomatic aspects of regional enteritis. *NY Med J* 1949; **49**: 2820–2824.

9. WOLF S, WOLF HG. *Human Gastric Function.* New York: Oxford University Press, 1947.

10. MARGOLIN SG. The behaviour of the stomach during psychoanalysis. A contribution to a method of verifying psychoanalytic data. *Psychoanalyt Q* 1951; **20**: 349–369.

11. ALMY TP, KERN F, JR, TULIN M. Alterations in colonic function in men under stress. *Gastroenterology* 1949; **12**: 425–436.

12. CRAIG TJ, BROWN GW. Life events, meaning and physical illness. In *Health Care and Human Behaviour* (Edited by STEPTOE A and MATHEWS A). New York: Academic Press, 1984.

13. BROWN GW. Meaning, measurement and stress. In *Stressfulness of Life Events: Their Nature and Effects* (Edited by DOHRENWEND BS and BP). London: John Wiley 1974.

14. BIRLEY JLT, CONNOLLY J. Life events and physical illness. In *Modern Trends in Psychosomatic Medicine Vol 3* (Edited by HILL OW). London: Butterworths, 1976.

15. COSTELLO CG. Social factors associated with depression: a retrospective community study. *Psychol Med* 1982; **12**: 329–339.

16. MURPHY E. Social origins of depression in old age. *Br J Psychiat* 1982; **141**: 135–142.

17. CONNOLLY J. Life events before myocardial infarction. *J Hum Stress* 1976; **2**: 3–17.

18. PENROSE RJJ. Life events before subarachnoid haemorrhage. *J Psychosom Res* 1972; **16**: 329–333.

19. MURPHY E, BROWN GW. Life events, psychiatric disturbance and physical illness. *Br J Psychiat* 1980; **136**: 326–338.

20. CREED F. Life events and appendicectomy. *Lancet* 1981; **1**: 381–385.

21. TENNANT C, SMITH A, BEBBINGTON P, HURRY J. The contextual threat of life events: The concept and its reliability. *Psychol Med* 1979; **9**: 525–528.

22. PARRY G, SHAPIRO DA, DAVIES L. Reliability of life event ratings: An independent replication. *Br J Clin Psychol* 1979; **20**: 133–134.

23. CHAUDRY NA, TRUELOVE SC. The irritable colon syndrome: a study of the clinical features, predisposing causes and prognosis in 130 cases. *Q J Med* 1962; **31**: 307–322.

24. HISLOP IG. Onset setting in inflammatory bowel disease. *Med J Aust* 1974; **1**: 981–984.

25. HILL OW, BLENDIS LM. Physical and psychological evaluation of non-organic abdominal pain. *Gut* 1967; **8**: 221–229.

26. PIPER DW, MCINTOSH JH, ARIOTTI DE, CALOGIURI JV, BROWN RW, SHY CM. Life events and chronic duodenal ulcer: a case control study. *Gut* 1981; **22**, 1011–1017.

27. THOMAS JH, GREIG M, PIPER DW. Chronic gastric ulcer and life events. *Gastroenterology* 1980; **78**: 905–911.

28. PIPER DW, GREIG M, SHINNERS J, THOMAS J, CRAWFORD J. Chronic gastric ulcer and stress: A comparison of an ulcer population with a control population regarding stressful events over a life time. *Digestion* 1978; **18**: 303–309.

29. MENDELOFF AI, MONK M, SIEGEL CI, LILIENFIELD A. Illness experience and life stresses in patients with irritable colons and with ulcerative colitis. *N Engl J Med* 1970; **282**: 14–17.

30. FELDMAN F, CANTOR D, SOLL S. Psychiatric study of a consecutive series of 34 patients with ulcerative colitis. *Br Med J* 1967; **3**: 14–17.

31. ALEXANDER F. *Psychosomatic Medicine.* New York: Norton, 1950.

32. ALEXANDER F, BACON C, WILSON GW, LEVEY HB, LEVINE M. The influence of psychologic factors upon gastrointestinal disturbances. *Psychoanalyt Q* 1934: **3**: 501–539.

33. STENBACH A. Gastric neurosis, pre-ulcer conflict and personality in duodenal ulcer. *J Psychosom Res* 1960; **4**, 282–296.

34. GROEN JJ. The psychosomatic specificity hypothesis for the etiology of peptic ulcer. *Psychotherap Psychosom* 1971; **19**: 295–309.

35. GROEN JJ. Social change and psychosomatic disease. In *Society, Stress and Disease Vol. 1* (Edited by LEVI L). London: Oxford University Press, 1971.

36. DAVIES DT, WILSON ATM. Observations on the life history of chronic peptic ulcer. *Lancet* 1937; **1**: 1354–1360.

37. DAVIES DT, WILSON ATM. Personal and clinical history in haematemesis and perforation. *Lancet* 1939; **3**: 723–727.

38. ALVAREZ WC. Ways in which emotions can affect the digestive tract. *J Am Med Assoc* 1929; **92**: 616–662.

39. DRAPER G, TOURAINE GA. The man environment unit and peptic ulcer. *Arch Intern Med* 1932; **49**: 616–662.

40. DUNBAR F. *Emotions and Bodily Change.* New York: Columbia University Press, 1947.

41. KAPP FT, ROSENBAUM M, ROMANO J. Psychological factors in men with peptic ulcers. *Am J Psychiat* 1947; **103**: 700–704.

42. KEZUR E, KAPP FT, ROSENBAUM M. Psychological factors in women with peptic ulcers. *Am J Psychiat* 1951; **108**: 368–373.

Psychosocial assets, life crisis and the prognosis of pregnancy

Katherine B. Nuckolls, John Cassel and Berton H. Kaplan

Department of Epidemiology, School of Public Health, University of North Carolina, Chapel Hill, NC, USA

Abstract

Nuckolls, K. B. (Yale University School of Nursing, New Haven, Conn. 06510), J. Cassel and B. H. Kaplan. Psychological assets, life crisis and the prognosis of pregnancy. *Am J Epidemiol* 95: 431–441, 1972.—This is a study of the relationships between psychosocial assets, social stresses as measured by a cumulative life change score and the prognosis of pregnancy. Psychosocial assets were measured early in pregnancy by a questionnaire (TAPPS) designed to assess the adaptive potential for pregnancy. At 32 weeks, subjects completed the Schedule of Recent Experience from which scores were calculated for life change during pregnancy and for the two years preceding it. Following delivery, the medical record was used to score each pregnancy as "normal" or "complicated." Complete data were obtained on 170 subjects. Taken alone, neither life change nor TAPPS scores were significantly related to complications. However, when these variables were considered conjointly, it was found that if the life change score was high both before and during pregnancy, women with high TAPPS scores (favorable psychosocial assets) had only one third the complication rate of women with low TAPPS scores. In the absence of high cumulative life change, there was no significant relationship between psychosocial assets and complications.

adaptation, psychological; pregnancy; pregnancy complications; psychosomatic medicine; social adjustment; stress

Attempts to document the role of psychosocial factors in the genesis of human disease and, in particular, in the disorders of pregnancy have yielded intriguing but often confusing or conflicting results. Despite the plethora of anecdotal and case study reports, the findings of carefully

Abbreviations: LCS, life change score; LCU, life change units; SRE, schedule of recent experiences; TAPPS, the adaptive potential for pregnancy.
Reprinted from Nuckolls, K. B., Cassel, J. and Kaplan, B. H. Psychosocial assets, life crisis and the prognosis of pregnancy. *American Journal of Epidemiology*, **95**, 431–41, 1972.

conducted epidemiologic or clinical investigations have tended to be ambiguous. This is in sharp contrast to the dramatic results which have been obtained with animal experiments (1–10). To some extent, this may be due to the methodological difficulties inherent in such studies, but to a larger extent it is probably a function of inadequacies in the current theoretical framework. A recent review of some of these theoretical issues (11) has identified one of the central problems to be the nature of the model of causation subscribed to (often implicitly) by the majority of such investigators. Conditioned by the model provided by the germ theory, we have become accustomed to thinking in mono-etiologic terms. Accordingly, much of the work concerned with social or psychological antecedents to disease has attempted to identify a particular situational set (usually labelled "stress" or "a stressor") as having a specific causal relationship to some clinical entity, following a model analogous to the relationship between the typhoid bacillus and typhoid fever. Further more, it is assumed that the only factors influencing this relationship will be the strength and duration of exposure to this source of "stress". Such a formulation would appear to be clearly at variance with some of the known evidence. The animal studies particularly would seem to indicate that variations in the social milieu (with all other factors—genetic stock, diet, temperature and sanitation—held constant) will lead to numerous pathologic conditions, including, for example, an increase in maternal and infant mortality rates, a reduced resistance to a wide variety of insults such as toxins, x-rays and microorganisms, an increase in the incidence of arteriosclerosis and of hypertension, and an increased susceptibility to various forms of neoplasia. Thus, rather than searching for a specific relationship between social factors and a particular disease or pathologic outcome, it might be more profitable to regard the role of such factors as enhancing susceptibility to disease in general. With that formulation, the specific manifestations of such increased susceptibility may not be a function of the particular social process under study but rather a function of the genetic constitutions of the exposed individuals and the nature of the physicochemical or microbiological insults encountered.

In addition, both animal and human studies indicate that the pathologic effects of any social process can be markedly modified by the availability of various sources of support (12–14). Therefore, to determine the harmful consequences of any postulated "stressful" situation, it would not be sufficient to attempt to measure only the strength and duration of the "stress"; rather the balance between the stressful situation and the nature and strength of the supportive or protective elements would need to be assessed.

Only a limited number of investigators have addressed themselves to conceptualizing and attempting to identify both deleterious and protective psychosocial processes. An approach that we have found useful is one developed by Holmes and his associates (15). Their approach to identifying "stressful" situations has been through the concept of the magnitude and importance of life changes.

Beginning in 1949, this research group began to study systematically the quality and quantity of life events observed to cluster at the time of illness onset. These events include changes in the family structure, marriage, occupations, friendship groups and other significant areas which are usually associated with some adaptive or coping behavior on the part of the individual. The term "life crisis" was coined to represent the occurrence of an extraordinary number of these changes in life adjustment clustered into one or two years. Through the use of a constant referent technique, a magnitude of significance was assigned to each of 43 life events. The resultant scale reflected the magnitude of change required in the ongoing life adjustment by each event, and the values were defined as life change units (LCU). An individual's total LCU score was calculated from his experience as reported on the Schedule of Recent Experiences (SRE), and it was found that the higher the quantitative estimate of life crisis, the greater the probability of an associated major health change occurring within the succeeding two years. Subsequent prospective studies (16) have borne out the initial findings showing illnesses to be preceded by clustering of life changes.

In an attempt to quantify the protective elements available to individuals, which they termed "psycho-social assets", Berle et al. (17) developed a guide to prognosis in stress diseases which Holmes and associates later used successfully as a prognostic instrument in a follow-up study of patients with tuberculosis (18).

The study here reported is an attempt to explore the degree to which psychosocial assets are protective, as well as the degree to which multiple life changes are detrimental to health. Thus, we have examined the relationship of an index of psychosocial assets to various health parameters of pregnancy and the puerperium, a life change score to these same conditions and, perhaps most importantly, the relationship of psychosocial assets to these health states in the presence and absence of high life change scores. By this latter type of analysis, we hoped to come closer to the formulation of the "balance" between the protective and the deleterious processes and the relationship of this balance to health status.

Outcome of pregnancy was chosen as the dependent variable partly for pragmatic reasons such as sample size, temporal predictability, and ease of data collection, and partly because of other advantages which it offers. Although not an illness per se, pregnancy is a health change which clearly challenges the adaptive capacity physiologically, psychologically and socially. It carries with it risks for a defined body of pathologic conditions, some of which may be considered as maladaptive responses. There is, in addition, a need for further research into the psychosocial variables which contribute to the prognosis of pregnancy. This is evidenced by the comparatively high infant mortality rate in this country and by the persistent incidence of certain complications of pregnancy which fail to yield to improvements in obstetrical skill. Although gross social factors are unquestionably the major contributors to the excess infant mortality in the United States, it seems reasonable to believe that other psychosocial factors may also affect the outcome of pregnancy.

Other researchers who have investigated the relationships of psycho-social factors to pregnancy have focused on either discrete complications like hyperemesis, toxemia or prematurity, or on a total "complication score" for the whole child-bearing episode. McDonald (19) in a review of the role of emotional factors in obstetrical complications summarizes these findings with the comment that "self-report of anxiety is to date the most discriminating behavioral measure for presaging complications." A number of retrospective studies have related stressful occurrences during pregnancy to difficult labor or untoward outcomes (20–25). Abramson (26) in a prospective study in Durban, South Africa, found a significant association between a woman's own report of stress during pregnancy and the development of her infant. Because we had no theoretical reason to believe that psychosocial assets or stress are specific to any one complication of pregnancy, it was decided to define the dependent variable "complications" as any untoward condition or outcome of pregnancy not related to an anatomical or other known maternal defect.

Method

The instruments

In keeping with the general approach of Berle et al. (17) and Holmes et al. (18), psychosocial assets were defined as any psychological or social factors which contribute to a woman's ability to adapt to her first pregnancy. We decided to measure them with a questionnaire from which a single index score could be derived representing the adaptive potential for pregnancy (TAPPS).

Details of the development of this instrument and the methods used to score it are available elsewhere (27). In summary, the score was derived from responses to questions designed to measure the subject's feelings or perceptions concerning herself, her pregnancy and her overall life situation including her relationships with her husband, her extended family and the community. Table 1 shows the factors tapped in each category of assets.

Table 1. *Factors tapped in each category of assets*

Self	Ego strength, loneliness, adaptability, trust, hostility, self esteem, crying, perception of health.
Marriage	Duration of marriage, marital happiness, concordance of age, religion.
Extended family	Relationship of subject with own parents, siblings, and in-laws. Confidence in emotional or economic support, if needed.
Social resources	Adjustment to community. Friendship patterns and support.
Definition of pregnancy	1. Extent to which pregnancy was desired and planned.
	2. Feelings about pregnancy and childbirth, confidence in physician, fear of labor.
	3. Anticipation of baby. Confidence in outcome.

Questions were classified into one or another of these categories as the questionnaire was developed. In scoring, the raw scores for each item were transformed to standard scores to equalize the variances and means. The standard scores were then summed to give category scores. The total score, TAPPS, is the sum of the category scores equally weighted.

The instrument was self-administered. In general, the format was such that responses could be checked on a 20-point scale, which, unlike the conventional multiple choice test, does not limit the subject to a few prestructured categories but allows answers to be placed along a broad continuum. Such a format has been used successfully by Jenkins and others (28, 29) to measure attitudes and beliefs about disease.

Life crisis was measured by the life change score (LCS) which was calculated from the Schedule of Recent Experience as developed by Holmes and Rahe (15). The form of the instrument used in this research provides for a summed score of the life changes which occurred in the two years before pregnancy, and a second score for more recent changes which occurred during pregnancy. The weights used to score the separate events were the same as those used in the work cited.

Scoring complications

Since any single complication of pregnancy is a relatively rare event, a prospective study requires a large sample in order to assure that the "desired" complication will appear with sufficient frequency. This is particularly true if the study population is not an exceptionally high risk group. Attempts to solve this problem usually result in the decision to use some measure of "all complications," conceptualizing them as derivatives of a common process (19, 30–33). Such measures do serve to optimize the variance of the dependent variable, but they present a difficult problem in scoring because there is a high degree of variability in the number, nature and severity of complications occurring in any single pregnancy.

In order to determine if there exist regular patterns of clustering of complications which could be ranked for severity by expert judges, we obtained data from the Collaborative Study by the Perinatal Research Branch, National Institute of Neurological Disease and Blindness, on all complications for 1000 white primigravidas[1]. Review of these data convinced us that apart from known syndromes, such as toxemia, identifiable cluster patterns do not occur, and that the reliability of a ranking procedure would be questionable. It was therefore decided to categorize the total course and outcome of each pregnancy as either "normal" or "complicated." Medical records were reviewed following delivery and all abnormal findings for each mother and infant were recorded using previously established criteria derived from a standard obstetrical text (34).

Since obstetrical care for the entire sample was provided by a limited number of physicians using the same standards for care and standardized record forms, the actual medical records were more reliable than would usually be found. A research assistant spot-schecked 10 of the records for the reliability of our coding. No errors were found for those 10 patients. Patients were classified as "complicated" if they had one or more of the following conditions:

- A systolic blood pressure during pregnancy of over 139 mm or a diastolic blood pressure of over 89 mm or a systolic elevation of more than 30 mm, any one of these in combination with proteinuria.
- Admission to the hospital for pre-eclampsia.
- Threatened abortion.
- Admission to the hospital for hyperemesis.
- Premature rupture of the membranes for more than 24 hours before delivery in the absence of cephalo-pelvic disproportion.
- Prolonged labor. First stage longer than 20 hours or the second stage longer than 150 minutes in the absence of cephalo-pelvic disproportion.
- Apgar rating of infant less than 7, or reported infant respiratory distress in the absence of cephalo-pelvic disproportion.

[1]The authors thank Dr. Zekin A. Shakhashiri, Assistant to the Chief, Perinatal Research Branch, National Institute of Neurological Disease and Blindness, for providing these data from that agency's continuing Collaborative Study on Cerebral Palsy, Mental Retardation and Other Neurological and Sensory Disorders of Infancy and Childhood.

- A systolic blood pressure of over 139 mm and/or a diastolic blood pressure of over 89 mm during both the labor and post-partum periods.
- Birthweight of less than 2500 grams.
- Abortion, stillbirth or neonatal death within the first three days.

With this definition, 96 or 47.1 per cent of the 204 patients were classified as "complicated." (The base for these figures includes 34 patients who were not included in the final analysis because their life change scores were not completed.) Of the 96 patients, only eight had single complications and only one was classified as "complicated" solely on the basis of blood pressure. This complication rate is comparable with the rate of 50.2 per cent found for the Collaborative Study sample using the foregoing criteria.

At first glance, these figures seem high but similar rates have been found in other studies. Heinstein (33) reports that in a sample of 156 gravidas, only 20 per cent were classified as having had no physical complications, either mild or severe, while 47 per cent were judged to have had mild complications and 33 per cent were thought to be serious. In other studies using similar classification schemes, Grim (32) categorized 122 out of 227 patients as "abnormal" and in McDonald's sample of 107 patients, 89 were classified as abnormal (19).

The sample

This study was conducted at a large military hospital. The subjects were white primigravidas, married to enlisted men, registered for obstetrical care prior to the 24th week of pregnancy. At the time of prenatal registration, the TAPPS questionnaire was administered to all women who met these criteria. The intake sample size was 340. Figure 1 is a flow diagram of intake and attrition.

The Schedule of Recent Experience was mailed to subjects during the 32nd week of their pregnancies and the medical records were reviewed following delivery and hospital discharge. Complete records were obtained for 170 subjects who delivered in the military hospital.

Attempts were made to follow-up all patients who were transferred before delivery by obtaining permanent addresses at the time of intake, maintaining a careful check on the clinic discharge book and, when a subject was transferred, sending a letter requesting the name of the physician who would deliver her. Modified data forms were mailed to these physicians. Responses from 88 per cent of the doctors contacted resulted in an additional 67 completed records. These were analyzed separately due to the possibility of varying criteria for complications and are not included in this discussion. In all, military transfer or discharge,

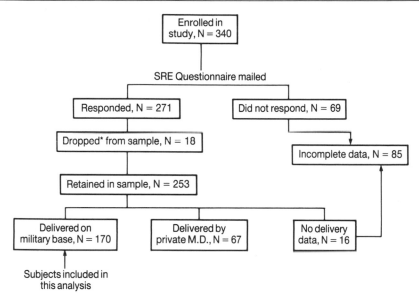

*Reasons for dropping from sample: twins, 5; not pregnant, 3; incomplete records, 4; previous illness, 1; previous miscarriage, 5.

Figure 1. Diagram of intake and attrition.

coupled with failure on the part of either the physician or the subject to provide follow-up data, accounted for the loss of 85 subjects. An additional 18 were dropped from the sample for reasons listed on figure 1.

As can be seen from tables 2, 3, 4 and 5 the original sample was quite homogeneous in terms of age, social clas, educational level, and duration of pregnancy. In order to determine whether or not there were any significant differences between those who were excluded from this analysis and those included, chi square tests for homogeneity for these characteristics were performed. No significant differences were found. In addition, as seen in table 6 (the mean and standard deviation of life change scores) and table 7 (the mean and standard deviation of TAPP scores), no significant differences were found between the two groups for the major independent variables. We are therefore reasonably sure that those subjects included in this analysis did not differ in any important respect from those lost or omitted.

Since no correlations between complications and age ($r = -.02$) and social class ($r = -.003$) occurred in this homogeneous sample, these factors were not controlled for in the final analyses (table 8). (Social class was scored for head of household of the woman's family of origin using Hollingshead's Two Factor Index of Social Class (35).)

Table 2. *Distribution of subjects by age at clinic admission*

Subjects	<18	18–19	20–24	25–29	>29	Total
No.	16	111	181	16	1	325
%	4.9	33.9	55.9	4.8	0.3	100.0

Table 3. *Distribution of subjects by social class as determined by occupation and education of head of household of subject's family orientation*

Subjects	Social class*					
	I	II	III	IV	V	Total
No.	4	13	53	164	91	325
%	1.2	4.0	16.3	50.4	28.0	100.0

*Hollingshead's Two Factor Index of Social Class (35).

Table 4. *Distribution of subjects by educational attainment*

Subjects	No. of years or type of schooling						
	<10	10–11	12	Technical	Some college	Bachelor Degree or +	Total
No.	9	45	165	47	51	8	325
%	2.7	13.9	50.7	14.5	15.7	2.5	100.0

Table 5. *Distribution of subjects by duration of pregnancy at clinic admission*

Subjects	Week of pregnancy				
	12	12–15	16–19	20–24	Total
No.	47	118	108	52	325
%	14.4	36.3	33.2	16.1	100.0

Table 6. *Range, mean and standard deviations of life change scores*

Life change scores	Delivered on military base, N = 170	Delivered by private M.D., N = 67	p
Before pregnancy			
Range	0–741	0–642	N.S.*
Mean	187.24	165.89	
S.D.	148.53	144.7	
During pregnancy			
Range	0–714	0–526	N.S.
Mean	188.78	204.75	
S.D.	114.39	109.82	
Total			
Range	70–1349	59–1091	N.S.
Mean	375.51	370.6	
S.D.	199.80	186.79	

*N.S. = not significant.

Table 7. *Mean and standard deviation of the adaptive potential for pregnancy score*

Sample	N	$\bar{X}$	S.D.	p
Delivered on military base	170	45.07	3.75	N.S.*
Delivered by private physician	67	44.41	3.60	N.S.

*Not significant.

Table 8. *Correlation of age and social class* with complications (N = 204†)*

Variable	r
Age	−.02
Social class	−.003

*Scored for head of household of woman's family of origin using Hollingshead Two Factor Index of Social Class (35).

†This correlation included 34 subjects for whom there were complete delivery records but no interim data.

Results

Table 9 shows the correlations between the life change scores, both before and during pregnancy, and complications of pregnancy, and the

Table 9. *Correlation of life change scores (LCS*) and TAPPS† with complications*

	r
LCS before pregnancy:	.003
LCS during pregnancy:	.07
Total LCS:	.05
TAPPS:	−.07

*N = 170.
†N = 204. Included 34 patients for whom there were no interim data.

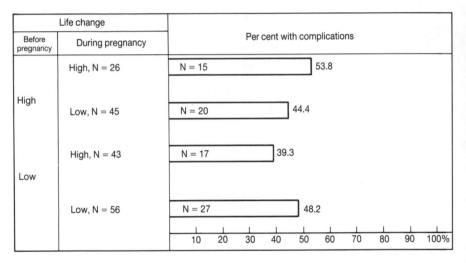

Figure 2. Comparison of percentage of patients with complications in four conditions of life change.

correlation between the TAPPS (psychosocial asset score) and complications. As can be seen from the table, none of the correlations attained even borderline significance. Similarly, figures 2 and 3 show no significant differences in the percentage of patients with complications given either high and low life change or high and low TAPPS scores. (Life change scores and TAPPS scores were divided at the means for the entire sample giving subsets with "high" and "low" scores for each variable.) Thus it is evident that, if considered separately, neither multiple life changes nor variations in psychosocial assets were related in this study to complications of pregnancy.

To test the extent to which the effect of multiple life changes might be modified by psychosocial assets, a contingency table was set up as shown in figure 4. In this figure it can be seen that in the presence of mounting

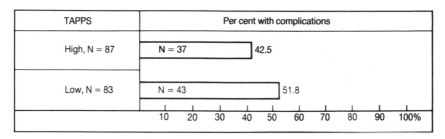

Figure 3. Comparison of percentage of patients with complications given high and low adaptive potential for pregnancy scores.

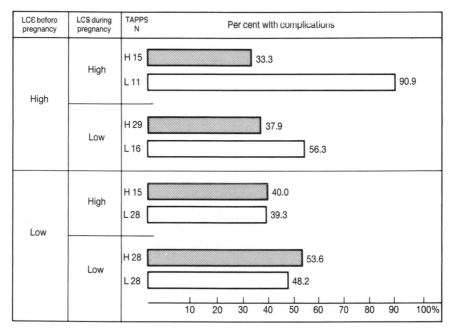

Figure 4. Comparison of percentage of patients with complications by high and low TAPPS scores, life change scores controlled. High—boxes with diagonal lines; low—clear boxes.

life change (life change scores high both before and during pregnancy), women with high psychosocial assets had only one-third the complication rate of women whose psychosocial assets were low. In the absence of such life changes, particularly for the period before pregnancy, the level of psychosocial assets was irrelevant, there being essentially no difference in the complication rate between those having high and low TAPPS scores.

Discussion

These findings, if replicated, could help to explain some of the discrepant results in the current literature. Taken alone, neither exposure to socially stressful situations nor the availability of multiple psychosocial assets will be consistently related to poor health states. Instead, the balance between these two processes will need to be assessed for an explanation of enhanced disease susceptibility. It should be emphasized further that we are not proposing this combination of high psychosocial stressors and low assets as the cause, or even *a* cause for any specific clinical entity, but rather propose that it may enhance susceptibility to a variety of environmental insults. As illustrated by the somewhat heterogeneous list of conditions we have included as complications, we suggest that the manifestations of such enhanced susceptibility will depend upon the nature of these environmental insults plus presumably the genetic constitution of the exposed subjects. Such a concept of generalized susceptibility would be consistent with the situation in the United States where it has recently been demonstrated that those regions of the country which have the highest death rates from cardiovascular disease (age, race, sex specific) also have higher than expected death rates from all causes, including cancer and infectious diseases (36). This illustration, of course, does not necessarily document that social processes are responsible for such an increased susceptibility, but does lend credence to the view that variations in generalized susceptibility may be a useful concept. Somewhat more direct evidence is provided by Christenson and Hinkle (37) whose data show that managers in an industrial company who, by virtue of their family background and educational experiences were least well prepared for the demands and expectations of executive industrial life, had the highest rate of *all* diseases—major as well as minor, physical as well as mental, long-term as well as short-term. It would also be consistent with the finding that widowed and divorced men, particularly of young ages, have from 3 to 5 times the death rate of married men of the same age from *every* cause of death (38).

As indicated earlier, this notion then casts serious doubt on the utility of specificity (as far as current clinical syndromes are concerned) in research concerned with psychosocial factors in disease etiology. Similar psychosocial factors may be related to different disease syndromes (depending upon the prevalent environmental factors and genetic make-up of the populations), and attempts to document and quantify the relevance of such factors will of necessity have to take this into account in the research design. Perhaps a more elegant and satisfactory approach to attempting to measure all disease manifestations in populations exposed to these psychosocial forces would be to standardize for the "manifestational" agents. To select populations all of whom have been exposed to the tubercle bacillus, for example, and determine whether the postulated psychosocial factors discriminate between those who develop and do not develop clinical disease. Alternatively, populations at high risk of developing myocardial infarction, by virtue of their "risk" factors, could be selected and a similar strategy employed.

Should such approaches be successful, the implications for intervention could be of considerable importance. By strengthening the psychosocial assets (a task which surely is not beyond human ingenuity), presumably we could reduce the incidence of illness and improve the quality of life.

Acknowledgements

The project was supported in part by Special Nurse Scientist Fellowship No. 1F4-NU-27, 066-01 Division of Nursing, Department of Health, Education and Welfare, USPHS. The authors express their appreciation to Dana Quade, Ph.D. and to Luther Talbert, M.D. for their assistance with this study and to the Departments of Obstetrics and Army Health Nursing at Womack Army Hospital, Fort Bragg, North Carolina for their interest and cooperation.

References

1. Ader R, Hahn EW: Effects of social environment on mortality to whole body x-irradiation in the rat. Psychol Rep 13: 214–215, 1963
2. Ader R, Kreutner A, Jacobs HL: Social environment, emotionality and alloxan diabetes in the rat. Psychosom Med 25: 60–68, 1963
3. Andervont HB: Influence of environment on mammary cancer in mice. J Natl Cancer Inst 4: 579–581, 1944
4. Calhoun JB: Population density and social pathology. Sci Am 206: 139, 1962
5. Christian JJ, Williamson HO: Effect of crowding on experimental granuloma formation in mice. Proc Soc Exp Biol Med 99: 385–387, 1958
6. Davis DE, Read CP: Effect of behavior on development of resistance in trichinosis. Proc Soc Biol Med 99: 269–272, 1958
7. Henry JP: Systematic arterial pressure as a measure of stressful social interaction. (Manuscript)
8. King JT, Lee YCP, Visscher MB: Single versus multiple cage occupancy and convulsion frequency in C_3H mice. Proc Soc Exp Biol Med 88: 661–663, 1955
9. Ratcliffe HL, Cronin MTI: Changing frequency of arteriosclerosis in mammals and birds at the Philadelphia Zoological Garden. Circulation 18: 41–52, 1959
10. Swinyard EA, Clark LD, Miyahara JT, et al: Studies on the mechanism of amphetamine toxicity in aggregated mice. J Pharmacol Exp Ther 132: 97–102, 1961
11. Symes SL, Reeder LG (editors): Proceedings of the National Workshop Conference on Socioenvironmental Stress and Cardiovascular Diseases— Phoenix, Arizona. Feb 14–16, 1966. Milbank Mem Fund Q 55: No. 2. 1967.

12. Bogdanoff MD, Klein R, Estes EH, et al: The physiologic response to conformity pressure in man. Ann Intern Med 57: 389–397, 1962
13. Conger JJ, Lawrey WL, Turrell ES: The role of social experience in the production of gastric ulcers in hooded rats placed in a conflict situation. J Abnorm Soc Psychol 57: 214–220, 1958
14. Henry JP, Meehand JP, Stephens PM: The use of psychosocial stimuli to induce prolonged hypertension in mice. Psychosom Med 29: 408–432, 1967
15. Holmes T, Rahe R: Life crisis and disease onset. Parts I, II, III. Unpublished research reports. Seattle, Washington: Department of Psychiatry, University of Washington School of Medicine, 1966
16. Rahe RH, Meyer M, Smith M, et al: Social stress and illness onset. J Psychosom Res 8: 35–44, 1964
17. Berle BB, Pinsky RH, Wolf S, et al: A Clinical Guide to Prognosis in Stress Diseases. JAMA 149: 1624–1627, 1952
18. Holmes TH, Joffe JR, Ketcham JW, et al: Experimental study of prognosis. J Psychosom Res 5: 235–252, 1961
19. McDonald RL: The role of emotional factors in obstetric complications, a review. Psychosom Med 30: 222–237, 1968
20. Brandon MWG: An epidemiological study of maladjustment in childhood. M.D. Thesis, University of Durham, 1960. *In* Childbearing. Edited by E Gruenberg. Baltimore, Williams and Wilkins, 1961
21. Gunter LM: Psychopathology and stress in the life experience of mothers of premature infants. Am J Obstet Gynecol 86: 333, 1963
22. Hetzel BS, Bruer B, Poidevin LOS: A survey of the relation between certain common antenatal complications in primiparae and stressful life situations during pregnancy. J Psychosom Res 5: 175–182, 1961
23. Scott EM, Thomson AM: A psychological investigation of primigravidae. J Obstet Gynecol 63: 1956
24. Stott DH: Physical and mental handicaps following a disturbed pregnancy. Lancet 1: 1006–1011, 1957
25. Stott DH: Some psychosomatic aspects of casualty in reproduction. J Psychosom Res 3: 42, 1958
26. Abramson JH, Singh AR, Moambo V: Antenatal stress and the baby's development. Arch Dis Child 36: 42–49, 1961
27. Nuckolls KB: Psychosocial Assets, Life Crisis and the Prognosis of Pregnancy. Ph.D. Dissertation, University of North Carolina at Chapel Hill, 1967
28. Jenkins DB: The semantic differential for health: A technique for mass beliefs about diseases. Public Health Rep 81: 549–558, 1966
29. Rosenstock IM, Hochbaum GM, Kegels SS: Determinants of Health Behavior. Presented at Golden White House Conference on Children and Youth, 1961
30. Erikson MT: Relationship between psychological attitudes during pregnancy and complications of pregnancy, labor, and delivery. Proc Am Psychological Assoc 1: 213–214, 1965
31. Werner E, Simonian K, Bierman JM, et al: Cumulative effect of perinatal complications and deprived environment on physical, intellectual, and social development of preschool children. Pediatrics 39: 490–505, 1967
32. Grim E, Venet WR: The relationship of emotional attitudes to the course and outcome of pregnancy. Psychosom Med 28: 34, 1966

33. Heinstein MI: Expressed attitudes and feelings of pregnant women and their relations to physical complications of pregnancy. Merrill-Palmer Q 13: 217–236, 1967
34. Eastman N, Hellman L: Williams Obstetrics. (13th rev ed) New York, Appleton-Century-Crofts, 1966
35. Hollingshead AB, Redlich FC: Social Class and Mental Illness. New York, John Wiley and Sons, 1958
36. Syme SL: Personal communication, 1968
37. Christenson WN, Hinkle LE Jr: Differences in illness and prognostic signs in two groups of young men. JAMA 177: 247–253, 1961
38. Kraus A, Lilienfeld A: Some epidemiologic aspects of the high mortality rate in the young widowed group. J Chronic Dis 10: 207–217, 1959

Section 2

Psychophysiological processes in disease

Readings

Pain mechanisms: a new theory.
R. Melzack and P. D. Wall. *Science*, **150**, 971–9, 1965.

Effects of coping behavior on gastric lesions in rats as a function of the complexity of coping tasks.
A. Tsuda, M. Tanaka, T. Nishikawa and H. Hirai. *Physiology and Behavior*, **30**, 805–8, 1983.

Social stress and atherosclerosis in normocholesterolemic monkeys.
J. R. Kaplan, S. B. Manuck, T. B. Clarkson, F. M. Lusso, D. M. Taub and E. W. Miller. *Science*, **220**, 733–5, 1983.

Mental stress and the induction of silent myocardial ischemia in patients with coronary artery disease.
A. Rozanski, C. N. Bairey, D. S. Krantz, J. Friedman, K. J. Resser, M. Morell, S. Hilton-Chalfen, L. Hestrin, J. Bietendorf and D. S. Berman. *New England Journal of Medicine*, **318**, 1005–12, 1988.

Depressed lymphocyte function after bereavement.
R. W. Bartrop, E. Luckhurst, L. Lazarus, L. G. Kiloh and R. Penny. *Lancet*, i, 834–6, 1977.

Psychological stress and susceptibility to the common cold.
S. Cohen, D. A. J. Tyrrell and A. P. Smith. *New England Journal of Medicine*, **325**, 606–12, 1991.

Introduction

Section 1 documented some of the empirically verified links between life stress, support and health. The question that arises is what are the processes through which factors in the psychosocial environment influence disease aetiology? Unless descriptive studies of clinical phenomena are coupled with a knowledge of mechanism, the study of psychosocial factors will remain outside the mainstream of biobehavioural research and understanding. The readings in Section 2 describe the psychophysiological processes linking behavioural stressors and emotional distress with disease aetiology. The papers highlight the importance of psychophysiological processes in several clinical conditions, including pain, gastrointestinal lesions, cardiovascular pathology and resistance to infection. These readings have been selected to illustrate the diverse research strategies that have proved valuable, and include the analysis of clinical phenomena (*Melzack and Wall*), acute and chronic stress studies with animals (*Tsuda et al.; Kaplan et al.*), short-term experiments with humans (*Rozanski et al.*) and the experience of life stress (*Bartrop et al.; Cohen et al.*).

The psychophysiological processes relevant to the aetiology and course of disease are complex. It is well established that noxious stimuli and challenging conditions may elicit a broad range of autonomic, neuroendocrine and immunological adjustments. Central to the stress response pattern are the pituitary-adrenocortical axis leading to the release of corticosteroids, and the sympathoadrenal pathway, stimulation of which results in sympathetic nervous activation and release of catecholamines from the adrenal medulla (Steptoe, 1990).

In relation to disease risk, at least three different types of psychophysiological process may be relevant:

(1) The first involves *psychophysiological hyperreactivity*, and is based on the notion that substantial physiological responses to behavioural stressors will, if repeated and sustained, lead directly to functional and structural organic changes indicative of pathology. The nature of the pathology will depend on the pattern of physiological response, the constitutional vulnerabilities of the individual, and concurrent factors such as nutritional state. The reading from *Tsuda et al.* illustrates this process in relation to gastric lesions, while *Kaplan et al.* indicate how it may be relevant to coronary atherosclerosis.

(2) A second pathway through which the psychophysiological responses influence health is by influencing *disease stability and progression*. Psychophysiological mechanisms are not only relevant to disease onset in a directly causal fashion, but may also affect the severity and stability of pathology that has already been diagnosed. For example, there is little evidence for psychosocial processes causing bronchial asthma, but numerous studies indicate that stressors may exacerbate the condition in susceptible patients (e.g. Goreczny *et al.*, 1988). Similarly, the stability of glucose metabolism in diabetics can be affected by life stress thorugh fluctuations in

neuroendocrine function, while the severity of chronic back pain may vary with the intensity of stress-induced paraspinal muscle tension (Hanson and Pichert, 1986; Flor and Turk, 1989). The impact of psychophysiological activation on pre-existing severe disease is vividly illustrated in *Rozanski et al.*'s study of myocardial ischaemia, while *Melzack and Wall* discuss central–peripheral interactions in relation to pain.

(3) The third psychophysiological process that is relevant to disease risk concerns alternations in *host vulnerability*. In these circumstances, physiological stress responses have no direct involvement in the pathological process at all, but act by reducing the person's resistance to invasive pathogens. The process may frequently involve the immune system, since stress-induced immunosuppression may increase probability of infections becoming established. The pathways related to this third mechanism are documented by *Bartrop et al.* and by *Cohen et al.*

It is important that these separate psychophysiological links with disease risk are recognised, since they are conceptually distinct and lead to different predictions concerning the impact of life stress on health (see Steptoe, 1991). Understanding the richness of psychophysiological processes relevant to health may help to account for the diverse associations that have been identified between psychosocial factors and illness.

The gate control theory of pain

Melzack and Wall's paper on pain mechanisms appeared in *Science* in 1965, and is a landmark in the recognition of higher nervous system involvement in what had hitherto been considered the purely 'physical' pathology of pain. The relevance of emotion and culture to pain experience has been recognised before (notably by Beecher, 1959), but what *Melzack and Wall* postulated was a physiological mechanism through which such influences might operate. This was a crucial link, and led through subsequent publications to a new integrative view of pain as a physiological system, complete with internal and external control loops, rather than as a simple ascending connectionist pathway (Melzack and Wall, 1982).

An important element of *Melzack and Wall*'s argument was the use of clinical phenomena such as causalgia to dispute the traditional linear model of pain as a primary sensation. Their theory hypothesised that the balance between large and small diameter nerve fibres determines the degree of spinal transmission of pain information. This was made possible by suggesting that the large fibres stimulate inhibitory interneurons in the substantia gelatinosa of the dorsal horn, while small fibres have a facilitatory effect. Subsequent work identified the facilitating nociceptor inputs with fine myelinated A-δ and unmyelinated c-fibres, and the inhibitory efferents with low threshold A-β fibres. The authors were then able to suggest how their theory accounted for pain phenomena such as hyperalgesia and referred pain that are not readily explained by simple linear models.

Melzack and Wall made further important advances in discounting the simple idea of a pain 'centre' in the brain. They proposed multiple pathways of transmission of pain information from the spinal cord. The distinction that has proved particularly valuable in subsequent research is between sensory and affective pathways, since it has become clear that the sensations associated with pain can be separated to some extent from the emotional distress that is elicited. Since the publication of the original gate control theory, much more has become known about the nociceptive fibres involved in pain conduction, the neurochemical mediators, and the intrinsic mechanisms of pain inhibition (Terman *et al.*, 1984; Rang *et al.*, 1991). The theory itself has undergone development, notably in the identification of distinct excitatory and inhibitory substantia gelatinosa interneurons instead of a single type of cell, both of which are susceptible to descending control from the brain (Wall, 1989). It is also acknowledged that cognitive and behavioural influences on pain are not all mediated by the spinal gate, but that other processes are involved. Nonetheless, the gate control theory forms the basis for much of the later development of integrative approaches to the study of pain that have called upon psychological and social as well as neurophysiological expertise.

Stress controllability and gastric lesions

Early studies of the mechanisms linking stress and disease often involved subjecting animals to severely traumatic conditions such as food deprivation, immobilisation and electric shock. Although physical pathology resulted, such experiments provided little information about the psychological factors involved. The reading from *Tsuda, Tanaka, Nishikawa and Hirai* goes beyond the simple documentation of stress effects on gastric lesions, and considers the controllability of aversive stimulation and the coping responses elicited. The impact of control over aversive stimulation on physical pathology has a chequered history. Early studies by Brady and co-workers (1958) indicated that monkeys with control over shock developed peptic ulcers. The analogy with decision makers was irresistible, so the studies became known as 'executive monkey' experiments. However, not only did these effects prove to be difficult to replicate (Folz and Miller, 1964), but later investigators found that animals exposed to adverse, uncontrollable events were even more vulnerable. Weiss (1977) developed the yoked control design in which two rats were paired for aversive stimulation. The difference was that while one animal was able to make a behavioural response to avoid or to escape the stimulation, the second was yoked to the first and was not able to control the stressor. Shock or noise of identical duration and intensity was therefore experienced by the two groups, and the only difference lay in the behavioural conting- ency of controllability. Using this paradigm, it was found that animals in the yoked, uncontrollable condition suffered higher levels of gastric lesions, increased corticosterone concentrations in the blood, and immune changes resulting in increased susceptibility to malignancy (see Steptoe, 1990).

The beneficial effect of controllability is illustrated in this reading by *Tsuda et al.* The study used operant learning techniques, with ex- perimental animals on contingencies in which they had to respond either twice or five times on a fixed ratio (i.e. two or five responses were always effective), or a variable ratio (the effective number of responses varied but averaged two or five). A 'Sidman' avoidance procedure was used, such that successful responding reset the delay before the next warning signal and shock. Rats that were able to avoid or to escape shock by responding on a simple schedule (e.g. two responses in a fixed ratio) developed less severe gastric lesions than their yoked partners. But the experiment goes further in showing that the effects of control are not always beneficial. Animals that could only avoid shock with a more complex task developed more severe pathology than their yoked partners. The experiment therefore suggests that the impact of control over stressful events depends on the difficulty and effort required to make successful responses. This interaction between the possibility of control and the effort involved in responding is a phenomenon that has emerged in human psychophysiological research as well (Öhman and Bohlin, 1989).

Another aspect of *Tsuda et al.*'s study that should be mentioned is that animals were food deprived prior to stress, and food and water deprived during the gruelling 24-hour session itself. Gastric pathology emerged through the interaction between these nutritional conditions and aversive stimulation, and not through the stress conflict alone. This illustrates the importance of underlying vulnerabilities when examining the impact of psychophysiological disturbances. Animal studies of this kind are important, since they permit documentation of psychophy- siological processes in disease under controlled conditions in which other sources of variation in pathology are eliminated.

Social stress and atherosclerosis

Atherosclerosis is the disease involving degeneration and thickening of artery walls leading to obstruction of the vessel lumen, and it underlies coronary artery disease, coronary (or ischaemic) heart disease and many forms of stroke. It is a condition that may develop insidiously for many years before reaching clinical significance. The reading from *Kaplan and co-workers* documents the influence of social stress on coronary atherosclerosis in monkeys, and is important for a number of reasons.

Firstly, the reading demonstrates the effects of a psychosocial manipulation on the development of objectively assessed changes in coronary vessel walls. This modification in coronary artery geometry is striking in that it implies a permanent anatomical change as opposed to a functional alteration in physiological processes. Moreover, this effect was achieved in monkeys fed a prudent low-fat diet, and not only in animals predisposed to atheroslcerosis through consumption of dietary fats. Differences in atherosclerosis between the high and low stress groups were not due to differences in cholesterol levels, body weight or blood pressure.

Secondly, the stress manipulation in this study involved the social challenge of colony reorganisation, rather than a trauma such as electric shock. This social manipulation may be ecologically more relevant than artificial laboratory stressors. The effects of social integration paralleled the results from *Berkman and Syme* in human populations (presented in Section 1), and suggests at least one of the mechanisms through which social support may influence health. The impact of the manipulation was corroborated by behavioural data showing more severe aggressive and submissive acts in the unstable groups, coupled with less affiliative behaviour. These data indicate that colony reorganisation was successful in disturbing social interactions between monkeys. Affiliative responses may be particularly important in reflecting poor social bonding, since other animal as well as human studies have documented the protective effects of intimate bonds (von Holst, 1986). Recently, it has been reported that monkeys in unstable social groups that are low in affiliative responses show suppressed mitogen-induced lymphocyte proliferation, and a diminution in immune responses that might further compromise health (Cohen *et al.*, 1992).

Finally, the coronary atherosclerosis data presented by *Kaplan et al.* illustrate wide individual differences in response. While animals in the unstable groups showed greater atherosclerosis on average, pathological responses were very variable. These differences may be related to social rank, with dominant males in unstable groups being particularly susceptible (Kaplan *et al.*, 1982). Moreover, the degree of atherosclerosis is correlated with the magnitude of heart rate responses to a standard stressor, so that animals which are more reactive psychophysiologically develop larger lesions (Manuck *et al.*, 1983). This result is interesting in that it has been shown that coronary artery obstruction progresses more rapidly in patients with high rather than low heart rates (Perski *et al.*, 1992). High heart rates may lead to extra stress on the branching points of the coronary artery tree, at precisely the locations at which lesions tend to develop (Strawn *et al.*, 1991).

Mental stress and cardiovascular responses

Studies involving animal models show how psychophysiological processes can influence the development of pathological responses. What is the evidence that similar processes are active in humans? Experimental psychophysiological studies are important, since they can be used to investigate disturbances of physiological reactivity in randomised groups where other sources of variance are eliminated. However, experiments with humans are inevitably limited to acute examinations of responses to brief stimuli. Work on laboratory stressors has expanded enormously over recent years, with studies with muscle tension in headache and back pain patients, pulmonary function in asthmatics, and gastrointestinal motility in patients with irritable bowel syndrome (Horton *et al.*, 1978; Kumar and Wingate, 1985; Flor and Turk, 1989).

Perhaps the most active field has been in cardiovascular research, with investigations of psychophysiological responsivity as it relates to the development of high blood pressure (hypertension) and coronary heart disease (Turner *et al.*, 1992). The reading from *Rozanski and his colleagues* describes the use of mental stress testing in the investigation of patients with coronary artery disease. The purpose was to discover whether acute stressors might induce episodes of transient ischaemia, in which the disruption of blood flow to the cardiac muscle leads to abnormalities in the function of the heart. Ischaemic episodes of this kind might be significant in the aetiology of coronary events such as myocardial infarction, ventricular fibrillation and sudden cardiac death.

The effects of acute stressors on blood pressure and heart rate is well recognised. *Rozanski et al.* utilised a range of tasks typical for this field of research, including mental arithmetic, the Stroop colour–word interference task and a simulated public speaking task. What was unusual was the introduction of sophisticated techniques for measuring myocardial function, so that effects on the heart could be studied directly. The results indicate that a proportion of patients do indeed show myocardial ischaemia during laboratory stressors. These responses are largely seen in predisposed individuals – patients with coronary artery disease as opposed to controls, and those who show ischaemic responses during physical exercise. Exercise increases the heart's demand for oxygen, but for some people the narrowing of their coronary arteries prevents this demand from being met adequately. *Rozanski et al.* found that ischaemic responses to mental stress occur at a lower heart rate and oxygen demand than with exercise, so that stress-induced responses are not simply due to the non-specific effect of demand exceeding supply. Spasm of the coronary arteries seems to be involved in producing the ischaemic effect (Yeung *et al.*, 1991).

Interestingly, few of the episodes of stress-induced ischaemia were accompanied by angina pain. Nor could patients who manifest these responses be distinguished on clinical characteristics such as symptoms, extent of coronary disease or use of medications. The reading thus appears to show the insidious but potentially catastrophic effects of mental stress on myocardial function in these patients. Considering the stimuli were relatively mild in relation to what might be experienced in real life, the implications are far-reaching (Steptoe and Tavazzi, 1994). It is notable that public speaking was the condition most likely to elicit ischaemic responses. This stimulus may have been more personally relevant than rather abstract tasks such as mental arithmetic.

It is difficult as yet to know whether reactions of this kind are important for cardiovascular morbidity, since few longitudinal trials have been conducted. Retrospective reports of the circumstances surrounding sudden cardiac death suggest that a proportion may result from stress-induced ischaemia or electrocardiographic abnormalities (Kamarck and Jennings, 1991). Moreover, longitudinal studies have shown that heightened cardiovascular responses to laboratory stressors may be related to future hypertension (Light *et al.*, 1992), while post-myocardial infarction patients with exaggerated reactivity may be at increased risk for later coronary events (Manuck *et al.*, 1992).

Immune function and stressful life events

Bartrop, Luckhurst, Lazarus, Kiloh and Penny's study of immune function following bereavement was one of the earlist systematic investigations in the burgeoning field of psychoneuroimmunology (Ader *et al.*, 1990). The notion that emotional factors might have an impact on immune function first emerged in animal stress experiments and with studies on the effects of brain lesions (Rasmussen, 1969). Subsequently, a number of human experimental studies have documented changes in lymphocyte function and natural killer cell activity in response to laboratory stressors (e.g. Bachen *et al.*, 1992; Sieber *et al.*, 1992). Since the significance of these acute responses is far from clear, many studies have investigated real-life stressors such as academic examinations, caring for disabled relatives, and marital disruption (e.g. Kiecolt-Glaser *et al.*, 1986, 1987).

Bartrop et al. studied a group of healthy men and women whose spouses had died from fatal injuries or illness. Tests were performed on the functional state of the immune system, and the ability of lympho-cytes to be transformed in the presence of mitogens. Lymphocyte function was found to be depressed at six but not at two weeks post-bereavement compared with controls, and the responsivity of the bereaved group was reduced between the two time periods. The authors argue that the emotional impact of bereavement developed over this period, and affected immune function in a progressive fashion. There were no differences in cell counts, and no hormonal effects that might account for the results.

Later studies have followed up men whose spouses have advanced breast cancer, and have found a suppression of immune function in the first two months following death in comparison with levels before bereavement (Schleifer *et al.*, 1983). There is some evidence that the suppression of immune function is related to depression, although studies of depressed patients have produced conflicting results (Stein *et al.*, 1991). The mechanisms responsible for the immune suppression reported in this reading are not clear. Psychophysiological pathways may be involved, but it is also possible that changes in health-related behaviours such as smoking, exercise and diet are relevant, since these have been associated with disturbances in immune function (Kusaka *et al.*, 1992).

Stress and vulnerability to infection

When the links between behaviour and immune dysfunction were first established, many investigators saw their primary clinical relevance in terms of cancer risk and progression. The supposed role of stress in cancer has a long history with studies of personality and life stress (Cooper and Watson, 1991). But despite some positive findings in relation to tumour recurrence (Ramirez *et al.*, 1989), the role of psychosocial factors in the development of cancer remains elusive (Fox, 1988). In addition, the involvement of immune processes in many types of cancer is a controversial topic in itself.

The more immediate implications of the data on psychoneuro-immunology can be seen for infectious illness. The immune system is the main line of defence against infectious organisms, so psychosocial processes that reduce immune competence may increase susceptibility to infection. Various studies have assessed the role of psychosocial factors in resistance to pathogens such as bacterial and viral upper respiratory tract infection and genital herpes recurrence in cross-sectional and longitudinal surveys. This literature, thoroughly reviewed by Cohen and Williamson (1991), suggests that stress may act as a co-factor in the pathogenesis of infectious disease. However, Cohen and Williamson (1991) have pointed out that it is difficult to distinguish the influence of stressors on susceptibility to infection, the development of symptoms, and the acknowledgement of frank illness. Moreover, stressors may operate by increasing exposure to pathogens (perhaps by altering habitual behaviour patterns) rather than by reducing resistance.

The reading from *Cohen, Tyrell and Smith* overcomes these methodological difficulties by examining the influence of stressors on susceptibility to experimentally administered respiratory rhinoviruses of the common cold. The authors exploited the unique facilities of the now disbanded Medical Research Council's Common Cold Unit, a research centre in which healthy volunteers took part in studies on the causes and treatment of colds. Cold viruses were administered experimentally, so the investigators were able to quantify the nature, timing and intensity of infective agents. The measurements of infection and illness and the assessment of possible confounding variables was extensive. Any differences in response are therefore most reasonably attributable to differences in susceptibility.

A consistent association was found betwen infection rates and a composite psychological stress index which included measures of life events, dysphoric mood and perceived stress. This effect persisted after controlling statistically for other factors known to influence vulnerability, and was not unique to any one virus. Equally importantly, stress was related to infection rate as well as to illness and symptoms. Subsequent analyses of these data suggest that the various elements of the psychological stress index are differentially associated with illness and infection. High levels of perceived stress and negative affect predict infection rates, while negative life events are not associated with infection *per se* but with the probability of illness among infected individuals (Cohen *et al.*, 1993*b*).

The relation between stress and infection did not appear to be mediated by health behaviours, although smoking and alcohol consumption are both associated with infection rates independently of stress levels (Cohen *et al.*, 1993*a*). Nor did the indices of immune status measured contribute to the link, although it is possible that more elaborate functional measures of immune response would throw light on mechanisms. The reading illustrates the advantages of behavioural scientists working with clinical researchers experienced in the biological aspects of disorders in order to delineate the influence of psychophysiological pathways on health.

References

Ader, R., Felten, D. L. and Cohen, N. (eds.) (1990). *Psychoneuroimmunology*, Second edition. New York: Academic Press.

Bachen, E. A., Manuck, S. B., Marsland, A. L., Cohen, S., Malkoff, S. B., Muldoon, M. F. and Rabin, B. S. (1992). Lymphocyte subset and cellular immune responses to a brief experimental stressor. *Psychosomatic Medicine*, **54**, 673–9.

Beecher, H. K. (1959). *Measurement of Subjective Responses*. Oxford: Oxford University Press.

Brady, J. V., Porter, R., Conrad, D. and Mason, J. (1958). Avoidance behavior and the development of gastro-duodenal ulcers. *Journal of the Experimental Analysis of Behavior*, **1**, 69–72.

Cohen, S. and Williamson, G. M. (1991). Stress and infectious disease in humans. *Psychological Bulletin*, **109**, 5–24.

Cohen, S., Kaplan, J. R., Kunnick, J. E., Manuck, S. B. and Rabin, B. S. (1992). Chronic social stress, affiliation, and cellular immune response in non-human primates. *Psychological Science*, **3**, 301–4.

Cohen, S., Tyrell, D. A. J., Russell, M. A. H., Jarvis, M. J. and Smith, A. P. (1993a). Smoking, alcohol consumption and susceptibility to the common cold. *American Journal of Public Health*, **83**, 1277–83.

Cohen, S., Tyrell, D. A. J. and Smith, A. P. (1993b). Negative life events, perceived stress, negative affect and susceptibility to the common cold. *Journal of Personality and Social Psychology*, **64**, 131–40.

Cooper, C. L. and Watson, M. (eds.) (1991). *Cancer and Stress: Psychological, Biological and Coping Studies*. Chichester: John Wiley.

Flor, H. and Turk, D. C. (1989). Psychophysiology of chronic pain: do chronic pain patients exhibit symptom-specific psychophysiological responses? *Psychological Bulletin*, **105**, 215–59.

Folz, E. L. and Miller, F. E. (1964). Experimental psychosomatic disease states in monkeys. I. Peptic ulcer 'executive monkeys'. *Journal of Surgical Research*, **4**, 445–53.

Fox, B. H. (1988). Epidemiologic aspects of stress, aging, cancer and the immune system. *Annals of the New York Academy of Sciences*, **521**, 16–28.

Goreczny, A. J., Brantley, P. J., Buss, R. R. and Waters, W. F. (1988). Daily stress and anxiety and their relation to daily fluctuations of symptoms in asthma and chronic obstructive pulmonary disease patients. *Journal of Psychopathology and Behavioral Assessment*, **10**, 259–67.

Hanson, S. L. and Pichert, J. W. (1986). Perceived stress and diabetes control in adolescents. *Health Psychology*, **5**, 439–52.

Horton, D. J., Suda, W. L., Kinsman, R. A., Souhrada, J. and Spector, S. L. (1978). Bronchoconstrictive suggestion in asthma: a role for airways hyperreactivity and emotions. *American Review of Respiratory Disorders*, **117**, 1029–38.

Kaplan, J. R., Manuck, S. B., Clarkson, T. B., Lusso, E. M. and Taub, D. M. (1982). Social status, environment and atherosclerosis in cynomolgus monkeys. *Arteriosclerosis*, **2**, 359–68.

Kamarck, T. and Jennings, J. R. (1991). Biobehavioral factors in sudden cardiac death. *Psychological Bulletin*, **109**, 42–75.

Kiecolt-Glaser, J. K., Glaser, R., Strain, E. C., Stout, J. C., Tarr, K. L., Holliday, J. E. and Speicher, C. E. (1986). Modulation of cellular immunity in medical students. *Journal of Behavioral Medicine*, **9**, 5–21.

Kiecolt-Glaser, J. K., Glaser, R., Shuttleworth, E. C., Dyer, C. S., Ogrocki, P. and Speicher, C. E. (1987). Chronic stress and immunity in family caregivers of Alzheimer's disease victims. *Psychosomatic Medicine*, **49**, 523–35.

Kumar, D. and Wingate, D. L. (1985). The irritable bowel syndrome. *Lancet*, **II**, 973–7.

Kusaka, Y., Kondou, H. and Morimoto, K. (1992). Healthy lifestyles are associated with higher natural killer cell activity. *Preventive Medicine*, **21**, 602–15.

Light, K. C., Dolan, C. A., Davis, M. R. and Sherwood, A. (1992). Cardiovascular responses to an active coping challenge as predictors of blood pressure patterns 10 to 15 years later. *Psychosomatic Medicine*, **54**, 217–30.

Manuck, S. B., Kaplan, J. R. and Clarkson, T. B. (1983). Behaviorally induced heart rate reactivity and atherosclerosis in cynomolgus monkeys. *Psychosomatic Medicine*, **45**, 95–108.

Manuck, S. B., Olsson, G., Hjemdahl, P. and Rehnquist, M. (1992). Does cardiovascular reactivity to mental stress have prognostic value in post infarction patients? A pilot study. *Psychosomatic Medicine*, **54**, 102–8.

Melzack, R. and Wall, P. D. (1982). *The Challenge of Pain*. Harmondsworth: Penguin.

Öhman, A. and Bohlin, G. (1989). The role of controllability in cardiovascular activation and cardiovascular disease: help or hindrance? In: *Stress, Personal Control and Health*, pp. 257–76. A. Steptoe and A. Appels (eds.). Chichester: John Wiley.

Perski, A., Olsson, G., Landou, C., de Faire, U., Theorell, T. and Hamsten, A. (1992). Minimum heart rate and coronary atherosclerosis: independent relations to global severity and rate of progression of angiographic lesions in men with myocardial infarction at a young age. *American Heart Journal*, **123**, 609–16.

Ramirez, A. J., Craig, T. K. J., Watson, J. P., Fentiman, I. S., North, W. R. S. and Rubens, R. D. (1989). Stress and relapse of breast cancer. *British Medical Journal*, **298**, 291–3.

Rang, H. P., Bevan, S. and Dray, A. (1991). Chemical activation of nociceptive peripheral neurones. *British Medical Bulletin*, **47**, 534–48.

Rasmussen, A. F. (1969). Emotions and immunity. *Annals of the New York Academy of Sciences*, **164**, 458–61.

Schleifer, S. J., Keller, S. E., Camerino, M., Thornton, J. C. and Stein, M. (1983). Suppression of lymphocyte stimulation following bereavement. *Journal of the American Medical Association*, **250**, 374–7.

Sieber, W. J., Rodin, J., Larson, L., Ortega, S., Cummings, N., Levy, S.,

Whiteside, T. and Herberman, R. (1992). Modulation of human natural killer cell activity by exposure to uncontrollable stress. *Brain, Behavior and Immunity*, **6**, 141–56.

Stein, M., Miller, A. H. and Trestman, R. L. (1991). Depression, the immune system, and health and illness. *Archives of General Psychiatry*, **48**, 171–7.

Steptoe, A. (1990). Psychobiological stress responses. In: *Stress and Medical Procedures*, pp. 3–24. M. Johnston and L. Wallace (eds.). Oxford: Oxford University Press.

Steptoe, A. (1991). The links between stress and illness. *Journal of Psychosomatic Research*, **35**, 633–44.

Steptoe, A. and Tavazzi, L. (1994). The mind and the heart. In: *Diseases of the Heart*, second edition. D. J. Julian, A. J. Camm, K. Fox, R. Hall and P. A. Poole-Wilson (eds.). London: W. B. Saunders, in press.

Strawn, W. B., Bondjers, G., Kaplan, J. R., Manuck, S. B., Schwenke, D. C., Hansson, G. K., Shively, C. A. and Clarkson, T. B. (1991). Endothelial dysfunction in response to psychosocial stress in monkeys. *Circulation Research*, **68**, 1270–9.

Terman, G. W., Shavit, Y., Lewis, J. W., Cannon, J. T. and Liebeskind, J. C. (1984). Intrinsic mechanisms of pain inhibition: activation by stress. *Science*, **226**, 1270–7.

Turner, J. R., Sherwood, A. and Light, K. C. (eds.) (1992). *Individual Differences in Cardiovascular Response to Stress*. New York: Plenum.

von Holst, D. (1986). Heart rate of tree shrews and its persistent modification by social contact. In: *Biological and Psychological Factors in Cardiovascular Disorders*, pp. 476–90. T. H. Schmidt, T. M. Dembroski and G. Blümchen (eds.). Berlin: Springer-Verlag.

Wall, P. D. (1989). Introduction. In: *Textbook of Pain*, pp. 1–18. 2nd edition, P. D. Wall and R. D. Melzack (eds.). Edinburgh: Churchill-Livingstone.

Weiss, J. M. (1977). Psychological and behavioral influences on gastrointestinal lesions in animal models. In: *Psychopathology: Experimental Models*, pp. 232–69. J. D. Maser and M. E. P. Seligman (eds.). San Francisco: W. H. Freeman.

Yeung, A. C., Vekshtein, V. I., Krantz, D. S., Vita, J. A., Ryan, T. J., Ganz, P. and Selwyn, A. P. (1991). The effect of atherosclerosis on the vasomotor response of coronary arteries to mental stress. *New England Journal of Medicine*, **325**, 1551–6.

Pain mechanisms: a new theory

Ronald Melzack and Patrick D. Wall

Dr. Melzack is associate professor in the department of psychology at McGill University, Montreal, Canada. Dr. Wall is professor in the department of biology at the Massachusetts Institute of Technology, Cambridge, USA

Abstract

A gate control system modulates sensory input from the skin before it evokes pain perception and response.

The nature of pain has been the subject of bitter controversy since the turn of the century (*1*). There are currently two opposing theories of pain: (i) specificity theory, which holds that pain is a specific modality like vision or hearing, "with its own central and peripheral apparatus" (*2*), and (ii) pattern theory, which maintains that the nerve impulse pattern for pain is produced by intense stimulation of nonspecific receptors since "there are no specific fibers and no specific endings" (*3*). Both theories derive from earlier concepts proposed by von Frey (*4*) and Goldscheider (*5*) in 1894, and historically they are held to be mutually exclusive. Since it is our purpose here to propose a new theory of pain mechanisms, we shall state explicitly at the outset where we agree and disagree with specificity and pattern theories.

Specificity theory

Specificity theory proposes that a mosaic of specific pain receptors in body tissue projects to a pain center in the brain. It maintains that free nerve endings are pain receptors (*4*) and generate pain impulses that are carried by A-delta and C fibers in peripheral nerves (*6*) and by the lateral spinothalamic tract in the spinal cord (*2*) to a pain center in the thalamus (*7*). Despite its apparent simplicity, the theory contains an explicit statement of physiological specialization and an implicit psychological assumption (*8, 9*). Consider the proposition that the skin contains "pain

Reprinted from Melzack, R. and Wall, P. D. Pain mechanisms: a new theory. *Science*, **150**, 971–9, 19 November 1965. © AAAS.

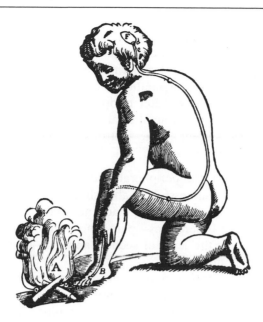

Fig. 1. Descartes' (*76*) concept of the pain pathway. He writes: "If for example fire (*A*) comes near the foot (*B*), the minute particles of this fire, which as you know move with great velocity, have the power to set in motion the spot of the skin of the foot which they touch, and by this means pulling upon the delicate thread *CC*, which is attached to the spot of the skin, they open up at the same instant the pore, *d.e.*, against which the delicate thread ends, just as by pulling at one end of a rope one makes to strike at the same instant a bell which hangs at the other end."

receptors." To say that a receptor responds only to intense, noxious stimulation of the skin is a physiological statement of fact; it says that the receptor is specialized to respond to a particular kind of stimulus. To call a receptor a "pain receptor," however, is a psychological assumption: it implies a direct connection from the receptor to a brain center where pain is felt (Fig. 1), so that stimulation of the receptor must always elicit pain and only the sensation of pain. This distinction between physiological specialization and psychological assumption also applies to peripheral fibers and central projection systems (*9*).

The facts of physiological specialization provide the power of specificity theory. Its psychological assumption is its weakness. As in all psychological theories, there is implicit in specificity theory the conception of a nervous system: and the model is that of a fixed, direct-line communication system from the skin to the brain. This facet of specificity theory, which imputes a direct, invariant relationship between stimulus and sensation, is examined here in the light of the clinical, psychological, and physiological evidence concerning pain.

Clinical evidence

The pathological pain states of causalgia (a severe burning pain that may result from a partial lesion of a peripheral nerve), phantom limb pain (which may occur after amputation of a limb), and the peripheral neuralgias (which may occur after peripheral nerve infections or degenerative diseases) provide a dramatic refutation of the concept of a fixed, direct-line nervous system. Four features of these syndromes plague patient, physician, and theorist (*8, 10*).

1) Surgical lesions of the peripheral and central nervous system have been singularly unsuccessful in abolishing these pains permanently, although the lesions have been made at almost every level (Fig. 2). Even after such operations, pain can often still be elicited by stimulation below the level of section and may be more severe than before the operation (*8, 10*).
2) Gentle touch, vibration, and other nonnoxious stimuli (*8, 10*) can trigger excruciating pain, and sometimes pain occurs spontaneously for long periods without any apparent stimulus. The fact that the thresholds to these stimuli are raised rather than lowered in causalgia and the neuralgias (*10*), together with the fact that referred pain can often be triggered by mild stimulation of normal skin (*8*), makes it unlikely that the pains can be explained by postulating pathologically hypersensitive "pain receptors."
3) The pains and new "trigger zones" may spread unpredictably to unrelated parts of the body where no pathology exists (*8, 11*).
4) Pain from hyperalgesic skin areas often occurs after long delays, and continues long after removal of the stimulus (*10*). Gentle rubbing, repeated pin pricks, or the application of a warm test tube may produce sudden, severe pain after delays as long as 35 seconds. Such delays cannot be attributed simply to conduction in slowly conducting fibers: rather, they imply a remarkable temporal and spatial summation of inputs in the production of these pain states (*8, 10*).

Psychological evidence

The psychological evidence fails to support the assumption of a one-to-one relationship between pain perception and intensity of the stimulus. Instead, the evidence suggests that the amount and quality of perceived pain are determined by many psychological variables (*12*) in addition to the sensory input. For example, Beecher (*13*) has observed that most American soldiers wounded at the Anzio beachhead "entirely denied pain from their extensive wounds or had so little that they did not want any medication to relieve it" (*13*, p. 165), presumably because they were

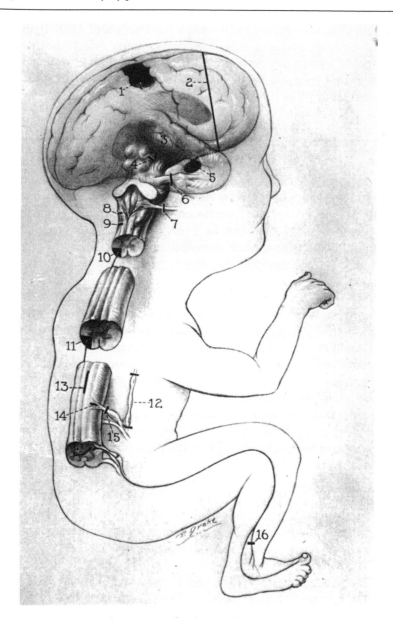

Fig. 2. MacCarty and Drake's (77) schematic diagram illustrating various surgical procedures designed to alleviate pain: 1, gyrectomy; 2, prefrontal lobotomy; 3, thalamotomy; 4, mesencephalic tractotomy; 5, hypophysectomy; 6, fifth-nerve rhizotomy; 7, ninth-nerve neurectomy; 8, medullary tractotomy; 9, trigeminal tractotomy; 10, cervical chordotomy; 11, thoracic chordotomy; 12, sympathectomy; 13, myelotomy; 14, Lissauer tractotomy; 15, posterior rhizotomy; 16, neurectomy.

overjoyed at having escaped alive from the battlefield (*13*). If the men had felt pain, even pain sensation devoid of negative affect, they would, it is reasonable to assume, have reported it, just as lobotomized patients (*14*) report that they still have pain but it does not bother them. Instead, these men "entirely denied pain." Similarly, Pavlov's (*15, 16*) dogs that received electric shocks, burns, or cuts, followed consistently by the presentation of food, eventually responded to these stimuli as signals for food and failed to show "even the tiniest and most subtle" (*15*, p. 30) signs of pain. If these dogs felt pain sensation, then it must have been nonpainful pain (*17*), or the dogs were out to fool Pavlov and simply refused to reveal that they were feeling pain. Both possibilities, of course, are absurd. The inescapable conclusion from these observations is that intense noxious stimulation can be prevented from producing pain, or may be modified to provide the signal for eating behavior.

Psychophysical studies (*18*) that find a mathematical relationship between stimulus intensity and pain intensity are often cited (*2, 13, 18, 19*) as supporting evidence for the assumption that pain is a primary sensation subserved by a direct communication system from skin receptor to pain center. A simple psychophysical function, however, does not necessarily reflect equally simple neural mechanisms. Beecher's (*13*) and Pavlov's (*15*) observations show that activities in the central nervous system may intervene between stimulus and sensation which may invalidate any simple psychophysical "law." The use of laboratory conditions that prevent such activities from ever coming into play reduces the functions of the nervous system to those of a fixed-gain transmission line. It is under these conditions that psychophysical functions prevail.

Physiological evidence

There is convincing physiological evidence that specialization exists within the somesthetic system (*9*), but none to show that stimulation of one type of receptor, fiber, or spinal pathway elicits sensations only in a single psychological modality. In the search for peripheral fibers that respond exclusively to high-intensity stimulation, Hunt and McIntyre (*20*) found only seven out of 421 myelinated A fibers, and Maruhashi *et al.* (*21*) found 13 out of several hundred. Douglas and Ritchie (*22*) failed to find any high-threshold C fibers, while Iggo (*23*) found a few. These data suggest that a small number of specialized fibers may exist that respond only to intense stimulation, but this does not mean that they are "pain fibers"—that they must always produce pain, and only pain, when they are stimulated. It is more likely that they represent the extreme of a continuous distribution of receptor-fiber thresholds rather than a special category (*24*).

Similarly, there is evidence that central-nervous-system pathways have specialized functions that play a role in pain mechanisms. Surgical lesions of the lateral spinothalamic tract (*2*) or portions of the thalamus (*25*) may, on occasion, abolish pain of pathological origin. But the fact that these areas carry signals related to pain does not mean that they comprise a specific pain system. The lesions have multiple effects. They reduce the total number of responding neurons; they change the temporal and spatial relationships among all ascending systems; and they affect the descending feedback that controls transmission from peripheral fibers to dorsal horn cells.

The nature of the specialization of central cells remains elusive despite the large number of single-cell studies. Cells in the dorsal horns (*24*, *26*) and the trigeminal nucleus (*27*) respond to a wide range of stimuli and respond to each with a characteristic firing pattern. Central cells that respond exclusively to noxious stimuli have also been reported (*28*, *29*). Of particular interest is Poggio and Mountcastle's (*28*) study of such cells in the posterior thalamus in anesthetized monkeys. Yet Casey (*30*), who has recently confirmed that posterior thalamic cells respond exclusively to noxious stimuli in the drowsy or sleeping monkey, found that the same cells also signaled information in response to gentle tactile stimulation when the animal was awake. Even if some central cells should be shown unequivocally to respond exclusively to noxious stimuli, their specialized properties still do not make them "pain cells." It is more likely that these cells represent the extreme of a broad distribution of cell thresholds to peripheral nerve firing, and that they occupy only a small area within the total multidimensional space that defines the specialized physiological properties of cells (*9*). There is no evidence to suggest that they are more important for pain perception and response than all the remaining somesthetic cells that signal characteristic firing patterns about multiple properties of the stimulus, including noxious intensity. The view that only the cells that respond exclusively to noxious stimuli subserve pain and that the outputs of all other cells are no more than background noise is purely a psychological assumption and has no factual basis. Physiological specialization is a fact that can be retained without acceptance of the psychological assumption that pain is determined entirely by impulses in a straight-through transmission system from the skin to a pain center in the brain.

Pattern theory

As a reaction against the psychological assumption in specificity theory, new theories have been proposed which can be grouped under the general heading of "pattern theory." Goldscheider (*5*), initially one of the champions of von Frey's theory, was the first to propose that stimulus intensity and central summation are the critical determinants of pain. Two kinds of theories have emerged from Goldscheider's concept; both recognize the concept of patterning of the input, which we believe (9) to be essential for any adequate theory of pain, but one kind ignores the facts of physiological specialization, while the other utilizes them in proposing mechanisms of central summation.

The pattern theory of Weddell (31) and Sinclair (3) is based on the earlier suggestion, by Nafe (17), that all cutaneous qualities are produced by spatiotemporal patterns of nerve impulses rather than by separate modality-specific transmission routes. The theory proposes that all fiber endings (apart from those that innervate hair cells) are alike, so that the pattern for pain is produced by intense stimulation for nonspecific receptors. The physiological evidence, however, reveals (9) a high degree of receptor-fiber specialization. The pattern theory proposed by Weddell and Sinclair, then, fails as a satisfactory theory of pain because it ignores the facts of physiological specialization. It is more reasonable to assume that the specialized physiological properties of each receptor-fiber unit— such as response ranges, adaptation rates, and thresholds to different stimulus intensities—play an important role in determining the characteristics of the temporal patterns that are generated when a stimulus is applied to the skin (9).

Other theories have been proposed, within the framework of Goldscheider's concept, which stress central summation mechanisms rather than excessive peripheral stimulation. Livingston (8) was perhaps the first to suggest specific neural mechanisms to account for the remarkable summation phenomena in clinical pain syndromes. He proposed that intense, pathological stimulation of the body sets up reverberating circuits in spinal internuncial pools, or evokes spinal cord activities such as those reflected by the "dorsal root reflex" (32), that can then be triggered by normally nonnoxious inputs and generate abnormal volleys that are interpreted centrally as pain. Conceptually similar mechanisms were proposed by Hebb (33) and Gerard (34), who suggested that hypersynchronized firing in central cells provides the signal for pain.

Related to theories of central summation is the theory that a specialized input-controlling system normally prevents summation from occurring, and that destruction of this system leads to pathological pain states. Basically, this theory proposes the existence of a rapidly conducting fiber system which inhibits synaptic transmission in a more slowly conducting system that carries the signal for pain. These two systems are identified as the epicritic and protopathic (7), fast and slow (35), phylogenetically new and old (36), and myelinated and unmyelinated (10) fiber systems. Under pathological conditions, the slow system establishes dominance over the fast, and the result is protopathic sensation (*7*), slow pain (*35*), diffuse burning pain (*36*), or hyperalgesia (*10*). It is important to note the transition from specificity theory (*7, 35, 36*) to the pattern concept: Noordenbos (*10*) does not associate psychological quality with each system but attributes to the rapidly conducting system the ability to modify the input pattern transmitted in the slowly conducting, multisynaptic system.

The concepts of central summation and input control have shown remarkable power in their ability to explain many of the clinical phenomena of pain. The various specific theoretical mechanisms that have been proposed, however, fail to comprise a satisfactory general theory of pain. They lack unity, and no single theory so far proposed is capable of integrating the diverse theoretical mechanisms. More important, these mechanisms have not received any substantial experimental verification. We believe that recent physiological evidence on spinal mechanisms, together with the evidence demonstrating central control over afferent input, provides the basis for a new theory of pain mechanisms that is consistent with the concepts of physiological specialization as well as with those of central summation and input control.

Gate control theory of pain

Stimulation of the skin evokes nerve impulses that are transmitted to three spinal cord systems (Fig. 3): the cells of the substantia gelatinosa in the dorsal horn, the dorsal-column fibers that project towards the brain, and the first central transmission (T) cells in the dorsal horn. We propose that (i) the substantia gelatinosa functions as a gate control system that modulates the afferent patterns before they influence the T cells; (ii) the afferent patterns in the dorsal column system act, in part at least, as a central control trigger which activates selective brain processes that influence the modulating properties of the gate control system; and (iii) the T cells activate neural mechanisms which comprise the action system responsible for response and perception. Our theory proposes that pain phenomena are determined by interactions among these three systems.

Gate control system

The substantia gelatinosa consists of small, densely packed cells that form a functional unit extending the length of the spinal cord. The cells connect with one another by short fibers and by the longer fibers of Lissauer's tract (*37, 38*), but do not project outside the substantia gelatinosa. Recent evidence (*39*) suggests that the substantia gelatinosa

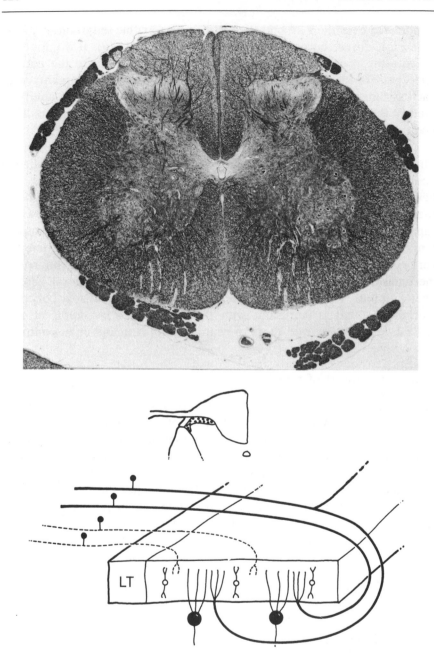

Fig. 3. (Top) A histological section of the cat spinal cord (lumbar region). (Middle) Cross section of the dorsal quadrant. The stippled region is the substantia gelatinosa. (Bottom) Main components of the cutaneous afferent system in the upper dorsal horn. The large-diameter cutaneous peripheral fibers are represented by thick lines running from the dorsal root and terminating in the region of the substantia gelatinosa; one of these, as shown, sends a branch toward the brain in the dorsal column. The finer peripheral fibers are

acts as a gate control system that modulates the synaptic transmission of nerve impulses from peripheral fibers to central cells.

Figure 4 shows the factors involved in the transmission of impulses from peripheral nerve to T cells in the cord. Recent studies (*39–41*) have shown that volleys of nerve impulses in large fibers are extremely effective initially in activating the T cells but that their later effect is reduced by a negative feedback mechanism. In contrast, volleys in small fibers activate a positive feedback mechanism which exaggerates the effect of arriving impulses. Experiments (*37, 39, 41*) have shown that these feedback effects are mediated by cells in the substantia gelatinosa. Activity in these cells modulates the membrane potential of the afferent fiber terminals and thereby determines the excitatory effect of arriving impulses. Although there is evidence, so far, for only presynaptic control, there may also be undetected postsynaptic control mechanisms that contribute to the observed input-output functions.

We propose that three features of the afferent input are significant for pain: (i) the ongoing activity which precedes the stimulus, (ii) the stimulus-evoked activity, and (iii) the relative balance of activity in large versus small fibers. The spinal cord is continually bombarded by incoming nerve impulses even in the absence of obvious stimulation. This ongoing activity is carried predominantly by small myelinated and unmyelinated fibres, which tend to be tonically active and to adapt slowly, and it holds the gate in a relatively open position. When a stimulus is applied to the skin, it produces an increase in the number of active receptor-fiber units as information about the stimulus is transmitted toward the brain. Since many of the larger fibres are inactive in the absence of stimulus change, stimulation will produce a disproportionate relative increase in large-fiber over small-fiber activity. Thus, if a gentle pressure stimulus is applied suddenly to the skin, the afferent volley contains large-fiber impulses which not only fire the T cells but also partially close the presynaptic gate, thereby shortening the barrage generated by the T cells.

If the stimulus intensity is increased, more receptor-fiber units are recruited and the firing frequency of active units is increased (*9, 24*). The resultant positive and negative effects of the large-fiber and small-fiber inputs tend to counteract each other, and therefore the output of the T cells rises slowly. If stimulation is prolonged, the large fibers begin to

Caption for Fig. 3 (cont.)

represented by dashed lines running directly into the substantia gelatinosa. The large cells, on which cutaneous afferent nerves terminate, are shown as large black spheres with their dendrites extending into the substantia gelatinosa and their axons projecting deeper into the dorsal horn. The open circles represent the cells of the substantia gelatinosa. The axons (not shown) of these cells connect them to one another and also run in the Lissauer tract (*LT*) to distant parts of the substantia gelatinosa. [From Wall (*37*).]

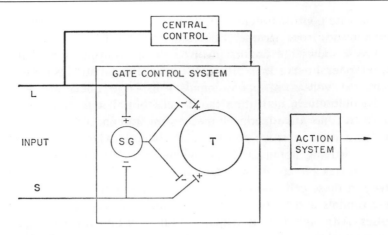

Fig. 4. Schematic diagram of the gate control theory of pain mechanisms: L, the large-diameter fibers; S, the small-diameter fibers. The fibers project to the substantia gelatinosa (SG) and first central transmission (T) cells. The inhibitory effect exerted by SG on the afferent fiber terminals is increased by activity in L fibers and decreased by activity in S fibers. The central control trigger is represented by a line running from the large-fiber system to the central control mechanisms; these mechanisms, in turn, project back to the gate control system. The T cells project to the entry cells of the action system. +, Excitation; –, Inhibition (see text).

adapt, producing a relative increase in small-fiber activity. As a result, the gate is opened further, and the output of the T cells rises more steeply. If the large-fiber steady background activity is artificially raised at this time by vibration or scratching (a maneuver that overcomes the tendency of the large fibers to adapt), the output of the cells decreases.

Thus, the effects of the stimulus-evoked barrage are determined by (i) the total number of active fibers and the frequencies of nerve impulses that they transmit, and (ii) the balance of activity in large and small fibers. Consequently, the output of the T cells may differ from the total input that converges on them from the peripheral fibers. Although the total number of afferent impulses is a relevant stimulus parameter, the impulses have different effects depending on the specialized functions of the fibers that carry them. Furthermore, anatomical specialization also determines the location and the extent of the central terminations of the fibers (*24, 41, 42*).

There are two reasons for believing that pain results after prolonged monitoring of the afferent input by central cells. First, threshold for shock on one arm is raised by a shock delivered as long as 100 milliseconds later to the other arm (*43*). Second, in pathological pain states, delays of pain sensation as long as 35 seconds after stimulation cannot be attributed to slow conduction in afferent pathways (*10*). We suggest, then, that there is temporal and spatial summation or integration of the arriving barrage by the T cells. The signal which triggers the action system responsible for pain experience and response occurs when the output of the T cells reaches or exceeds a critical level. This critical level of firing, as we have seen, is determined by the afferent barrage that actually impinges on the T cells and has already undergone modulation by substantia gelatinosa activity. We presume that the action system requires a definite time period for integrating the total input from the T cells. Small, fast variations of the temporal pattern produced by the T cells might be ineffective, and the smoothed envelope of the frequency of impulses—which contains information on the rate of rise and fall, the duration, and the amplitude of firing—would be the effective stimulus that initiates the appropriate sequence of activities in the cells that comprise the action system.

Central control trigger

It is now firmly established (*44*) that stimulation of the brain activates descending efferent fibers (*45*) which can influence afferent conduction at the earliest synaptic levels of the somesthetic system. Thus it is possible for central nervous system activities subserving attention, emotion, and memories of prior experience to exert control over the sensory input. There is evidence (*44*) to suggest that these central influences are mediated through the gate control system.

The manner in which the appropriate central activities are triggered into action presents a problem. While some central activities, such as anxiety or excitement, may open or close the gate for all inputs at any site on the body, others obviously involve selective, localized gate activity. Men wounded in battle may feel little pain from the wound but may complain bitterly about an inept vein puncture (*13*). Dogs that repeatedly receive food immediately after the skin is shocked, burned, or cut soon respond to these stimuli as signals for food and salivate, without showing any signs of pain, yet howl as normal dogs would when the stimuli are applied to other sites on the body (*16*). The signals, then, must be identified, evaluated in terms of prior conditioning, localized, and inhibited *before* the action system is activated. We propose, therefore, that there exists in the nervous system a mechanism, which we shall call the central control trigger, that activates the particular, selective brain processes that exert control over the sensory input (Fig. 4). There are two known systems that could fulfill such a function, and one or both may play a role.

The first is the dorsal column–medial lemniscus system. The largest and most rapidly conducting A fibers which enter the spinal cord send short branches to the substantia gelatinosa, and long central branches directly to the dorsal column nuclei. Fibers from these nuclei form the medial lemniscus, which provides a direct route to the thalamus and thence to the somatosensory cortex. The striking characteristics of this system are that information is transmitted rapidly from the skin to the cortex, that separation of signals evoked by different stimulus properties and precise somatotopic localization are both maintained throughout the system (*46*), and that conduction is relatively unaffected by anesthetic drugs (*47*). Traditionally, the dorsal column system is supposed to carry two-point discrimination, roughness discrimination, spatial localization, tactile threshold, and vibration (*48*). Complex discrimination and localization, however, are not a modality; they represent decisions based on an analysis of the input. Indeed, the traditional view is questionable in the light of Cook and Browder's (*49*) observation that surgical section of the dorsal columns produced no permanent change in two-point discrimination in seven patients.

The second candidate for the role of central control trigger is the dorsolateral path (*50*), which originates in the dorsal horn and projects, after relay in the lateral cervical nucleus, to the brain stem and thalamus. This system has small, well-defined receptive fields (*51*) and is extremely fast; in spite of having one additional relay, it precedes the dorsal column–medial lemniscus volley in the race to the cortex (*52*).

Both these systems, then, could fulfill the functions of the central control trigger. They carry precise information about the nature and location of the stimulus, and they conduct so rapidly that they may not only set the receptivity of cortical neurons for subsequent afferent volleys but may, by way of central-control efferent fibers, also act on the gate control system. Part, at least, of their function, then, could be to activate selective brain processes that influence information which is still arriving over slowly conducting fibers or is being transmitted up more slowly conducting pathways.

Action system

Pain is generally considered to be the sensory adjunct of an imperative protective reflex (*53*). Pain, however, does not consist of a single ring of the appropriate central bell, but is an ongoing process. We propose, then, that once the integrated firing-level of T cells exceeds a critical preset level, the firing triggers a sequence of responses by the action system.

Sudden, unexpected damage to the skin is followed by (i) a startle response; (ii) a flexion reflex; (iii) postural readjustment; (iv) vocalization; (v) orientation of the head and eyes to examine the damaged area; (vi) autonomic responses; (vii) evocation of past experience in similar situations and prediction of the consquences of the stimulation; (viii) many other patterns of behavior aimed at diminishing the sensory and affective components of the whole experience, such as rubbing the damaged area, avoidance behavior, and so forth.

The perceptual awareness that accompanies these events changes in quality and intensity during all this activity. This total complex sequence is hidden in the simple phrases "pain response" and "pain sensation." The multiplicity of reactions demands some concept of central mechanisms which is at least capable of accounting for sequential patterns of activity that would allow the complex behavior and experience characteristic of pain.

The concept of a "pain center" in the brain is totally inadequate to account for the sequences of behavior and experience. Indeed, the concept is pure fiction, unless virtually the whole brain is considered to be the "pain center," because the thalamus (*7, 25*), the limbic system (*54*), the hypothalamus (*55*), the brain-stem reticular formation (*56*), the parietal cortex (*57*), and the frontal cortex (*14*) are all implicated in pain perception. Other brain areas are obviously involved in the emotional and motor features of the behavior sequence. The idea of a "terminal center" in the brain which is exclusively responsible for pain sensation and response therefore becomes meaningless.

We propose, instead, that the triggering of the action system by the T cells marks the beginning of the sequence of activities that occur when the body sustains damage. The divergence of afferent fibers going to the dorsal horns and the dorsal column nuclei marks only the first stage of the process of selection and abstraction of information. The stimulation of a single tooth results in the eventual activation of no less than five distinct brain-stem pathways (*58*). Two of these pathways project to cortical somatosensory areas I and II (*59*), while the remainder activate the thalamic reticular formation and the limbic system (*60*), so that the input has access to neural systems involved in affective (*54*) as well as sensory activities. It is presumed that interactions occur among all these systems as the organism interacts with the environment.

We believe that the interactions between the gate control system and the action system described above may occur at successive synapses at any level of the central nervous system in the course of filtering of the sensory input. Similarly, the influence of central activities on the sensory input may take place at a series of levels. The gate control system may be set and reset a number of times as the temporal and spatial patterning of the input is analyzed and acted on by the brain.

Adequacy of the theory

The concept of interacting gate control and action systems can account for the hyperalgesia, spontaneous pain, and long delays after stimulation characteristic of pathological pain syndromes. The state of hyperalgesia would require two conditions: (i) enough conducting peripheral axons to generate an input that can activate the action system (if, as in the case of leprosy, all components of the peripheral nerve are equally affected, there is a gradual onset of anesthesia), and (ii) a marked loss of the large peripheral nerve fibers, which may occur after traumatic peripheral-nerve lesions or in some of the neuropathies (*61*), such as post-herpetic neuralgia (*10*). Since most of the larger fibers are destroyed, the normal presynaptic inhibition of the input by the gate control system does not occur. Thus, the input arriving over the remaining myelinated and unmyelinated fibers is transmitted through the unchecked, open gate produced by the C-fiber input.

Spatial summation would easily occur under such conditions. Any nerve impulses, no matter how they were generated, which converge on the central cells would contribute to the output of these cells. These mechanisms may account for the fact that nonnoxious stimuli, such as gentle pressure, can trigger severe pain in patients suffering causalgia, phantom limb pain, and the neuralgias. The well-known enhancement of pain in these patients during emotional disturbance and sexual excitement (*62*) might be due to increased sensory firing [as a result of an increased sympathetic outflow (*63, 64*)] which is unchecked by presynaptic inhibition. Conversely, the absence of small fibers in the dorsal roots in a patient with congenital insensitivity to pain (*65*) suggests that the mechanisms for facilitation and summation necessary for pain may be absent.

Spontaneous pain can also be explained by these mechanisms. The smaller fibers show considerable spontaneous activity, which would have the effect of keeping the gate open. Low-level, random, ongoing activity would then be transmitted relatively unchecked (because of the predominant loss of A fibers), and summation could occur, producing spontaneous pain in the absence of stimulation. This is a possible mechanism for the pains of anesthesia dolorosa and the "spontaneous" pains which develop after peripheral-nerve and dorsal-root lesions. Because the total number of peripheral fibers is reduced, it may take considerable time for the T cells to reach the firing level necessary to trigger pain responses, so perception and response are delayed. This same mechanism can also account for post-ischemic pressure-block hyperesthesia and for the delays in sensation of as much as 10 seconds which occur when the large peripheral fibers fail to conduct (*66*).

We propose that the A-fiber input normally acts to prevent summation from occurring. This would account for Adrian's (*67*) failure to obtain pain responses in the frog from high-frequency air blasts which fired peripheral nerves close to their maximum firing rate, in an experiment meant to refute the view that summation of the effects of noxious stimuli is important for pain. It is now clear that the air blasts would tend to fire a high proportion of the low-threshold A fibers, which would exert presynaptic inhibition on the input by way of the gate control system; thus the impulses would be prevented from reaching the T cells where summation might occur. The double effect of an arriving volley is well illustrated by the effects of vibration on pain and itch. Vibration activates fibers of all diameters, but activates a larger proportion of A fibers, since they tend to adapt during constant stimulation, whereas C-fiber firing is maintained. Vibration therefore sets the gate in a more closed position. However, the same impulses which set the gate also bombard the T cell and therefore summate with the inputs from noxious stimulation. It is observed behaviorally (*26, 68*) that vibration reduces low-intensity, but enhances high-intensity, pain and itch. Similar mechanisms may account for the fact that amputees sometimes obtain relief from phantom limb pain by tapping the stump gently with a rubber mallet (*69*), whereas heavier pressure aggravates the pain (*8*).

The phenomena of referred pain, spread of pain, and trigger points at some distance from the original site of body damage also point toward summation mechanisms, which can be understood in terms of the model. The T cell has a restricted receptive field which dominates its "normal activities." In addition, there is a widespread, diffuse, monosynaptic input to the cell, which is revealed by electrical stimulation of distant afferents (*41*). We suggest that this diffuse input is normally inhibited by presynaptic gate mechanisms, but may trigger firing in the cell if the input is sufficiently intense or if there is a change in gate activity. Because the cell remains dominated by its receptive field, anesthesia of the area to which the pain is referred, from which only spontaneous impulses are originating, is sufficient to reduce the bombardment of the cell below the threshold level for pain. The gate can also be opened by activities in distant body areas, since the substantia gelatinosa at any level receives inputs from both sides of the body and (by way of Lissauer's tract) from the substantia gelatinosa in neighboring body segments. Mechanisms such as these may explain the observations that stimulation of trigger points on the chest and arms may trigger anginal pain (*70*), or that pressing other body areas, such as the back of the head, may trigger pain in the phantom limb (*11*).

The sensory mechanisms alone fail to account for the fact that nerve lesions do not always produce pain and that, when they do, the pain is usully not continuous. We propose that the presence or absence of pain is determined by the balance between the sensory and the central inputs to the gate control system. In addition to the sensory influences on the gate control system, there is a tonic input to the system from higher levels of the central nervous system which exerts an inhibitory effect on the sensory input (*44, 71*). Thus, any lesion that impairs the normal downflow of impulses to the gate control system would open the gate. Central nervous system lesions associated with hyperalgesia and spontaneous pain (*7*) could have this effect. On the other hand, any central nervous system condition that increases the flow of descending impulses would tend to close the gate. Increased central firing due to denervation supersensitivity (*72*) might be one of these conditions. A peripheral nerve lesion, then, would have the *direct* effect of opening the gate, and the *indirect* effect, by increasing central firing and thereby increasing the tonic descending influences on the gate control system, of closing the gate. The balance between sensory facilitation and central inhibition of the input after peripheral-nerve lesion would account for the variability of pain even in cases of severe lesion.

The model suggests that psychological factors such as past experience, attention, and emotion influence pain response and perception by acting on the gate control system. The degree of central control, however, would be determined, in part at least, by the temporal–spatial properties of the input patterns. Some of the most unbearable pains, such as cardiac pain, rise so rapidly in intensity that the patient is unable to achieve any control over them. On the other hand, more slowly rising temporal patterns are susceptible to central control and may allow the patient to "think about something else" or use other stratagems to keep the pain under control (*73*).

The therapeutic implications of the model are twofold. First, it suggests that control of pain may be achieved by selectively influencing the large, rapidly conducting fibers. The gate may be closed by decreasing the small-fiber input and also by enhancing the large-fiber input. Thus, Livingston (*74*) found that causalgia could be effectively cured by therapy such as bathing the limb in gently moving water, followed by massage, which would increase the input in the large-fiber system. Similarly, Trent (*75*) reports a case of pain of central nervous system origin which could be brought under control when the patient tapped his fingers on a hard surface. Conversely, any manipulation that cuts down the sensory input lessens the opportunity for summation and pain, within the functional limits set by the opposing roles of the large- and small-fiber systems. Second, the model suggests that a better understanding of the pharmacology and physiology of the substantia gelatinosa may lead to new ways of controlling pain. The resistance of the substantia gelatinosa to nerve-cell stains suggests that its chemistry differs from that of other neural tissue. Drugs affecting excitation or inhibition of substantia gelatinosa activity may be of particular importance in future attempts to control pain.

The model suggests that the action system responsible for pain perception and response is triggered after the cutaneous sensory input has been modulated by both sensory feedback mechanisms and the influences of the central nervous system. We propose that the abstraction of information at the first synapse may mark only the beginning of a continuing selection and filtering of the input. Perception and response involve classification of the multitude of patterns of nerve impulses arriving from the skin and are functions of the capacity of the brain to select and to abstract from all the information it receives from the somesthetic system as a whole (7–9). A "modality" class such as "pain," which is a linguistic label for a rich variety of experiences and responses, represents just such an abstraction from the information that is sequentially re-examined over long periods by the entire somesthetic system.

References and notes

1. K. M. Dallenbach, *Amer. J. Physiol.* **52**, 331 (1939): K. D. Keele, *Anatomies of Pain* (Blackwell, Oxford, 1957).
2. W. H. Sweet, *Handbook Physiol.* **1**, 459 (1959).
3. D. C. Sinclair, *Brain* **78**, 584 (1955).
4. M. von Frey, *Ber. Kgl. Sächs. Ges. Wiss.* **46**, 185 (1894); *ibid.*, p. 283.
5. A. Goldscheider, *Ueber den Schmerz in physiologischer und klinischer Hinsicht* (Hirschwald, Berlin, 1894).
6. G. H. Bishop, *Physiol. Rev.* **26**, 77 (1946); A-delta fibers are the smallest myelinated fibers, C fibers are the unmyelinated fibers, in peripheral nerve.
7. H. Head, *Studies in Neurology* (Keegan Paul, London, 1920).
8. W. K. Livingston, *Pain Mechanisms* (Macmillan, New York, 1943).
9. R. Melzack and P. D. Wall, *Brain* **85**, 331 (1962).
10. W. Noordenbos, *Pain* (Elsevier, Amsterdam, 1959).
11. B. Cronholm, *Acta Psychiat. Neurol. Scand. Suppl.* **72**, 1 (1951).
12. W. K. Livingston, *Sci. Amer.* **88**, 59 (1953); R. Melzack, *ibid.* **204**, 41 (1961); T. X. Barber, *Psychol. Bull.* **56**, 430 (1959).
13. H. K. Beecher, *Measurement of Subjective Responses* (Oxford Univ. Press, New York, 1959).
14. W. Freeman and J. W. Watts, *Psychosurgery in the Treatment of Mental Disorders and Intractable Pain* (Thomas, Springfield, Ill., 1950).
15. I. P. Pavlov, *Conditioned Reflexes* (Milford, Oxford, 1927).
16. —, *Lectures on Conditioned Reflexes* (International Publishers, New York, 1928).
17. J. P. Nafe, in *Handbook of General Experimental Psychology*, C. Murchison, Ed. (Clark Univ. Press, Worcester, Mass., 1934).
18. J. D. Hardy, H. G. Wolff, H. Goodell, *Pain Sensations and Reactions* (Williams and Wilkins, Baltimore, 1952).

19. C. T. Morgan, *Introduction to Psychology* (McGraw-Hill, New York, 1961).
20. C. C. Hunt and A. K. McIntyre, *J. Physiol. London* **153**, 88, 99 (1960).
21. J. Maruhashi, K. Mizaguchi, I. Tasaki, *ibid.* **117**, 129 (1952).
22. W. W. Douglas and J. M. Ritchie, *ibid.* **139**, 385 (1957).
23. A. Iggo, *ibid.* **143**, 47 (1958).
24. P. D. Wall, *J. Neurophysiol.* **23**, 197 (1960).
25. V. H. Mark, F. R. Ervin, P. I. Yakovlev, *Arch. Neurol.* **8**, 528 (1963).
26. P. D. Wall and J. R. Cronly-Dillon, *ibid.* **2**, 365 (1960).
27. P. D. Wall and A. Taub, *J. Neurophysiol.* **25**, 110 (1962); L. Kruger and F. Michel, *Exp. Neurol.* **5**, 157 (1962).
28. G. F. Poggio and V. B. Mountcastle, *Bull. Johns Hopkins Hosp.* **106**, 226 (1960).
29. G. M. Kolmodin and C. R. Skoglund, *Acta Physiol. Scand.* **50**, 337 (1960); G. Gordon, S. Landgren, W. A. Seed, *J. Physiol. London* **158**, 544 (1960); J. S. Eisenman, S. Landgren, D. Novin, *Acta Physiol. Scand. Suppl.* **214**, 1 (1963).
30. K. L. Casey, "A search for nociceptive elements in the thalamus of the awake squirrel monkey," paper read at the 16th Autumn meeting of the American Physiological Society, Providence, R.I., 1964.
31. G. Weddell, *Annu. Rev. Psychol.* **6**, 119 (1955).
32. D. H. Barron and B. H. C. Matthews, *J. Physiol. London* **92**, 276 (1938).
33. D. O. Hebb, *The Organization of Behavior* (Wiley, New York, 1949).
34. R. W. Gerard, *Anesthesiology* **12**, 1 (1951).
35. T. Lewis, *Pain* (Macmillan, New York, 1942).
36. G. H. Bishop, *J. Nervous Mental Disease* **128**, 89 (1959).
37. P. D. Wall, *Progr. Brain Res.* **12**, 92 (1964).
38. J. Szentagothai, *J. Comp. Neurol.* **122**, 219 (1964).
39. P. D. Wall, *J. Physiol. London* **164**, 508 (1963); L. M. Mendell and P. D. Wall, *ibid.* **172**, 274 (1964).
40. P. D. Wall, *J. Neurophysiol.* **22**, 205 (1959); *J. Physiol. London* **142**, 1 (1958).
41. L. M. Mendell and P. D. Wall, *Nature* **206**, 97 (1965).
42. D. G. Whitlock and E. R. Perl, *Exp. Neurol.* **3**, 240 (1961).
43. A. M. Halliday and R. Mingay, *Quart. J. Exp. Psychol.* **13**, 1 (1961).
44. K. E. Hagbarth and D. I. B. Kerr, *J. Neurophysiol.* **17**, 295 (1954).
45. H. G. J. M. Kuypers, W. R. Fleming, J. W. Farinholt, *Science* **132**, 38 (1960); A. Lundberg, *Progr. Brain Res.* **12**, 197 (1964).
46. V. B. Mountcastle, in *Sensory Communication*, W. A. Rosenblith, Ed. (Massachusetts Institute of Technology, Cambridge, 1961).
47. J. D. French, M. Verzeano, W. H. Magoun, *A.M.A. Arch. Neurol. Psychiat.* **69**, 519 (1953); F. P. Haugen and R. Melzack, *Anesthesiology* **18**, 183 (1957).
48. T. C. Ruch and J. F. Fulton, *Medical Physiology and Biophysics* (Saunders, Philadelphia, 1960).
49. A. W. Cook and E. J. Browder, *Arch. Neurol.* **12**, 72 (1965).
50. F. Morin, *Amer. J. Physiol.* **183**, 245 (1955).
51. E. Oswaldo-Cruz and C. Kidd, *J. Neurophysiol.* **27**, 1 (1964).
52. U. Norrsell and P. Voerhoeve, *Acta Physiol. Scand.* **54**, 9 (1962).
53. C. S. Sherrington, in *Textbook of Physiology*, E. A. Schäfer, Ed. (Pentland, Edinburgh, 1900).

54. J. V. Brady, *Handbook Physiol.* 3, 1529 (1960).
55. W. R. Hess, *Diencephalon: Autonomic and Extrapyramidal Functions (Grune, New York, 1954).*
56. J. M. R. Delgado, *J. Neurophysiol.* 18, 261 (1955); R. Melzack, W. A. Stotler, W. K. Livingston, *ibid.* 21, 353 (1958).
57. P. Schilder and E. Stengel, *A.M.A. Arch. Neurol. Psychiat.* 25, 598 (1931).
58. D. I. B. Kerr, F. P. Haugen, R. Melzack, *Amer. J. Physiol.* 183, 253 (1955).
59. R. Melzack and F. P. Haugen, *ibid.* 190, 570 (1957).
60. W. J. H. Nauta and H. G. J. M. Kuypers, in *Reticular Formation of the Brain,* H. H. Jasper *et al.,* Eds. (Little, Brown, Boston, 1958).
61. W. Blackwood, W. H. McMenemey, A. Meyer, R. M. Norman, D. S. Russell, *Greenfield's Neuropathology* (Arnold, London, 1963).
62. W. R. Henderson and G. E. Smyth, *J. Neurol. Neurosurg. Psychiat.* 11, 88 (1948).
63. K. E. Chernetski, *J. Neurophysiol.* 27, 493 (1964).
64. J. Doupe, C. H. Cullen, G. Q. Chance, *J. Neurol. Neurosurg. Psychiat.* 7, 33 (1944).
65. A. G. Swanson, G. C. Buchan, E. C. Alvord, *Arch. Neurol.* 12, 12 (1965).
66. D. C. Sinclair and J. R. Hinshaw, *Brain* 74, 318 (1951).
67. E. D. Adrian, *The Basis of Sensation: The Action of Sense Organs* (Christophers, London, 1928).
68. R. Melzack, P. D. Wall, A. Z. Weisz, *Exp. Neurol.* 8, 35 (1963); R. Melzack and B. Schecter, *Science* 147, 1047 (1965).
69. W. R. Russell and J. M. K. Spalding, *Brit. Med. J.* 2, 68 (1950).
70. H. Cohen, *Trans. Med. Soc. London* 64, 65 (1944).
71. A. Taub, *Exp. Neurol.* 10, 357 (1964).
72. G. W. Stavraky, *Supersensitivity following Lesions of the Nervous System* (Univ. of Toronto Press, Toronto, 1961); S. K. Sharpless, *Annu. Rev. Physiol.* 26, 357 (1964).
73. R. Melzack, A. Z. Weisz, L. T. Sprague, *Exp. Neurol.* 8, 239 (1963).
74. W. K. Livingston, *Ann. N.Y. Acad. Sci.* 50, 247 (1948).
75. S. E. Trent, *J. Nervous Mental Disease* 123, 356 (1956).
76. R. Descartes, "L'Homme" (Paris, 1644), M. Foster, transl., in *Lectures on the History of Physiology during the 16th, 17th and 18th Centuries* (Cambridge Univ. Press, Cambridge, England, 1901).
77. C. S. MacCarty and R. L. Drake, *Proc. Staff Meetings Mayo Clinic* 31, 208 (1956).

78. This study was supported in part by contract SD-193 from the Advanced Research Projects Agency, U.S. Department of Defense (to R.M.); and in part by the Joint Services Electronics Program under contract DA36-039-AMC-03200(E), the Bell Telephone Laboratories, Inc., the Teagle Foundation, Inc., the National Science Foundation (grant GP-2495), the National Institutes of Health (grants MH-04737-05 and NB-04897-02), the National Aeronautics and Space Administration (grant NsG-496), and the U.S. Air Force (ASD contract AF33 (615)-1747).

Effects of coping behavior on gastric lesions in rats as a function of the complexity of coping tasks

Akira Tsuda, Masatoshi Tanaka, Tadashi Nishikawa and
Hisashi Hirai

*Department of Pharmacology, Kurume University School of Medicine,
Kurume 830; Department of Psychology, Sophia University, Tokyo 102,
Japan*

Abstract

TSUDA, A., M. TANAKA, T. NISHIKAWA AND H. HIRAI. *Effects of
coping behavior on gastric lesions in rats as a function of the complexity of coping
tasks*. PHYSIOL BEHAV **30**(5) 805–808, 1983,—In fixed ratio (FR) 2 coping task
condition, experimental rats which could avoid and/or escape shock by emitting a
disk-pulling operant response developed less stomach ulceration than did yoked
"helpless" rats which had exactly the same shock but which had no control over
shock. In variable ratio (VR) 5 coping task condition, however, the experimental
rats developed more lesions than did the matched yoked rats. Neither the VR 2-
nor the FR 5-experimental group was significantly different from its yoked group.
Ulceration of non-shock control group was negligible compared to experimental
and yoked rats in each of the four coping task conditions. The level of complexity or difficulty of coping response tasks required has a detrimental effect
on ulcerogenesis for "coping" experimental rats. The effectiveness of a coping
behavior covaries with the nature or ease of the coping tasks in a stressful
situation.

Coping behavior   Coping task   Controllability   Helplessness   Gastric lesions

Weiss [13] has demonstrated that although being able to acquire a simple
avoidance/escape response to turn off shock reduces the development of
gastric ulceration for "coping" rats when the coping task is simple,

ulceration is exacerbated if the coping task involves conflict. Tsuda and Hirai [10] have also reported that by changing the values of a fixed ratio (FR) schedule for the coping tasks, it is possible to reverse the normally beneficial effects of having control over shock.

Research to date suggests that gastric ulcer severity may be etiologically related to the two factors of controllability of shock and the coping tasks required to cope with it [8]. However, because very few studies have manipulated the complexity or difficulty of the coping tasks, the extent to which the beneficial effects of controllability are compounded by the degree of coping task complexity or difficulty is not clear.

The present study was undertaken to examine the effects of shock controllability on the development of gastric lesions in rats after extended exposure to the avoidance/escape procedure with either simple or hard coping task. Controllability was tested by allowing some animals access to an operant response, which either postponed or terminated shock as compared to other animals which did not have access to this operant controlling response. The complexity of the coping task conditions was manipulated by either requiring a low number of responses (2) for reinforcement (i.e., shock termination) or a high number of responses (5) for reinforcement, and by changing the nature of the coping task schedules (fixed ratio, FR, or variable ratio, VR).

We assumed that the complexity of the coping task conditions probably might have a functional relationship with the nature of the coping response required to terminate a shock (e.g., a required frequency of the operant response). Should it be the case, an easy task condition was defined as performing the FR 2 operant response, as opposed to a hard task which was defined as performing the VR 5 operant response.

Method

Animals and apparatus

One hundred and thirty-two male naive Wistar-strain rats, 8 weeks old (approximately 230 g) at the beginning of the study, were used as subjects. All animals were housed in groups in an animal colony room with constant temperature ($24 \pm 1°C$) and humidity ($50 \pm 10\%$). The room lights were on between 0800 and 2000 hr.

The apparatus consisted of three individual clear Plexiglas chambers ($9 \times 19.5 \times 20$ cm), which were modelled after those used by Weiss [12], were placed in sound-proof boxes. The end walls were at an angle, and the top fitted across the rat's back in such a way that the rat could not turn around in the chamber. A 2-cm diameter stainless disk manipulandum (0.3 cm thick) was suspended 6.5 cm from the ceiling into the chamber and situated in front of the rat's nose. The disk, when pulled by the experimental rat, activated a switch allowed the experimental rat to escape or avoid shock delivered to the tail. The force required to pull was roughly 20 g.

Shock from a constant-current shocker was delivered to two copper clips (1.3×0.3 cm) which were attached to the tails of all three animals. The tail electrodes of the experimental rat and yoked rat were wired in series with the shock source. The control rat's tail electrodes were not connected to the shock circuit. The auditory signal (1250 Hz, 80 dB) originated from an oscillator and was delivered through a speaker attached to the inside of each sound-proof box. The sequence of stimulus presentations was controlled by an automatic pattern generator. The number of disk-pulling responses and shock pulses administered were continuously recorded with digital counters.

Procedure

Animals were deprived of food, but not water for 48 hr prior to the beginning of the stress session, and were randomly assigned to one of three treatment groups (N = 11 per group): one being designated as the experimental group, which controlled shock with its disk-pulling response; another as the yoked group, which received the identical shock as the experimental partner rat but could not control shock by its own response; and the third as the non-shock control group.

Coping task condition

Each triplet was subsequently randomly assigned to one of four coping task conditions according to designated avoidance/escape contingencies by the discriminated Sidman procedure: FR 2, FR 5, VR 2 or VR 5 schedule. This produced eleven matched triplets for each coping task conditions. The contingency of response and signal or shock in these different coping task conditions was as follows: whenever the experimental rat pulled the disk the designated number of times (2, 5, 1–3 on average 2 or 1–9 on average 5 responses, respectively) in order to avoid or escape shock, the next shock was postponed for 100 sec.

Stress-session procedure

The avoidance/escape procedure used a train of shock pulses with a shock-shock interval of 1.5 sec and a pulse duration of 1.0 sec. The auditory signal was activated for 10 sec before the occurrence of shock.

The response-shock interval was 100 sec. A response by the experimental rat reset the shock mechanism and delayed the onset of shock by 100 sec. The shock intensity was initially set at 1.0 mA until the first 3 hr and increased gradually over a 21 hr period to a maximum of 2.5 mA. In all four coping task conditions, experimental rats were given a standard avoidance/escape procedure (i.e., FR 1 contingency) which lasted for the first 3 hr, since a pilot study revealed that naive rats sometimes failed to learn the VR 5 disk-pulling response for the termination of shock if such prior trials were not provided. From the fourth hour onward, an accumulation of each predetermined number of coping responses could terminate or postpone either the shock or the signal in each of these conditions. A stress-session started at 1000 hr and lasted for 24 hr. Animals did not have access to food and water throughout a session.

Assessment of gastric lesions

At the end of the stress session, animals were quickly sacrificed by decapitation and their stomachs were examined for presence and degree of gastric lesions by a scorer who was blind with respect to the rat's treatment condition. The rating procedure, slight modified from rating scales reported by Fujiwara and Mori [3], was as follows: a score of "0" was given to no change, "1" to small hemorrhagic points and edemas, "2" to one or two small (smaller than 2 mm in diameter) mucosal defects, "3" to many small mucosal defects, "4" to one or two large (greater than 2 mm in diameter) mucosal defects and "5" to many large mucosal defects.

Statistical analysis

All statistical comparisons on the data of gastric lesions were made using a group (experimental, yoked or control group) by the coping task schedule (FR or VR) by ratio for reinforcement (2 or 5) factorial analysis of variance (at least $p < 0.05$) and subsequent Tukey's pairwise comparisons ($\alpha = 0.05$). The statistical evaluations of the behavioral measurements were performed as follows: the Wilcoxon's T-test (at least $p < 0.05$, two-tailed) for matched subjects was used for comparisons between experimental, yoked and control groups within the same coping task conditions. The Mann-Whitney's U-test (at least $p < 0.05$, two-tailed) was used for comparisons between groups that were not of the same coping task condition.

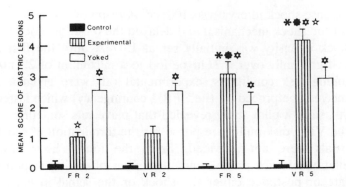

Fig. 1. The mean (±SEM) severity score of gastric lesions for the experimental, yoked and control groups in the fixed ratio (FR) 2, variable ratio (VR) 2, FR 5 and VR 5 coping task conditions. ✻ Differs significantly ($p < 0.05$) from FR 2-experimental group. ✿ Differs significantly ($p < 0.05$) from VR 2-experimental group. ✿ Differs significantly ($p < 0.05$) from respective control group. ☆ Differs significantly ($p < 0.05$) from respective yoked group.

Results

Gastric lesions

Figure 1 shows the degree of gastric lesions severity for each group. An analysis of variance revealed a significant group effect, ratio effect and interaction effect of group and ratio. But a schedule main effect was not significant. Tukey pairwise comparisons revealed that experimental rats in each of the FR 2 and VR 2 conditions had significantly less severe lesions than did experimental rats in each of the FR 5 and VR 5 conditions. The experimental rats in FR 2 condition did not differ significantly from the VR 2-experimental rats, nor did the FR 5-experimental rats differ from the VR 5-experimental rats. Yoked rats exhibited similar severity of gastric lesions irrespective of different coping task conditions.

Gastric lesions were not found in non-shock control rats. Consequently, all other treatment groups had significantly more lesions than these control rats, excluding the FR 2- and VR 2-experimental groups. Comparisons within each of the four coping task conditions showed that although experimental rats in the FR 2 condition had significantly fewer lesions than their matched FR 2-yoked rats, the VR 5-experimental rats had significantly more gastric lesions than their matched VR 5-yoked rats. In the FR 2 and FR 5 conditions, experimental rats did not significantly differ from yoked rats.

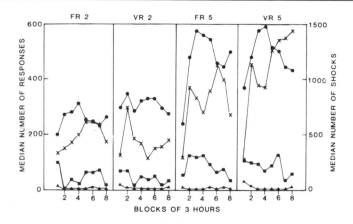

Fig. 2. The median number of disk-pulling responses by experimental (—●—), yoked (—■—) and control (—▲—) groups, and shock pulses (—x—) received by shocked groups during a 24-hr discriminated Sidman procedure across 3-hr blocks in FR 2, VR 2, FR 5 and VR 5 coping task conditions.

Disk-pulling behavior and number of shock pulses

Experimental rats made significantly more disk-pulling responses than did yoked or control rats, and the yoked rats responded significantly more than the control rats. This relationship, which is illustrated in Fig. 2, occurred in all coping task conditions. The number of responses was significantly greater for each of FR 5- and VR 5-experimental rats when compared with FR 2- or VR 2-experimental rats. The yoked group demonstrated a similar number of responses in all conditions. The control rats also emitted a similar pattern of a low number of response across all conditions.

The amount of shock received by both shocked groups was affected by different coping task conditions. As depicted in Fig. 2, there were significant differences between both of the FR 2 and VR 2 conditions and both of the FR 5 and VR 5 conditions. These two ratio conditions, however, did not significantly differ from each other. The number of shock presentations over the 24-hr stress session did differ. There were significantly more shocks presented during the second 3-hr block as compared to the first 3-hr block and this significant increase in shocks occurred in all the coping task conditions exclusive of the FR 2 condition. In addition, there was a substantial rise in number of shocks received between block 4 to 6 in FR 5 condition and block 4 to last in VR 5 coping condition.

Discussion

The present experiment used response frequency or schedule in examining effects of coping task complexity or difficulty on gastric pathology. Although rats which could avoid or escape shock by pulling a disk manipulanda twice (FR 2) developed less gastric lesions than did their shock yoked rats, the rats which could control shock by pulling the disk average five (VR 5) exhibited more gastric damage than did their yoked rats. Furthermore, the degree of gastric lesions in the yoked rats was the same irrespective of whether the coping task was simple or complex. The present study, thus verified the hypothesis that the severity of stress pathology for "coping" rats covaried with the complexity or difficulty of coping task conditions, as suggested by Maier *et al.* [4], Miller [5], Moran and Lewis-Smith [7] and Sligman and Beagley [9]. The results from this experiment are generally in agreement with other research studies on "coping," "helplessness" and ulcer development [1, 2, 6, 10, 11, 12].

Differences in the extent of gastric lesions did not appear in the FR versus VR schedules, but the ratio requirement of either 2 or 5 did produce differences in ulcer severity. Theoretically, although the VR schedule should contain an obscured contingency between response and shock termination as compared with the FR schedule, no obvious difference was found in the production of gastric damage. "Coping" experimental rats exposed to either FR 5 or VR 5 coping task condition displayed significantly more gastric lesions than did experimental rats exposed to either FR 2 or VR 2 condition.

The value "2" of the ratio in FR and VR schedules was presumed to be less complex or require less effort as compared with the ratio "5" of these schedules. The FR 2 coping task condition contained a clear contingency between response and shock termination, while the FR 5 or VR 5 task involved a highly degraded contingency, which in turn, may be an important factor in producing differences in gastric lesions between the ratio "2"-coping rats and the ratio "5"-coping rats.

The behavioral data revealed that there was a substantial rise in number of shock received between block 4 to 6 in FR 5 and block 4 to last in VR 5 condition. These results are interpreted as a striking evidence of "losing control" in both FR 5 and VR 5 conditions. When the FR 5- or VR 5-experimental animals exhibited physical fatigue due to depletion of energy reserves by food and water deprivation and stress-induced enhancement of glucose utilization, the complexity or difficulty of the FR 5- or VR 5-coping task became a vivid construct applied to these animals at this stage of their tasks.

The data from the amount of shock received by experimental and yoked rats are problematic. There was a progressive increase in severity of gastric lesions in the experimental rats as the amount of shock increased from the FR 2 to VR 5 coping task. The difference in terms of the degree of gastric pathology between the FR 2- or VR 2-experimental rats and the FR 5- or VR 5-experimental rats might be caused by differences in the amount of shock. This possibility, however, is unlikely in light of the fact that the yoked rats, which received exactly the same number, intensity and duration of shock as did the experimental rats, showed no differences in gastric lesions within all four coping task conditions. A progressive increase in gastric lesions in the coping-experimental rats did not likely arise from a difference in the amount of shock pulses, but rather the difference in the complexity level of the coping task required.

Indeed, the present investigation apparently support that the notion of the response-produced feedback hypothesis [12, 14], indicating that the amount of gastric damage is inversely proportional to the amount of relevant feedback produced by successful coping responses, as a critical variable in determining stress effects of coping behavior. In conclusion, both factors of controllability of shock and the complexity or difficulty of the coping task required seem to be important for causing gastric ulcerogenesis.

Acknowledgements

We are grateful to Prof. Nobuyuki Nagasaki of the Department of Pharmacology, Kurume University School of Medicine, for his valuable comments on an earlier version of the manuscript. We also wish to thank Dr. Gary B. Glavin of the Department of Psychology, University of Winnipeg, Canada, for stimulating discussion.

This work was supported by the Association for the Advancement of Sciences of Japan for a Postgraduate Scholarship to one of the authors (A. Tsuda).

References

1. Barbaree, H. E. and R. K. Harding. Free-operant avoidance behavior and gastric ulceration in rats. *Physiol Behav* 11: 269–271, 1973.
2. Guile, M. N. and N. B. McCutcheon. Prepared responses and gastric lesions in rats. *Physiol Psychol* 8: 480–482, 1980.
3. Fujiwara, M. and J. Mori. Experimental stress ulcer and biogenic amines. *Saishin Igaku* 25: 2058–2067, 1970.
4. Maier, S. F., R. W. Albin and T. Testa. Failure of learn to escape shock in rats previously exposed to inescapable shock depends on nature of escape response. *J Comp Physiol Psychol* 85: 581–592, 1973.
5. Miller, N. E. Effects of learning on gastrointestinal functions. *Clin Gastroenterol* 6: 533–546, 1977.
6. Mott, S. A., R. P. Cebulla and J. M. Crabtree. Instrumental control and ulceration in rats. *J Comp Physiol Psychol* 71: 405–410, 1970.

7. Moran, P. W. and M. Lewis-Smith. Learned helplessness and response difficulty. *Bull Psychon Soc* **13**: 250–252, 1979.
8. Murison, R., E. Isaksen and H. Ursin. "Coping" and gastric ulceration in rats after prolonged active avoidance performance. *Physiol Behav* **27**: 345–348, 1981,
9. Seligman, M. E. P. and G. Beagley. Learned helplessness in the rat. *J Comp Physiol Psychol* **88**: 534–541, 1975.
10. Tsuda, A. and H. Hirai. Effects of the amount of required coping response tasks on gastrointestinal lesions in rats. *Jpn Psychol Res* **17**: 119–132, 1975.
11. Tsuda, A., M. Tanaka, H. Hirai and W. P. Pare, Effects of coping behavior on gastric lesions in rats as a function of predictability of shock. *Jpn Psychol Res* **25**: in press, 1983.
12. Weiss, J. M. Effects of coping behavior in different warning signal conditions on stress pathology in rats. *J. Comp Physiol Psychol* **77**: 1–13, 1971.
13. Weiss, J. M. Effects of punishing the coping response (conflict) on stress pathology in rats. *J Comp Physiol Psychol* **77**: 14–21, 1971.
14. Weiss, J. M. Effects of coping behavior with and without a feedback signal on stress pathology in rats. *J Comp Physiol Psychol* **77**: 22–30, 1971.

Social stress and atherosclerosis in normocholesterolemic monkeys

Jay R. Kaplan, Stephen B. Manuck, Thomas B. Clarkson, Frances M. Lusso, David M. Taub and Eric W. Miller

Arteriosclerosis Research Center, Bowman Gray School of Medicine, Wake Forest University, Winston-Salem, North Carolina 27103, USA; Department of Psychology, University of Pittsburgh, Pittsburgh, Pennsylvania 15260, USA; Yemassee Primate Center, Yemassee, South Carolina 29945, USA

Abstract

Socially stressed adult male cynomolgus monkeys (*Macaca fascicularis*) fed a low fat, low cholesterol diet developed more extensive coronary artery atherosclerosis than unstressed controls. Groups did not differ in serum lipids, blood pressure, serum glucose, or ponderosity. These results suggest that psychosocial factors may influence atherogenesis in the absence of elevated serum lipids. Psychosocial factors thus may help explain the presence of coronary artery disease (occasionally severe) in people with low or normal serum lipids and normal values for the other "traditional" risk factors.

The initiation and progression of coronary artery atherosclerosis is often associated with increased concentrations of lipids in the serum (*1*). Despite this association, many individuals develop severe atherosclerotic lesions while having low serum lipid concentrations, and others develop far more atherosclerosis than would be expected on the basis of a modest evaluation of serum lipids (*2*). Work with animal models suggests that some of this variability may be explained by the influence of hypertension and immunologic injury to arteries, (*3, 4*). Yet, much additional variability in atherosclerosis lesion extent remains unexplained, suggesting the existence of other pathogenic mechanisms among normocholesterolemic

Reprinted from Kaplan, J. R., Manuck, S. B., Clarkson, T. B., Lusso, F. M., Taub, D. M. and Miller, E. W. Social stress and atherosclerosis in normocholesterolemic monkeys. *Science*, **220**, 733–5, 13 May 1983, © AAAS.

individuals. In recent years, psychosocial variables have been linked increasingly to ischemic heart disease in human beings (5) and psychosocial manipulations have been shown to exacerbate atherosclerosis in cholesterol-fed cynomolgus monkeys, rabbits, and swine (6–8). At present, though, it is unclear whether psychosocial manipulations are capable of promoting atherogenesis in normocholesterolemic animals and, by implication, in human beings with low or normal serum cholesterol concentrations. The purpose of the present investigation was to provide an initial test of this hypothesis. Our results demonstrate that socially stressed monkeys fed a low fat, low cholesterol diet developed more extensive intimal lesions in the coronary arteries than control animals living under unstressed conditions. Moreover, the differences in lesion extent observed here were not associated with elevations or group differences in serum lipids, blood pressure, serum glucose, or ponderosity.

The experimental animals were 30 male, cynomolgus monkeys (*Macaca fascicularis*), imported as adults from Malaysia and the Philippine Islands. They were assigned to two experimental conditions (designated the "stressed" and "unstressed" conditions), and within each condition ($N = 15$), the monkeys were divided randomly into three, five-member groups. During the study, all groups were housed separately in identical pens measuring 2.0 by 3.2 by 2.5 m. The experiment lasted 21 months, after which all animals were killed and necropsied.

Throughout the study the monkeys were fed a "prudent" diet, modeled on the current recommendations of the American Heart Association; this diet contained almost no cholesterol (0.05 mg of cholesterol per calorie) and was low in saturated fats (9). Blood samples for determination of total serum cholesterol and high-density lipoprotein cholesterol (HDLC) concentrations were taken approximately once per month over the course of the study. Other physiologic variables associated with atherosclerosis were measured at regular intervals; these variables included systolic and diastolic blood pressure (bimonthly), fasting serum glucose concentration (semiannually) and ponderosity (the ratio of body weight to body length) (semiannually). All monkeys were sampled in the morning, under ketamine restraint and following a suitable fast (*10*).

To create a significantly stressful social environment, we periodically altered group memberships in the stressed condition by redistributing animals among the three affected groups. The monkeys were redistributed once every 12 weeks in the first year of the study and once every 4 weeks in the following 9 months. Unlike the stressed animals, group memberships among monkeys assigned to the unstressed, or control condition, remained constant throughout the 21-month experiment.

Reorganization of groups was selected as a means of inducing stress in the present study because previous reports had indicated that introduction of strangers fosters a high degree of social instability in macaques (*11*). In an attempt to further enhance competition and social uncertainty, an ovariectomized female with an estrogen-containing capsule implanted under the skin was also placed into each of the stressed groups for the last 2 weeks of each 4-week reorganization during the final 9 months of the study. Finally, to document behavioral effects associated with these experimental manipulations, we recorded the frequencies of aggressive, submissive, and affiliative acts. These data were obtained by means of a focal sampling technique in which each animal was observed for 195 15-minute periods (*10*).

At the time of necropsy, the heart was removed and the coronary arteries were perfused with 10 percent neutral buffered Formalin at a pressure of 100 mmHg. Fifteen tissue blocks (each 3 mm in length) were then cut perpendicularly to the long axis of the coronary arteries. Five of these were serial blocks taken from the left circumflex, five from the left anterior descending, and five from the right coronary artery. Two sections were cut from each block and stained with either hematoxylin and eosin or Verhoeff Van Gieson stains. Upon projection of the Verhoeff Van Gieson-stained sections (at ×440 magnification), two measures of atherosclerosis were calculated with the use of a Zeiss MOP III Image Analyzer. The first measurement was of the total area occupied by intima or intimal lesion (termed intimal area). The second measure, intimal thickness, was calculated as the maximum distance obtaining at any one point between the internal elastic lamina and the lumen of the artery.

For the present analysis, the extent of coronary artery atherosclerosis in each monkey was expressed as a mean intimal area (in square millimeters) and mean intimal thickness (in millimeters) of 15 sections of coronary artery. The area measures for all monkeys are depicted in Fig. 1. Substantial differences in coronary artery atherosclerosis were observed between the stressed and unstressed conditions, with stressed animals having larger intimal areas relative to controls ($P < .002$, Mann-Whitney U test) (*12*). Maximum intimal thickness was highly correlated with intimal area ($\rho = .73$, $P < .001$) and was also significantly greater in stressed than control animals ($P < .02$, Mann-Whitney U test).

The arterial lesions of each monkey were also graded for extent of change. One of three grades was assigned to each coronary artery upon the consensus of five investigators who did not know the animals' experimental conditions. The grades recorded were 0 for no intimal changes; 1 for intimal changes present but characterized by fatty streaks only (that is, foam cells); and 2 for fatty streaks that had progressed to small plaques with smooth muscle cell profileration. Among animals in the stressed condition, 11 of 15 monkeys received grade 2 on one or more

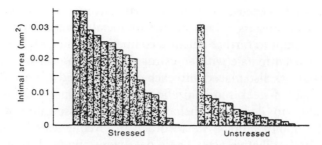

Fig. 1. Area occupied by intimal lesion in stressed and unstressed monkeys; bars represent individual animals. Early mortality resulted in the loss of one animal from the unstressed condition.

coronary arteries, whereas only 4 of 14 unstressed animals had lesions of similar extent. This difference in the distribution of relatively advanced lesions (that is, plaque) between the stressed and unstressed conditions was statistically significant ($\chi^2 = 4.16$, $P < .05$).

Animals in the two conditions also differed behaviorally. Stressed and unstressed monkeys had similar rates of aggressive and submissive behaviors (expressed as incidents per hour) over the course of the experiment (Table 1). Yet the proportions of all agonistic encounters involving both direct, contact aggression (for example, biting, grabbing, slapping) and extreme forms of submission (for example, fleeing, cowering, grimacing) were significantly greater in the periodically reorganized groups (Table 1). Likewise, stressed animals spent significantly less time huddling affiliatively (that is, in passive body contact). These findings suggest that the redistribution of group members fostered a high degree of tension among animals in the stressed condition, promoting a greater proportion of overt fights and interfering with the development of social bonds.

The effects of the psychosocial manipulation on coronary artery atherosclerosis apparently are not due to concomitant differences among other physiologic variables commonly associated with atherosclerosis. Comparisons of the two conditions (by t-tests) revealed no significant differences between the stressed and unstressed monkeys on measures of total serum cholesterol [157 ± 20 mg/dl (mean $\pm$ standard error) and 146 ± 22 mg/dl, respectively] or HDLC concentrations (57 ± 11 mg/dl; 59 ± 13 mg/dl), systolic (89 ± 7 mmHg; 88 ± 9 mmHg) or diastolic (56 ± 6 mmHg; 53 ± 6 mmHg) blood pressure, fasting blood glucose concentration (59 ± 4 mg/dl; 58 ± 6 mg/dl), or ponderosity (1.79 ± 0.26 kg/cm; 1.84 ± 0.15 kg/cm).

The present study provides evidence that psychosocial stress promotes atherogenesis in normocholesterolemic, normotensive monkeys, thus

Table 1. *Behavioral characteristics of the stressed and unstressed groups*

Group	Rate of aggression*	Percentage with severe aggression	Rate of submission	Percentage with severe submission	Percentage of time in affiliation
Stressed ($N = 15$)	5.16	30.0	6.59	27.0	21.0
Unstressed ($N = 14$)	6.69	20.0	7.10	19.0	26.0
Probability†	N.S.	<.05	N.S.	<.05	<.05

*Median rates of performance per hour per monkey, as determined by focal samples.
†Tests of significance by Mann-Whitney U test (two-tailed).

identifying a possible variable in the pathogenesis of atherosclerosis among some "low risk" individuals in human populations. Though it is unclear what mechanisms may mediate behavioral influences on the development of atherosclerosis, we believe the present results may be attributable, in part, to effects of repeated arterial injury. For example, there is a close resemblance between the histological characteristics of lesions reported here (intimal smooth muscle cell proliferation with intra- and extracellular lipid accumulation) and those seen after repeated mechanical injury to arteries among normocholesterolemic rabbits (*13*). Also, an experimental stressor (electric tail shock) has been shown to result in endothelial injury in normocholesterolemic rats (*14*). Albeit speculative, several investigators have suggested that such arterial injury may result, in turn, from hormonal (for example, cortisol, catecholamine) and hemodynamic alterations commonly observed in response to laboratory and social stressors (*15*).

Reorganization of group memberships in the present experiment resulted in proportionately more displays of intensely aggressive behavior among animals assigned to the stressed condition. In a prior investigation involving hypercholesterolemic cynomolgus monkeys, periodic group reorganization also led to increased contact aggression and to greater atherosclerosis (*16*). It is interesting that a high "potential for hostility" represents, among humans, a central component of the type A (coronary-prone) behavior pattern (*17*). Moreover, independent of its association with type A behavior, hostility has been found associated with extent of angiographically documented coronary artery atherosclerosis (*18*). Although these findings reflect only descriptive behavioral similarities, it is noteworthy that aspects of the present data are consistent with studies of psychosocial factors among human beings.

References and notes

1. National Heart, Lung, and Blood Institute, *NIH Pub. No. 81-2034* (1981).
2. L. Solberg, S. Enger, I. Hjermann, A. Helgeland, I. Holme, P. Leren, J. Strong, in *Atheroslcerosis V.* A. Gotto, L. Smith, B. Allen, Eds. (Springer-Verlag, New York, 1980), p. 57; L. Carlson in *Metabolic Risk Factors in Ischemic Cardiovascular Disease*, L. Carlson and B. Pernow, Eds. (Raven, New York, 1982), p. 1.
3. H. McGill, M. Frank, J. Geer, *Arch. Pathol.* **71**, 96 (1961).
4. C. Minick, G. Murphy, W. Campbell, Jr., *J. Exp. Med.* **124**, 635 (1966); T. Clarkson and N. Alexander, *J. Clin. Invest.* **65**, 15 (1980).
5. C. Jenkins, *Annu. Rev. Med.* **29**, 543 (1978).
6. J. Kaplan, S. Manuck, T. Clarkson, F. Lusso, D. Taub, *Arteriosclerosis* **2**, 359 (1982).
7. R. M. Nerem, M. J. Levesque, J. F. Cornhill, *Science* **208**, 1475 (1980).
8. H. Ratcliffe, H. Luginbuhl, W. Schnarr, K. Chacko, *J. Comp. Physiol. Psychol.* **68**, 385 (1969).
9. Each 100 g of diet contained 8.0 g of casein, 8.0 g of lactalbumin, 35.0 g of wheat flour, 6.0 g of dextrin, 5.0 g of sucrose, 4.5 g of applesauce, 7.0 g of lard, 1.2 g of safflower oil, 3.0 g of beef tallow, 0.37 g of dried egg yolk, 15.37 g of alphacel, 4.0 g of Hegsted salt mixture, and 2.56 g of vitamin mixture.
10. For reliabilities of measurement and methods for collecting and analyzing behavioral, pathologic, and physiologic data, see (*6*).
11. I. Bernstein, T. Gordon, R. Rose, *Folia Primatol.* **21**, 90 (1974).
12. All tests of significance were two-tailed.
13. S. Moore, *Lab. Invest.* **29**, 478 (1973).
14. D. Gordon, J. Guyton, M. Karnovsky, *ibid.* **45**, 14 (1981).
15. J. Herd, in *Perspectives on Behavioral Medicine*, S. Weiss, J. Herd, B. Fox, Eds. (Academic Press, New York, 1981), p. 55; R. B. Williams, Jr., J. D. Lane, C. M. Kuhn, W. Melosh, A. D. White, S. M. Schanberg, *Science* **218**, 483 (1982).
16. See J. Kaplan *et al.* (*6*). In the previous experiment exacerbated atherosclerosis was observed only in the stressed animals that were socially dominant. Because hierarchical relationships in the stressed group were somewhat less stable in the current investigation, here we were unable to identify similarly well-differentiated dominant and subordinate animals. Nevertheless, 2 of 15 monkeys housed in the stressed condition clearly retained dominant positions throughout the experiment; as in the previous study, these had the most extensive coronary artery atherosclerosis (see Fig. 1).
17. M. Friedman, *Pathogenesis of Coronary Artery Disease* (McGraw-Hill, New York, 1969).
18. R. Williams, T. Haney, K. Lee, Yi-Hong Kong, J. Blumenthal, R. Whalen, *Psychosom. Med.* **42**, 539 (1980).
19. Supported in part by grants from the National Heart, Lung, and Blood Institute (HL 14164 and RO1 HL 26561) and R. J. Reynolds Industries, Inc.

Mental stress and the induction of silent myocardial ischemia in patients with coronary artery disease

Alan Rozanski, MD, C. Noel Bairey, MD, David S. Krantz, PhD, John Friedman, MD, Kenneth J. Resser, MS, Marie Morell, PhD, Sally Hilton-Chalfen, BS, Lisa Hestrin, MPH, James Bietendorf, CRRT and Daniel S. Berman, MD

From the Division of Cardiology, Department of Medicine, and the Department of Nuclear Medicine, Cedars-Sinai Medical Center, University of California at Los Angeles School of Medicine, USA; the Department of Medical Psychology, Uniformed Services University of the Health Sciences, Bethesda, Md, USA; and the Department of Psychology, University of California at Los Angeles, USA

Abstract

To assess the causal relation between acute mental stress and myocardial ischemia, we evaluated cardiac function in selected patients during a series of mental tasks (arithmetic, the Stroop color–word task, simulated public speaking, and reading) and compared the responses with those induced by exercise. Thirty-nine patients with coronary artery disease and 12 controls were studied by radionuclide ventriculography.

Of the patients with coronary artery disease, 23 (59 percent) had wall-motion abnormalities during periods of mental stress and 14 (36 percent) had a fall in ejection fraction of more than 5 percentage points. Ischemia induced by mental stress was symptomatically "silent" in 19 of the 23 patients with wall-motion abnormalities (83 percent) and occurred at lower heart rates than exercise-induced ischemia ($P < 0.05$). In contrast, we observed comparable elevations in arterial pressure during ischemia induced by mental stress and ischemia induced by exercise. A personally relevant, emotionally arousing speaking task induced more frequent and greater regional wall-motion abnormalities than did less specific cognitive tasks causing mental stress ($P < 0.05$). The magnitude of cardiac dysfunction induced by the speaking task was similar to that induced by exercise.

Reprinted from Rozanski, A., Bairey, C. N., Krantz, D. S., Friedman, J., Resser, K. J., Morell, M., Hilton-Chalfen, S., Hestrin, L., Bietendorf, J. and Berman, D. S. Mental stress and the induction of silent myocardial ischemia in patients with coronary artery disease. *New England Journal of Medicine*, **318**, 1005–12, 1988.

Personally relevant mental stress may be an important precipitant of myocardial ischemia – often silent – in patients with coronary artery disease. Further examination of the pathophysiologic mechanisms responsible for myocardial ischemia induced by mental stress could have important implications for the treatment of transient myocardial ischemia. (N Engl J Med 1988; 318:1005–12.)

Recent research indicates that transient myocardial ischemia is common in patients with coronary artery disease. It usually occurs without symptoms,[1–5] at low heart rates,[3–7] and has a circadian rhythm that parallels changes in heart rate, blood, pressure, and the release of catecholamines.[7,8] Other evidence suggests that mental stress – like physical stress – may be associated with myocardial ischemia.[9,10] It is currently unknown whether ischemia is a direct consequence of mental activities or a spontaneous or independent phenomenon. Laboratory studies involving the provocation of myocardial ischemia by mental stress are needed to confirm such a causal relation.

Studies involving positron-emission tomography have demonstrated that a wide variety of physiologic stimuli, including physical exercise,[11] exposure to cold temperature,[11] smoking,[12] and nonspecific forms of mental stress,[13] can induce transient ischemia in selected patients with coronary artery disease. These studies have not determined whether nonspecific mental arousal or specific forms of mental stress (e.g., anxiety-provoking stress) induce myocardial ischemia. Delineation of this issue could have important implications for both understanding the mechanisms of transient ischemia and developing new therapeutic interventions. Accordingly, we studied the comparative pathophysiologic effects of different forms of mental stress in a group of patients with coronary artery disease. We used radionuclide ventriculography, a sensitive and widely available method of assessing ischemia.

Methods

Patient population

We chose two groups of patients for testing. The group with coronary artery disease consisted of 39 patients (35 men and 4 women; mean age, 61.5 years; age range, 39 to 84) who had either previously confirmed coronary artery disease (demonstrated by angiography or myocardial infarction) or a high pretest probability of coronary artery disease according to analysis of age, sex, symptoms, and results of exercise tests.[14] Thirty-three of these patients had angiographically documented coronary artery disease – 25 within one year of testing. Each of the six uncatheterized patients in this group had a high pretest probability of coronary disease. A control group consisted of 12 patients (11 men; mean age, 48.5 years; age range, 28 to 70) with a low (<5 percent) probability of coronary disease according to serial Bayesian analysis.[15] Patients with noncoronary heart disease were not included in the study.

Test protocol

Testing was usually performed betwen the hours of 11 a.m. and 5 p.m. Patients were asked to refrain from taking beta-blocking medication for 48 hours before testing, calcium-channel blockers for 24 hours before testing, and long-acting nitrates on the day of testing. Testing was performed in the nine patients who did not comply with this request, however (four did not comply at their physicians' request, and five did not follow instructions adequately). After giving written informed consent, the patients were injected with technetium-99m–labeled (in vitro) red cells. When imaging was performed during mental-stress testing, the patients were positioned with the upper torso semierect (i.e., at approximately a 45-degree angle); when imaging was performed during bicycle exercise, the patients were upright.

Relaxation phase

After an initial 5-minute left anterior oblique radionuclide ventriculogram was obtained, each patient was asked to relax for 12 to 15 minutes with the room lights off. At the end of this period, two additional 2-minute base-line resting studies were obtained.

Mental-task phase

Patients performed a series of four tasks involving mental stress, each lasting three to five minutes, with a rest period of seven minutes between tasks. Serial two-minute radionuclide ventriculograms were obtained at the end of each rest period and during the performance of each task, beginning 30 to 60 seconds after the starting time. Patients rated each task according to six factors (interest, tension, anger, anxiety, mental arousal, and degree of challenge) on a 5-point scale, ranging from 1 (none) to 5 (very much). The four mental tasks are described below.

Mental arithmetic Each patient was instructed to subtract serial 7s from a four-digit number for five minutes, as quickly and as accurately as possible, and was prompted periodically to increase speed and accuracy. This task is a standard cognitive mental challenge.

Stroop color–word task   Like the arithmetic task, this one is a cognitive challenge involving an element of frustration.[16] Each patient was shown a rapidly changing series of slides for three minutes. The slides displayed the names of colors (e.g., green), each written in letters of a nonmatching color (e.g., blue). The patients were required to state out loud the color used for the word display rather than the word itself.

Simulated public speaking   This task was chosen to be more personally relevant and emotionally arousing – hence, a more natural stress inducer. Patients were asked to give a five-minute speech in front of two observers. They were instructed to talk specifically and honestly about personal faults or undesirable habits with which they were dissatisfied.

Reading   This task was introduced into the series of stress-inducing tasks after the testing of the eighth recruited patient was completed. Each patient was given a prose passage on a neutral topic to read out loud for three minutes. Performed after the speech task, this task was designed to assess the physiologic influence of impersonal speech that is not emotionally arousing.

Exercise phase

After the mental tasks, each patient was positioned on an upright bicycle ergometer, and another imaging study at rest was obtained. Patients performed graded exercise, with workload increases of 200 kp·m (2000 J) per minute every three minutes. Patients exercised to the point of exhaustion or marked chest pain. Radionuclide imaging was performed during the last two minutes of each three-minute stage of exercise and immediately after exercise.

Data acquisition

R-wave–synchronized, multiple-gated equilibrium radionuclide ventriculography was performed at 20 frames per cycle with use of a mobile gamma camera equipped with a 1/4-inch sodium iodide crystal and an all-purpose collimator.[17] Imaging was performed with the camera positioned in the left anterior oblique angle that best separated the left and right ventricles. The two-minute imaging (used throughout the study) resulted in approximately 100,000 counts per frame. Cardiac rhythm, ST segments, and heart rate were continuously monitored. During mental tasks, blood pressure was monitored at two-minute intervals with use of an automated blood-pressure cuff; during exercise, it was monitored at three-minute intervals with use of a standard mercury sphygmomanometer.

Data interpretation

The left ventricular ejection fraction and segmental wall motion were determined for each resting condition and intervention. A computer operator blinded to the clinical data determined ejection-fraction values, using light-pen assignment of end-diastolic, end-systolic, and background regions.[17] Decreases in the ejection fraction were considered significant when peak values decreased by more than 5 percentage points during stress – a value above the variability expected in repeated calculations of the ejection fraction.[18,19] Segmental wall motion was assessed visually through observation of a continuous-loop video display of the images after algorithms were applied to achieve spatial and temporal smoothing of the data. The video format involved an eight-image display (two rows of four images) in which the first two images were initial resting images and the subsequent six were images obtained either during or before a task and intermixed in random order. Wall motion was scored according to the consensus of two of us who are experienced observers, who viewed the images concurrently. The observers were blinded to the clinical data and did not know which images represented control studies and which task studies. The mental-task studies were interpreted before the exercise studies. For wall-motion scoring, the left ventricle was divided into five segments (two septal, one apical, and two posterolateral), each graded on a 5-point scale: 3 (normal wall motion), 2 (mild hypokinesis), 1 (moderate to severe hypokinesis), 0 (akinesis), and -1 (dyskinesis).[18] The reliability of wall-motion scoring was excellent among 84 randomly selected images (420 segments) read twice by our observers during the interpretation of 33 patient studies: agreement was 88 percent (weighted kappa, mean [±SE] 0.86 ± 0.02).[20] Segmental wall motion was considered to have worsened when the peak score decreased $\geqslant 1$ from both the initial base-line score and the immediately preceding resting score.

Electrocardiographic ST-segment depression was measured at 0.08 second from the J point, with an abnormal response defined as $\geqslant 1$ mm of induced horizontal or downsloping, or $\geqslant 1.5$ mm of upsloping, ST-segment depression.

Exercise-redistribution thallium scintigraphy

Twenty-seven of the 39 patients with coronary disease underwent tomographic (23 patients) or planar (4 patients) exercise-redistribution thallium-201 scintigraphy during the three months before mental-stress testing. All had one or more reversible thallium-perfusion defects. These defects were designated either anterior or posterior,[21,22] and their locations were compared with those of the worst wall-motion abnormalities induced by mental stress.

Coronary arteriography

Selective coronary cineangiography was performed in multiple views with use of the Judkins technique. Serious stenosis was considered present when there was a narrowing of the diameter of a major coronary vessel by ≥50 percent. The presence and location of regional wall-motion abnormalities and coronary stenoses were compared, as described elsewhere,[23] in the 25 patients who had undergone angiography within one year of testing.

Statistical analysis of data

The distribution of categorical variables were compared with use of the chi-square or Fisher's exact test. Variables between the tasks were compared on complete data sets with use of Friedman's analysis of variance for repeated measures.[24,25] Adjusted pairwise comparisons were made with Tukey's procedure applied to the ranks. For continuous or ordinal variables, samples were compared with use of the t-test or Wilcoxon signed-rank test (for dependent samples) or the t-test or Wilcoxon rank-sum test (for independent samples). Analysis of the difference in the frequency of wall-motion abnormality between the tasks was performed with use of Cochran's test.[25] The significance level for all tests (two-tailed) was 0.05. Since the reading task was added after the testing of the eighth patient, analyses of variance were performed with and without this task; the results were essentially the same. P values based on the test results for the larger patient sample (reading task excluded) are reported.

Results

Segmental wall-motion responses

Wall-motion abnormalities developed in 29 of the 39 patients with coronary disease (74 percent) during exercise and in 21 of those 29 patients (72 percent) during mental stress. Figure 1 shows still-frame scintigraphic images of worsening of wall motion during a mental task. Of the 10 patients with normal wall motion during exercise, 2 had dysfunction induced by a mental task; the peak heart rate during exercise in both

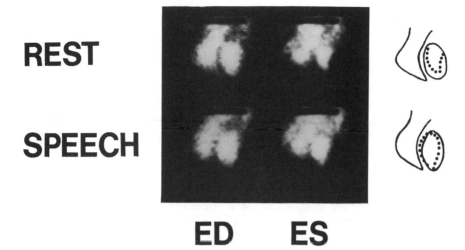

Figure 1. Comparative left anterior oblique scintigrams in a patient who had worsening of left ventricular segmental wall motion while speaking about feelings of personal stress concerning his problems in caring for his family. The images shown were obtained during rest (top) and during the speaking task (bottom). Shown are the end-diastolic (ED) images (left), end-systolic (ES) images (middle), and superimposed ED and ES edges (right). During speech, frank dyskinesis (abnormal outward motion during systole) developed in the septum.

these patients was less than 85 percent of the maximal predicted rate. Four others with normal wall motion during exercise also had less than 85 percent of the maximal predicted heart rate. Two of the 12 control patients had wall-motion abnormalities, induced in one patient by exercise and in the other by a mental task.

Perfusion imaging and angiographic correlations

Of the 23 patients with coronary disease who had wall-motion abnormalities during mental stress (Group 1), 17 underwent thallium testing. Among these 17, reversible thallium defects corresponded with the location of mental-stress–induced wall-motion abnormalities that developed within a single vascular distribution (10 patients) and with the location of the most severe wall-motion abnormality if it developed in multiple vascular distributions (the other 7 patients). Wall-motion abnormalities induced by mental stress always occurred within the distribution of stenosed coronary arteries in the 18 Group 1 patients who underwent coronary angiography.

Clinical predictors

We divided the patients with coronary disease into two groups according to their responses to mental tasks. The 23 patients (59 percent) with wall-motion abnormalities during mental tasks were assigned to Group 1, and the 16 (41 percent) without such abnormalities to Group 2. The clinical characteristics of the two groups are shown in Table 1. There were no statistically significant differences between the groups with respect to these characteristics, although patients in Group 2 had a somewhat lower frequency of typical angina and were somewhat more likely to have never experienced chest pain. Among the 29 patients with exercise-induced wall-motion abnormalities, a small inverse relation was noted between the magnitude of a mental-stress–induced wall-motion abnormality and the stage of exercise at which a wall-motion abnormality first occurred (Spearman's rho = -0.43).

Comparison of tasks

Figure 2 shows the frequency and magnitude of wall-motion abnormalities that occurred in the 21 patients from Group 1 who had abnormalities both during one or more mental tasks and during exercise. Both the frequency and magnitude of wall-motion abnormalities induced by the speech task significantly exceeded those of the abnormalities induced by the other mental tasks ($P < 0.05$). The magnitude of abnormality induced during speech was not significantly different from that induced during exercise (P not significant).

Responses of left ventricular ejection fraction

Table 2 shows the ejection-fraction changes that occurred during mental tasks and exercise in the two groups of patients with coronary disease and in the control group. Ejection-fraction responses varied widely during mental stress, ranging from a decrease of 21 percent to an increase of 6 percent among the patients with coronary disease. Decreases in ejection fraction of more than 5 percentage points occurred during 22 mental tasks in 14 of the 39 patients with coronary disease (36 percent) but during no tasks in the control patients ($P = 0.005$). Regional wall-motion abnormalities were observed during 19 of the 22 tasks (86 percent) associated with a decline in ejection fraction of more than 5 percentage points.

Chest pain and electrocardiographic abnormality

The induction of chest pain or electrocardiographic abnormalities during mental tasks occurred exclusively in association with the worsening of

Table 1. *Characteristics of the patients with coronary artery disease who did and did not have wall-motion abnormalities (WMA) during mental tasks*

	Group 1 – WMA present (N = 23)	Group 2 – WMA absent (N = 16)
Age (yr, mean ±SD)	63.1 ± 11.9	59.1 ± 11.3
Characteristic	*No. of patients(%)*	
Symptom class		
Typical angina	14 (61)	6 (38)
Atypical angina	3 (13)	3 (19)
Nonanginal pain	2 (9)	0 (0)
Asymptomatic	4 (17)	7 (44)
Chest-pain frequency		
Never	4 (17)	7 (44)
≤1 Episode/day	14 (61)	6 (40)
2 to 3 Episodes/day	5 (22)	1 (7)
>3 Episodes/day	0 (0)	1 (7)
Precipitants of chest pain		
None	4 (17)	7 (44)
Exercise only	9 (39)	4 (25)
Mental stress only	1 (4)	1 (6)
Both mental stress and exercise	9 (39)	4 (25)
Long-term anti-ischemia drugs		
None	5 (22)	3 (19)
Nitrates	2 (9)	3 (19)
Calcium blockers	9 (39)	6 (38)
Beta-blockers*	5 (22)	2 (13)
Calcium and beta-blockers*	2 (9)	2 (13)
Taking drugs during testing (n = 9)	7†	2
Angiographic extent of coronary disease		
3 Vessels or left main vessel	7 (47)	4 (40)
2 Vessels	4 (27)	4 (40)
1 Vessel	4 (27)	2 (20)

*P not significant for the frequency and magnitude of wall-motion abnormalities induced by mental stress in eight patients who stopped taking beta-blockers, as compared with those not receiving or still taking beta-blockers.

†Two patients taking beta-blockers, four taking calcium blockers, and one taking both.

wall motion. These abnormalities were relatively infrequent, however. There was electrocardiographic evidence of ischemia in only 6 of the 23 Group 1 patients (23 percent), and chest pain occurred in only 4 (17 percent). Like the worsening of wall motion, the ischemic electrocardiographic responses occurred more commonly and with greater magnitude

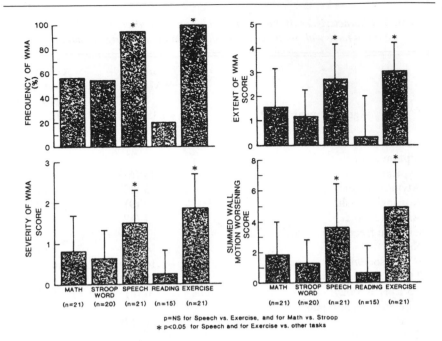

Figure 2. Exercise-induced wall-motion abnormalities (WMA) and their worsening in 21 group 1 patients with coronary disease. The top left graph illustrates the comparative frequency of wall-motion abnormalities (vertical axis) during each of the mental tasks and exercise (horizontal axis). The other three graphs summarize three indexes of wall-motion worsening for each of the mental tasks and exercise. The score for the extent of WMA (vertical axis, top right graph) represents the number of left ventricular segments in which worsening of wall motion occurred during stress. The score for the severity of WMA (vertical axis, bottom left graph) represents the change in score for the segment demonstrating the greatest degree of worsening. Summed wall-motion worsening (vertical axis, bottom right graph) integrates the extent and severity of the indexes. It represents the difference in the summed wall-motion score for the five left ventricular segments between rest and the performance of each task. Each bar represents the mean value ±SD. The wall-motion abnormalities induced by the speech task were more frequent, extensive, and severe than those associated with the other mental tasks and were comparable to those induced by exercise.

during the speech task (Fig. 3), as did chest pain (in four patients during the speech task and in one during the arithmetic task).

Heart rate and blood-pressure responses

The hemodynamic responses during the mental tasks and exercise in the Group 1 patients with coronary disease are shown in Figure 4. Although the heart rate increased during the mental tasks, the magnitude of the increase was much less than that during exercise ($P < 0.05$ for exercise vs.

Table 2. *Ejection-fraction changes in all groups of patients**

Patient Group	Arithmetic	Stroop	Speech	Reading†	Exercise
Controls (n = 12)	1.4 ± 4.6% [−5 to +9%] (12)	0.4 ± 2% [−3 to +4%] (11)	−1.1 ± 2.9% [−4 to +6%] (12)	1.1 ± 3.2% [−4 to +7%] (12)	11.6 ± 8%‡ [+4 to +20%] (12)
Patients with CAD§					
Group 1 (n = 23)	−1.8 ± 5.7% [−21 to +5%] (23)	−4.3 ± 5.4% [−20 to +2%] (21)	−5.0 ± 5.7%¶ [−17 to +6%] (23)	0.4 ± 2.3% [−3 to +5%] (16)	−2.0 ± 9.7% [−26 to +13%] (23)
Group 2 (n = 16)	0.5 ± 3.3% [−4 to +6%] (16)	0.3 ± 3.2% [−5 to +6%] (16)	−0.1 ± 3.5% [−6 to +6%] (16)	−0.1 ± 2.7% [−5 to +4%] (14)	3.4 ± 9.0% [−10 to +20%] (16)

*Plus–minus values represent means ± SD. Values in brackets represent ranges, and those in parentheses indicate numbers of patients.
†Excluded from analyses of variance.
‡P < 0.05 as compared with all mental tasks.
§CAD denotes coronary artery disease.
¶P < 0.05 as compared with the arithmetic task.

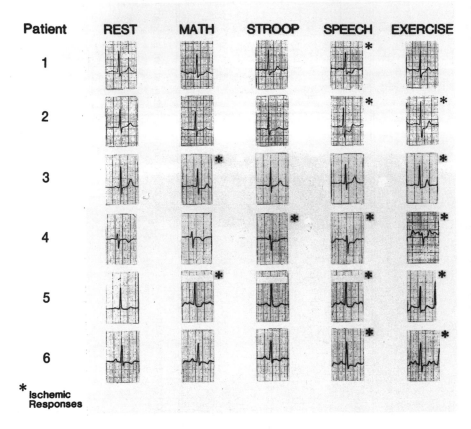

Figure 3. The electrocardiograms obtained during rest, mental tasks, and exercise in the six group 1 patients with an ischemic electrocardiographic response during one or more mental tasks. Note that an ischemic response occurred more frequently during the speaking task. The different electrocardiographic responses during speech and exercise in Patient 1 (2-mm downsloping ST-segment depression vs. none, respectively) occurred despite a slightly higher heart rate during exercise, exemplifying the variable heart-rate threshold for ischemia during mental stress and exercise.

each mental task). In contrast, the difference between elevations of systolic blood pressure during mental tasks and during exercise was relatively small (P not significant for each mental task vs. exercise), and the response of diastolic blood pressure during mental tasks was greater (P < 0.05 for arithmetic and for speech vs. exercise). There were only minor differences in the hemodynamic responses during the mental tasks.

In 10 patients from Group 1, the onset of an exercise-induced wall-motion abnormality occurred after the first stage of exercise. In these patients, an accurate heart-rate and blood-pressure threshold for the development of exercise-induced ischemia could be determined. During

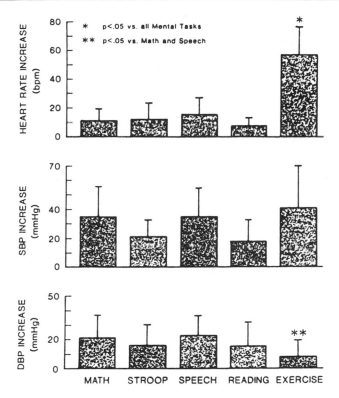

Figure 4. Differences from control levels in the mean heart rate (top graph), systolic blood pressure (SBP) (middle graph), and diastolic blood pressure (DBP) (lower graph) in the group 1 patients during each of the four mental tasks and exercise.

mental tasks, both the mean peak (±SD) heart rate (64 ± 6 vs. 94 ± 16, $P < 0.001$) and double product ($11,297 \pm 1875$ vs. $17,465 \pm 3484$, $P = 0.001$) were markedly lower than the exercise thresholds for ischemic onset. In contrast, comparable systolic blood pressure (176 ± 27 vs. 190 ± 19 mm Hg, $P = 0.19$) combined with significantly higher diastolic blood pressure (109 ± 10 vs. 97 ± 11 mm Hg, $P < 0.05$) resulted in mean arterial blood pressures that were similar during mental tasks and the threshold for exercise-induced ischemia (131 ± 13 vs. 128 ± 8 mm Hg, $P = 0.45$).

Task ratings

Although the speech task clearly induced more ischemic abnormalities, the patients did not report affective differences. They tended to rate the math, Stroop color–word, and speech tasks as similarly tension-producing, anxiety-provoking, arousing, and challenging (P not significant, according to analysis of variance for each affective rating). In contrast, the patients viewed the reading task as significantly less stressful (P < 0.05 for each affective rating vs. that for other tasks).

Discussion

Our results suggest a causal association between acute mental stress and myocardial ischemia – often silent – in patients with coronary artery disease. Thus, 23 of our 39 patients with coronary disease (59 percent) had cardiac wall-motion abnormalities during mental stress at levels designed to simulate those encountered in daily life. Remarkably, the magnitude of abnormality induced by the most potent mental stress was not significantly different from that induced by vigorous exercise in the same patients. These data are particularly important because they may help to explain the link between mental stress and the occurrence of catastrophic cardiac events in patients with coronary artery disease – a link that has been observed but not understood for many years.[26–32]

Neither symptoms nor other historical variables were indicators that certain patients with coronary disease would have myocardial ischemia during mental stress. Such ischemia occurred in patients with no symptoms as well as in those with typical angina. Among the patients with exercise-induced ischemia, we observed a wide range of responses to mental stress, from the absence of abnormalities to abnormalities exceeding in magnitude those induced by exercise.

Our results emphasize the importance of using a sensitive tool to measure the effects of mental stress in the laboratory. In our study, radionuclide ventriculography was much more sensitive in detecting mental-stress–induced ischemia than electrocardiography, which has been used alone in most previously reported laboratory studies.[33–35] Radionuclide ventriculography is a common imaging technique that can be used to compare a patient's responses during serial mental-stress stimuli and stages of exercise after a single injection of radioactive material. Although it is not generally available, positron-emission tomography may also be used to assess myocardial ischemia during a variety of mentally stressful activities.[13]

A question could be raised about whether the ventriculographic abnormalities induced by mental stress represent myocardial ischemia. In patients with known coronary artery disease, in whom the prevalence of myocardial ischemia is high, a positive result in a test with moderately high sensitivity and specificity is very likely to indicate myocardial ischemia.[36,37] The ischemic causation of the mental-stress–induced segmental wall-motion abnormalities in our study is indicated both by their anatomical correspondence with thallium-perfusion defects and by the occurrence of these abnormalities within the distribution of stenosed coronary arteries. Declines in ejection fraction of more than 5 percentage points were probably also ischemic in origin, since they were highly associated with regional wall-motion abnormalities. Such decreases in ejection fraction were not observed in any control patient. The worsening of wall motion in one control during mental tasks and in another during exercise probably represents false positive responses.[36,37]

Recent ambulatory electrocardiographic studies have suggested that transient myocardial ischemia occurs more frequently during periods of mental stress.[9,10] The similarities in the characteristics of transient ischemia between those observed during ambulatory monitoring and those observed during laboratory-induced mental stress are striking: during both, the ischemia is predominantly "silent" (i.e. the patients have no chest pain) and occurs at heart rates well below the threshold for ischemia during exercise testing.[3-7]

Possible pathophysiologic mechanisms

Although the heart rate at the onset of ischemia was lower during mental stress than during exercise, the myocardial oxygen demand may be higher during mental stress than this single factor suggests. There were substantial increases in systolic and diastolic blood pressure during mental stress, elevating the afterload to levels observed during exercise. Mental stress also induces catecholamine secretion,[38-40] which has direct effects on myocardial contractility. Unrecognized factors such as the rate of the rise in catecholamine levels, possibly more rapid during mental stress than during exercise, have not been addressed as determinants of myocardial oxygen demand. With respect to coronary blood supply, transient vasoconstriction in stenosed coronary arteries has been observed during both mental stress[41] and exercise.[42] Whether this vasoconstriction is greater with either form of stress has not been evaluated.

Comparison of mental-stress inducers

An important element of our study design was the use of a series of inducers of mental stress. They were designed to determine whether nonspecific arousal provided by all the stress inducers or specific forms of mental stress (e.g., arithmetic or more emotionally charged public speaking) were as likely to induce myocardial ischemia in patients with coronary disease. We found that the personally relevant public-speaking task produced the most frequent and greatest abnormality according to all markers of ischemia. The specific psychological features of this task may account for its greater ability to induce ischemia: both public speaking and emotional recall are potent forms of stress.[43,44] The pathophysiologic links between specific mental tasks and ischemia may relate to levels of catecholamine and cortisol, which have been found to be higher in some states of mental arousal (e.g., apprehension and uncertainty) than in others.[10,32,38,39]

Since the public-speaking task followed the arithmetic and Stroop tasks, we cannot exclude the possibility that a task-ordering effect was partly responsible for these observations. This is unlikely, however, since in 9 of the 23 patients with wall-motion abnormalities induced by mental stress (39 percent), an abnormal response to one mental task was followed by a lesser response during a subsequent task, despite the generally similar hemodynamic responses. Moreover, the reading task, which followed the speech task, elicited virtually no ischemic response.

Implications

The clinical implications of our findings are potentially far-reaching. Whereas previous reports of transient myocardial ischemia during ambulatory electrocardiography suggested the existence of "spontaneous" myocardial ischemia, our results point toward a possible causal link between such episodes and mental stress occurring in daily life. Accordingly, variations in the stress of daily life may be an important determinant of the unexplained variability in the frequency of transient myocardial ischemia during serial ambulatory monitoring. Mental stress can also lower ventricular fibrillatory thresholds and promote ventricular ectopy.[45-49] Since mental stress may occur more frequently than stress from exercise in daily life, it could represent an important and largely unrecognized factor in the precipitation of more severe clinical coronary events.

Acknowledgements

Supported in part by a grant to Dr. Rozanski from the Health and Behavior Network of the John D. and Catherine T. MacArthur Foundation, a Specialized Centers of Research grant (17651) from the National Institutes of Health, and a Uniformed Services University of the Health Sciences research protocol (R07233). During this study, Dr. Rozanski was the Midcareer Sabbatical Fellow of the MacArthur Research Network on the Determinants and Consequences of Health-Damaging and Health-Promoting Behavior.

We are indebted to Dr. James Forrester for his review and suggestions regarding the manuscript; to Drs. Judith Rodin, Herbert Weiner, David Shapiro, and other members of the MacArthur Foundation Research Network on Health and Behaviour for their advice; to Drs. Charles Kleeman, Andrew Baum, and Alan Waxman, and to Norma Cousins; to Ceia Collins, M.S., for programming,

Dwana Williams, Malcolm Smith, and Susanna Montes for word processing, and Lance Laforteza for illustrations.

References

1. Stern S, Tzivoni D. Early detection of silent ischaemic heart disease by 24-hour electrocardiographic monitoring of active subjects. Br Heart J 1974; 36:481–6.
2. Allen RD, Gettes LS, Phalan C, Avington MD. Painless ST-segment depression in patients with angina pectoris; correlation with daily activities and cigarette smoking. Chest 1976; 69:467–73.
3. Schang SJ Jr, Pepine CJ. Transient asymptomatic S-T segment depression during daily activity. Am J Cardiol 1977; 39:396–402.
4. Deanfield JE, Maseri A, Selwyn AP, et al. Myocardial ischaemia during daily life in patients with stable angina: its relation to symptoms and heart rate changes. Lancet 1983; 2:753–8.
5. Cecchi AC, Dovellini EV, Marchi F, Pucci P, Santoro GM, Fazzini PF. Silent myocardial ischemia during ambulatory electrocardiographic monitoring in patients with effort angina. J Am Coll Cardiol 1983; 1:934–9.
6. Carboni GP, Celli P, D'Ermo M, Santoboni A, Zanchi E. Combined cardiac cinefluoroscopy, exercise testing and ambulatory ST-segment monitoring in the diagnosis of coronary artery disease: a report of 104 symptomatic patients. Int J Cardiol 1985; 9:91–101.
7. Quyyumi AA, Mockus L, Wright C, Fox KM. Morphology of ambulatory ST segment changes in patients with varying severity of coronary artery disease: investigation of the frequency of nocturnal ischaemia and coronary spasm. Br Heart J 1985; 53:186–93.
8. Rocco MB, Barry J, Campbell S, et al. Circadian variation of transient myocardial ischemia in patients with coronary artery disease. Circulation 1987; 75:395–400.
9. Rebecca GS, Wayne RR, Campbell S, et al. Transient ischemia in coronary disease is associated with mental arousal during daily life. J Am Coll Cardiol 1986; 7:239. abstract.
10. Freeman LJ, Nixon PG, Sallabank P, Reaveley D. Psychological stress and silent myocardial ischemia. Am Heart J 1987; 114:477–82.
11. Deanfield JE, Shea M, Ribiero P, et al. Transient ST-segment depression as a marker of myocardial ischemia during daily life. Am J Cardiol 1984; 54:1195–1200.
12. Deanfield JR, Shea MJ, Wilson RA, Horlock P, de Landsheere CM, Selwyn AP. Direct effects of smoking on the heart: silent ischemic disturbances of coronary flow. Am J Cardiol 1986; 57:1005–9.
13. Deanfield JE, Kensett M, Wilson RA, et al. Silent myocardial ischemia due to mental stress. Lancet 1984; 2:1001–4.
14. Diamond GA, Forrester JS, Hirsch M, et al. Application of conditional probability analysis to the clinical diagnosis of coronary artery disease. J Clin Invest 1980; 65:1210–21.
15. Rozanski A, Diamond GA, Forrester JS, Berman DS, Morris D, Swan HJC.

Alternative referent standards for cardiac normality: implications for diagnostic testing. Ann Intern Med 1984; 101:164–71.

16. Stirling, N. Stroop interference: an input and an output phenomenon. Q J Exp Psychol 1979; 31:121–32.

17. Rozanski A, Berman D, Gray R, et al. Preoperative prediction of reversible myocardial asynergy by postexercise radionuclide ventriculography. N Engl J Med 1982; 307:212–6.

18. Maddahi J, Berman DS, Diamond GA, Shah PK, Gray RJ, Forrester JS. Evaluation of left ventricular ejection fraction and segmental wall motion by multiple-gated equilibrium cardiac blood pool scintigraphy. In: Cady LD Jr, ed. Computer techniques in cardiology. New York: Marcel Dekker, 1978:389–416.

19. Folland ED, Hamilton GW, Larson SM, Kennedy JW, Williams DL, Ritchie JL. The radionuclide ejection fraction: a comparison of three radionuclide techniques with contrast angiography. J Nucl Med 1977; 18:1159–66.

20. Fleiss JL. Statistical methods for rates and proportions. 2nd ed. New York: John Wiley, 1981:217–25.

21. Prigent FM, Maddahi J, Garcia E, et al. Thallium-201 stress-redistribution myocardial rotational tomography: development of criteria for visual interpretation. Am Heart J 1985; 109:274–81.

22. Reisman S, Berman D, Maddahi J, Swan HJ. The severe stress thallium defect: an indicator of critical coronary stenosis. Am Heart J 1985; 110:128–34.

23. Morris DD, Rozanski A, Berman DS, Diamond GA, Swan HJC. Noninvasive prediction of the angiographic extent of coronary artery disease after myocardial infarction: comparison of clinical, bicycle exercise electrocardiographic, and ventriculographic parameters. Circulation 1984; 70:192–201.

24. Conover WJ. Practical nonparametric statistics. 2nd ed. New York: John Wiley, 1980:144–70, 299–305.

25. Lehmann EL. Nonparametrics: statistical methods based on ranks. San Francisco, Calif.: Holden-Day, 1975:260–8.

26. Williams J, Edwards G, John Hunter's last pupil. Ann R Coll Surg Engl 1968; 42:69–70. [Quoted in JAMA 1968; 204:806.]

27. Engel GL. Sudden and rapid death during psychological stress. Folklore or folk wisdom? Ann Intern Med 1971; 74:771–82.

28. Greene WA, Goldstein S, Moss AJ. Psychological aspects of sudden death: a preliminary report. Arch Intern Med 1972; 129:725–31.

29. Rahe RH, Romo M, Bennett L, Siltanen P. Recent life changes, myocardial infarction, and abrupt coronary death: studies in Helsinki. Arch Intern Med 1974; 133:221–8.

30. Myers A, Dewar HA. Circumstances attending 100 sudden deaths from coronary artery disease with coroner's necropsies. Br Heart J 1975; 37:1133–43.

31. Dimsdale JE. Emotional causes of sudden death. Am J Psychiatry 1977; 134:1361–6.

32. Krantz DS, Manuck SB. Acute psychophysiologic reactivity and risk of cardiovascular disease: a review and methodologic critique. Psychol Bull 1984; 96:435–64.

33. Schiffer F, Hartley LH, Schulman CL, Abelmann WH. The quiz electrocar-

diogram: a new diagnostic and research technique for evaluating the relation between emotional stress and ischemic heart disease. Am J Cardiol 1976; 37:41–7.

34. Specchia G, de Servi S, Falcone C, et al. Mental arithmetic stress testing in patients with coronary artery disease. Am Heart J 1984; 108:56–63.

35. DeBusk RF, Taylor CB, Agras WS. Comparison of treadmill exercise testing and psychologic stress testing soon after myocardial infarction. Am J Cardiol 1979; 43:907–12.

36. Berman DS, Rozanski A, Knoebel SB. The detection of silent ischaemia: cautions and precautions. Circulation 1987; 75:101–5.

37. Rozanski A, Berman DS. Silent myocardial ischemia. I. Pathophysiology, frequency of occurrence, and approaches toward detection. Am Heart J 1987; 114:615–26.

38. Mason JW. Emotion as reflected in patterns of endocrine integration. In: Levi L, ed. Emotions: their parameters and measurement. New York: Raven Press, 1975:143–81.

39. Frankenhaeuser M. Experimental approaches to the study of catecholamines and emotion. In: Levi L, ed. Emotions: their parameters and measurement. New York: Raven Press, 1975; 209–34.

40. Dimsdale JE, Moss J. Plasma catecholamines in stress and exercise. JAMA 1980; 243:340–2.

41. Rebecca G, Wagner R, Zebede T, et al. Pathogenetic mechanisms causing transient myocardial ischemia with mental arousal in patients with coronary artery disease. Clin Res 1986; 34:338A. abstract.

42. Gordon JB, Zebede J, Wayne RR, Mudge GH, Ganz P, Selwyn AP. Coronary constriction with exercise: possible role for endothelial dysfunction and alpha tone. Circulation 1986; 74:Suppl 2:II–481. abstract.

43. Taggart P, Carruthers M, Somerville W. Electrocardiogram, plasma catecholamines and lipds, and their modification by oxyprenolol when speaking before an audience. Lancet 1973; 2:341–6.

44. Sigler LH. Emotion and atherosclerotic heart disease. 1. Electrocardiographic changes observed on the recall of past emotional disturbances. Br J Med Psychol 1967; 40:55–64.

45. Stevenson IP, Duncan CH, Wolf S, Ripley HS, Wolff HG. Life situations, emotions, and extrasystoles. Psychosom Med 1949; 11:257–72.

46. Lown B, Verrier R, Corbalan R. Psychologic stress and threshold for repetitive ventricular response. Science 1973; 182:834–6.

47. Reich P, DeSilva RA, Lown B, Murawski BJ. Acute psychological disturbances preceding life-threatening ventricular arrhythmias. JAMA 1981; 246:233–5.

48. Skinner JE, Lie JT, Entman ML. Modification of ventricular fibrillation latency following coronary artery occlusion in the conscious pig: the effects of psychological stress and beta-adrenergic blockade. Circulation 1975; 51:656–67.

49. Tavazzi L, Zotti AM, Rondanelli R. The role of psychologic stress in the genesis of lethal arrhythmias in patients with coronary artery disease. Eur Heart J 1986; 7:Suppl A:99–106.

Depressed lymphocyte function after bereavement

R. W. Bartrop, E. Luckhurst, L. Lazarus, L. G. Kiloh and
R. Penny

*Department of Immunology and Garvan Institute for Medical Research,
St. Vincent's Hospital; Department of Medicine and School of Psychiatry,
University of New South Wales; and New South Wales Institute of
Psychiatry, Sydney, Australia*

Summary

During 1975 twenty-six bereaved spouses took part in a detailed prospective
investigation of the effects of severe stress on the immune system. T and B cell
numbers and function, and hormone concentrations were studied approximately 2
weeks after bereavement and 6 weeks thereafter. The response to phytohæmagglutinin was significantly depressed in the bereaved group on the second occasion,
as was the response to concanavalin A at 6 weeks. There was no difference in T
and B cell numbers, protein concentrations, the presence of autoantibodies and
delayed hypersensitivity, and in cortisol, prolactin, growth hormone, and thyroid
hormone assays between the bereaved group and the controls. This is the first
time severe psychological stress has been shown to produce a measurable
abnormality in immune function which is not obviously caused by hormonal
changes.

Introduction

Cell and tissue changes are known to be part of a non-specific response to
stressful stimuli.[1] Stressful physical stimuli in rodents increased their
susceptibility to infection.[2] These findings implied modification of the
immune response, and were attributed to the effects of adrenal corticosteroids. Recent work extending these studies to other species has
implicated the action of other hormones,[3] possibly mediated via lymphocyte receptors.[4]

The experiments in the NASA Skylab Programme,[5] which demonstrated depression of lymphocyte transformation and rosette formation on

Reprinted from Bartrop, R. W., Luckhurst, E., Lazarus, L., Kiloh, L. G. and
Penny, R. Depressed lymphocyte function after bereavement. *Lancet*, i, 834-6,
1977.

the day of splashdown, appear to be the only prospective studies of the effects of stress on the immune system of healthy people. Retrospective investigations of bereavement and other severely stressful situations have been claimed to show an association between stress and many diseases,[6] including diabetes mellitus, coronary-artery disease, ulcerative colitis, rheumatoid arthritis, lupus erythematosus, and schizophrenia. Claims for an increased mortality after conjugal bereavement are controversial. Bereavement is a life event resulting in great distress or the need for considerable adaptation.[7] We determined prospectively the behavioural, endocrinological, and immunological consequences of bereavement.[8]

Methods

Subjects.—Arrangements were made in our group of hospitals for one of us (R. B.) to provide a counselling service for the surviving spouses of patients either fatally injured or who had died from illness. Twenty-six people between the ages of 20 and 65 years[9] were interviewed for the study.

Control group.—This group consisted of twenty-six hospital staff members (not bereaved within the previous 24 months) who were matched for age, sex, and race with a bereaved spouse.

Design of study.—The service and the study were explained to the spouse on the first visit. Further contact was maintained with all families either directly or through ministers of religion or social workers. The first blood-samples were taken 1–3 weeks after bereavement (sample 1) and the second samples obtained 6 weeks later (sample 2). Control subjects had blood-samples taken at the same times for identical laboratory testing.

Physical health.—Each individual received a standardised questionnaire and was excluded if there was a history of recent infection, allergic diathesis, or blood dyscrasia.

Stimulation with mitogens.—Peripheral-blood mononuclear cells were isolated on 'Ficoll-Hypaque'[10] and lymphocyte transformation tests were performed as described elsewhere.[11] Response to phytohæmagglutinin (P.H.A.) was assessed at doses of 10, 20, 100, 200 μg/ml, and to concanavalin A at doses of 1, 5, and 50 μg/ml.

Lymphocyte markers.—E and EAC rosette-forming lymphocytes were detected by methods previously reported.[11]

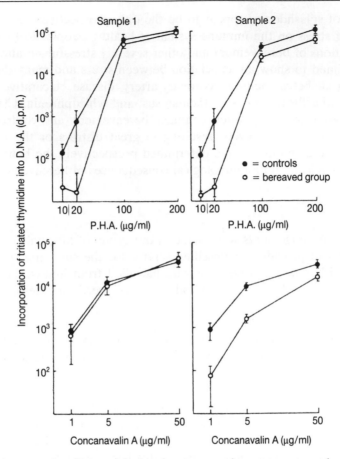

Geometric mean values (±s.e.m.) for lymphocyte responsiveness to P.H.A. and concanavalin A in control and bereaved groups.

Serum-protein concentrations.—Serum protein electrophoresis was performed with a Beckman microzone system. Radial immunodiffusion methods were used to measure serum IgG, IgA, IgM, and α_2-macroglobulin.

Autoantibodies.—Sera were tested for antinuclear factor, mitochondrial, and smooth-muscle antibodies by immunofluorescence techniques. The R.A. latex test was performed for rheumatoid factor.

Delayed skin hypersensitivity.—Twelve bereaved spouses and fourteen control subjects had skin tests with dermatophyton O, streptokinase-streptodornase, mumps antigen, and purified protein derivative of tuberculin.

Hormone assays.—The following were measured by standard radioimmunoassays: thyroxine and triiodothyronine, growth hormone, and cortisol; and prolactin was assayed by a modification of the standard radioimmunoassay with reagents provided by N.I.H. (U.S.A.).

Statistical analysis.—Results of tests of cell-mediated immunity were expressed as the geometric mean (±s.e.m.) values as reported elsewhere.[12] Statistical analysis was carried out by means of the Wilcoxon rank sum test (Mann-Whitney).

Results

Lymphocyte transformation test.—The results of the lymphocyte transformation tests on samples 1 and 2 with p.h.a. and concanavalin A are shown in the accompanying figure. Responses to doses of 10 and 20 µg/ml p.h.a. in sample 2 were strikingly different in the bereaved and control groups ($p < 0.05$). In addition, there was a significant difference between samples 1 and 2 of the spouse group at a dose of 100 µg/ml p.h.a. [. . .] At 6 weeks (sample 2) responsiveness to doses of 5 and 50 µg/ml of concanavalin A in the bereaved group was significantly less than in the control group ($p < 0.05$). In addition, the responsiveness of lymphocytes in samples 1 and 2 of the bereaved group was significantly different at doses of 5 and 50 µg/ml concanavalin A.

Other measures of T and B cell function.—There was no significant difference between the bereaved and control groups in terms of T and B cell numbers, serum protein electrophoresis, immunoglobulins, α_2-macroglobulin concentrations, the presence of autoantibodies, and delayed hypersensitivity.

Hormone assays.—Mean serum concentrations of thyroxine, triiodothyronine, cortisol, prolactin, and growth hormone were no different in the bereaved and control groups.

Discussion

This is the first prospective study of immunological function in healthy people under great psychological stress. We demonstrated that T-cell function was significantly depressed after bereavement (sample 2) in the absence of a change in T-cell numbers as tested by E rosetting. We have not demonstrated abnormal B-cell function, as measured by IgG, IgA, and IgM concentrations, after bereavement, nor any differences in B-cell numbers between the bereaved and control groups, as tested by the EAC rosetting scheme.

Hamburg et al. reported that concentrations of adrenocortical, adrenomedullary, and thyroid hormones were raised for weeks or months at times of great stress and seemed to correlate directly with the degree of distress and inversely with the ability to cope.[3] We did not demonstrate any significant difference in hormone concentrations between the two groups in either sample 1 or sample 2. This would tend to exclude these hormones as mediators of the T-cell functional abnormality that we demonstrated.

A detailed endocrinological analysis was not attempted in the bereaved group, a single blood-sample being used for hormone assays. An extended study will include a more detailed investigation of hormonal responses rather than isolated blood estimations and this will be particularly pertinent in the case of cortisol, but we also intend to continue investigation of other hormones.

For the first time, we have shown prospectively that severe psychological stress can produce a measurable abnormality in immune function. The origin of the defect in T-cell function is being investigated and a more extensive analysis of B-cell function is required. This may give a clue to the genesis of suggested stress-related diseases which have an immunological basis.

References

1. Selye, H. *A Rev. Med.* 1951, **2**, 327.
2. Gisler, R. H., Bussard, A. E., Mazie, I. C., Hess, R. *Cell Immun.* 1971, **2**.
3. Hamburg, D. A., Hamburg, B. A., Barchas, J. D. *in* Emotions: Their Parameters and Measurement (edited by L. Levi); p.232. New York, 1974.
4. Bourne, H. R., Lichtenstein, L. M., Melmon, K. L., Henney, C. S., Weinstein, Y., Shearer, G. M. *Science*, 1974, **184**, 19.
5. Kimzey, S. L. *Acta Astronautica*, 1974, **127**, 1.
6. Solomon, G. F., Amkraut, A. A. *Front Radiat. Ther. Onc.* 1972, **7**, 84.
7. Tennant, C., Andrews, G. *Aust. N.Z. J. Psychiat.* 1976, **10**, 27.
8. Amkraut, A. A., Solomon, G. F. *Int. J. Psychiat. Med.* 1974, **5**, 541.
9. Foad, B. S. I., Adams, L. E., Yamauchi, Y., Litwin, A. *Clin. exp. Immun.* 1974, **17**, 657.
10. Boyum, A. *Scan. J. clin. Lab. Invest.* 1968, **21**, suppl. 97, p. 51.
11. Cooper, D. A., Petts, V., Luckhurst, E., Biggs, J. C., Penny, R. *Br. J. Cancer*, 1975, **31**, 550.
12. Ziegler, J. B., Hansen, P., Penny, R. *Clin. Immun. Immunopath.* 1975, **3**, 451.

Psychological stress and susceptibility to the common cold

Sheldon Cohen, PhD, David A. J. Tyrrell, MD and
Andrew P. Smith, PhD

*From the Department of Psychology, Carnegie Mellon University,
Pittsburgh (S. C.); the Medical Research Council Common Cold Unit,
Salisbury, United Kingdom (D. A. J. T.); and the Health Psychology
Research Unit, University of Wales College of Cardiff, Cardiff,
United Kingdom (A. P. S.)*

Abstract

Background. It is not known whether psychological stress suppresses host resistance to infection. To investigate this issue, we prospectively studied the relation between psychological stress and the frequency of documented clinical colds among subjects intentionally exposed to respiratory viruses.

Methods. After completing questionnaires assessing degrees of psychological stress, 394 healthy subjects were given nasal drops containing one of five respiratory viruses (rhinovirus type 2, 9, or 14, respiratory syncytial virus, or coronavirus type 229E), and an additional 26 were given saline nasal drops. The subjects were then quarantined and monitored for the development of evidence of infection and symptoms. Clinical colds were defined as clinical symptoms in the presence of an infection verified by the isolation of virus or by an increase in the virus-specific antibody titer.

Results. The rates of both respiratory infection (P < 0.005) and clinical colds (P < 0.02) increased in a dose–response manner with increases in the degree of psychological stress. Infection rates ranged from approximately 74 percent to approximately 90 percent, according to levels of psychological stress, and the incidence of clinical colds ranged from approximately 27 percent to 47 percent. These effects were not altered when we controlled for age, sex, education, allergic status, weight, the season, the number of subjects housed together, the infectious status of subjects sharing the same housing, and virus-specific antibody status at base line (before challenge). Moreover, the associations observed were similar for all five challenge viruses. Several potential stress–illness mediators, including smoking, alcohol consumption, exercise, diet, quality of sleep, white-cell counts,

Reprinted from Cohen, S., Tyrrell, D. A. J. and Smith, A. P. Psychological stress and susceptibility to the common cold. *New England Journal of Medicine*, **325**, 606–12, 1991.

and total immunoglobulin levels, did not explain the association between stress and illness. Similarly, controls for personality variables (self-esteem, personal control, and introversion–extraversion) failed to alter our findings.

Conclusions. Psychological stress was associated in a dose–response manner with an increased risk of acute infectious respiratory illness, and this risk was attributable to increased rates of infection rather than to an increased frequency of symptoms after infection. (N Engl J Med 1991; 325:606–12.)

Stressful life events are commonly believed to suppress host resistance to infection. When demands imposed by events exceed a person's ability to cope, a psychological stress response composed of negative cognitive and emotional states is elicited.[1] Psychological stress, in turn, is thought to influence immune function through autonomic nerves innervating lymphoid tissue[2,3] or hormone-mediated alteration of immune cells.[4,5] Stress may also alter immune responses through the adoption of coping behaviors such as increased smoking and alcohol consumption.[6]

There is substantial evidence that stressful life events and perceived stress are associated with changes in immune function.[7–9] Although psychological stress is often described as suppressing immune response, the implications of stress-induced immune changes for susceptibility to disease have not been elucidated.[10,11]

There is some direct evidence from previous studies that psychological stress increases the risk of verified acute infectious respiratory illness.[12–14] These studies, however, did not control for the possible effects of stressful events on exposure to infectious agents (as opposed to their effects on resistance) or provide evidence about other behavioral and biologic mechanisms through which stress might influence a person's susceptibility to infection. Moreover, the literature on this topic is not entirely consistent; several studies have failed to find a relation between stress and respiratory disease.[15,16]

We present data from a prospective study of the association between psychological stress and susceptibility to the common cold. Healthy persons were assessed for degree of stress and then experimentally exposed to one of five cold viruses (394 subjects) or placebo (26 subjects). The association between stress and the development of biologically verified clinical disease was examined with use of control for base-line (prechallenge) serologic status, the identity of the challenge virus, allergic status, weight, the season, the number of subjects housed together, the infectious status of any subjects sharing housing, and various demographic factors. In further analyses we tested the possibility that a relation between stress and susceptibility to illness could be attributed to differences in health practices or differences in base-line white-cell counts or total antibody levels. A final analysis investigated the possibility that differences in personality rather than environmental factors causing stress might account for the association between stress and clinical colds.

Methods

The subjects were 154 men and 266 women who were residents of Britain and who volunteered to participate in trials at the Medical Research Council's Common Cold Unit (CCU) in Salisbury. All reported on their applications that they had no chronic or acute illness and were taking no regular medication; all were judged to be in good health after clinical and laboratory examination on their arrival at the unit. Pregnant women were excluded. The subjects' ages ranged from 18 to 54 years (mean [±SD], 33.6 ± 10.6). Sixty-three percent of the subjects were women. Twenty-two percent had not completed their secondary education, 51 percent had completed secondary school but did not attend a university, and 27 percent had spent at least one year at a university. The subjects were reimbursed for their travel expenses and received free meals and accommodations during the study. The trial was approved by the Harrow District Ethical Committee, and informed consent was obtained from each subject after the nature and possible consequences of the study were fully explained.

Procedures

During their first two days at the CCU, the subjects underwent a thorough medical examination, completed a series of questionnaires related to behavior, psychological stress, personality, and health practices and had blood drawn for immune assessments and measurement of cotinine (a biochemical indicator of smoking) in serum. Subsequently, the subjects were given nasal drops containing a low infectious dose of one of five respiratory viruses – rhinovirus type 2 (n = 86), type 9 (n = 122), or type 14 (n = 92), respiratory syncytial virus (n = 40), or coronavirus type 229E (n = 54) – or saline drops (n = 26). The viral doses were intended to resemble those common in person-to-person transmission and to result in illness rates between 20 and 60 percent. For two days before and seven days after the viral challenge, the subjects were quarantined in large apartments (alone or with one or two others). Starting two days before the viral challenge and continuing through six days after the challenge, each subject was examined daily by a clinician who used a standard checklist of respiratory signs and symptoms.[17] Examples of items on the checklist are sneezing, watering of the eyes, nasal stuffiness, nasal obstruction, postnasal discharge, sinus pain, sore throat, hoarseness, cough, and sputum. The number of facial tissues used daily by each subject was also counted. Approximately 28 days after the challenge, a second serum sample was collected by the subjects' own physicians and shipped to the CCU for serologic testing. All the investigators were blinded to the subjects' psychological status and to whether they had received virus or saline drops.

Psychological-stress index

Three measures of psychological stress were used: the number of major stressful life events judged by the subject as having had a negative impact on his or her psychological state in the past year, the degree to which the subject perceived that current demands exceeded his or her ability to cope, and an index of current negative affect. The list of major stressful life events contained events that might have occurred in the life of the subject (41 items) or those of others close to the subject (26 items). The events were taken from the List of Recent Experiences compiled by Henderson et al.[18] and were chosen because of their potential negative impact and their relatively high frequency in population studies. The score on this life-events scale was the number of events during the previous 12 months that the subject reported as having had a negative impact on his or her life. The 10-item Perceived Stress Scale[19] was used to assess the degree to which situations in life were perceived as stressful (reliability, $\alpha = 0.85$).[20] Items on the Perceived Stress Scale were designed to measure the degree to which the subjects felt their lives were unpredictable, uncontrollable, and overwhelming. Finally, the negative-affect scale included 15 items from Zevon and Tellegen's list of negative emotions[21]: "distressed," "nervous," "sad," "angry," "dissatisfied with self," "calm" (scored negatively), "guilty," "scared," "angry at yourself," "upset," "irritated," "depressed," "hostile," "shaky," and "content" (scored negatively). Each subject was asked to indicate the intensity of each feeling during the past week on a five-point scale ranging from 0 to 4 (reliability, $\alpha = 0.84$).

All three stress scales formed a single principal component with loadings of 0.66, 0.86, and 0.86, providing evidence that the scales measured a common underlying concept.[22] An index combining the three measures was therefore used as an indicator of the degree of psychological stress experienced by the subjects (stress index). Because life events were not distributed normally, an index based on normalized scores was not appropriate. Instead, the index was created by calculating the quartiles for each scale and summing the quartile ranks for each subject (assigning a value of 1 for the lowest quartile and 4 for the highest); the resulting stress index ranged from 3 to 12. The quartiles divided the subjects into groups with the values 0, 1 through 2, 3 through 4, and 5 through 14 for the life-events scale; 0 through 10, 11 through 14, 15 through 18, and 19 through 33 for the Perceived Stress Scale; and 0 through 7, 8 through 13, 14 through 20, and 21 through 49 for the negative-affect scale. The index scores were approximately normally distributed. In all cases, a higher score indicated a greater degree of stress.

Viral isolates and virus-specific antibody levels

Nasal-wash samples were collected for viral isolation before inoculation and on days 2 through 6 after inoculation. They were mixed with broth and stored in aliquots at −70°C. Rhinoviruses were detected in O-HeLa cells, respiratory syncytial virus in HEp-2 cells, and coronavirus in the C-16 strain of continuous human fibroblast cells. When a characteristic cytopathic effect was observed in the tissue culture, fluids were transferred to further cultures and tests were performed to identify the virus. The identity of rhinoviruses and coronaviruses was confirmed by neutralization tests with specific rabbit immune serum, and that of respiratory syncytial virus by immunofluorescent staining of culture cells.

Levels of neutralizing antibodies and of specific antiviral IgA and IgG were determined before and 28 days after the challenge. Neutralizing antibodies (for rhinoviruses only) were determined by neutralizing tests with homologous virus.[23] The results were recorded as the highest dilution showing neutralization, and a fourfold increase was regarded as significant. Suitable neutralizing tests were not available for respiratory syncytial virus and coronavirus.

Specific IgA and IgG levels for rhinoviruses,[24] coronavirus,[25] and respiratory syncytial virus[25] were determined by enzyme-linked immunosorbent assay. This test detects antibody that correlates with neutralization titers, is associated with resistance to infection, and increases in response to infection.[23]

Infections and clinical colds

A subject was deemed infected if virus was isolated after the challenge or if there was a significant increase over base-line levels in the virus-specific serum antibody titer (i.e., a fourfold increase in neutralizing antibody [rhinoviruses]) or an increase in the IgG or IgA level of more than 2 SD above the mean for the unchallenged subjects (all viruses). Eighty-two percent of the subjects who received virus (325 subjects) were infected. Five subjects who received saline (19 percent) were also infected. We attributed infections in the saline (placebo) group to transmission of virus from infected subjects to others housed in the same apartments. Control for person-to-person transmission was included in the data analysis.

At the end of the trial, a physician judged the severity of each subject's cold on a scale ranging from none (0) to severe (4). Ratings of mild cold (2) or more were considered positive clinical diagnoses. The subjects also rated the severity of their colds on the same scale. The clinical diagnosis was in agreement with the subject's rating in 94 percent of the cases. The subjects were classified as having clinical colds if they both had evidence of infection and were given the diagnosis of a clinical cold. Of the 394 subjects who received virus, 38 percent (148) had clinical colds. None of the 26 subjects who received saline had a cold.

Seven subjects with positive clinical diagnoses but no indication of infection were excluded from the sample because we assumed the illness was caused by exposure to another virus before the trial. Analyses including these seven subjects resulted in conclusions identical to those reported here.

Standard control variables

We used a series of control variables that might provide alternative explanations for the relation between stress and illness. These include serologic status for the experimental virus before the challenge, age, sex, education, allergic status, weight, the season, the number of subjects housed together, whether a subject housed in the same apartment was infected, and the identity of the challenge virus.

Serologic status was defined as positive when a subject had a base-line neutralizing antibody titer above 2 for rhinoviruses and a base-line antibody level greater than the sample median for coronavirus or respiratory syncytial virus. Forty-three percent of the subjects were seropositive before the challenge: 55 percent for rhinovirus type 2, 48 percent for rhinovirus type 9, 20 percent for rhinovirus type 14, 50 percent for respiratory syncytial virus, and 50 percent for coronavirus.

Because age was not normally distributed, it was scored categorically as above or below the median: 18 through 33 years or 34 through 54 years. Education levels were classified on an 8-point scale ranging from no schooling (0) to a doctoral degree (8), as reported by the subjects. Allergic status was determined on the basis of the subjects' answers to questions about allergies to food, drugs, or other allergens. Subjects who reported any allergy were defined as allergic. A ponderal index (the weight divided by the cube of the height) was used to control for subjects' weight. We used the number of hours of daylight on the first day of the trial as a continuous measure of the season. The number of daylight hours is correlated ($r = 0.80$, $P < 0.001$) with the average temperature on the same day. Control for the possibility that person-to-person transmission rather than viral challenge might be responsible for infections or clinical colds was also included. Because person-to-person transmission would have been possible only if a subject sharing the same housing had been infected by the viral challenge, a control variable indicated whether or not any subject sharing the same housing was infected. Finally, the challenge virus was a categorical variable indicating the experimental virus to which a subject was exposed.

Measures of health practice

Health practices – including smoking, alcohol consumption, exercise, quality of sleep, and dietary practices – were assessed as possible factors linking stress and susceptibility. Cotinine measured in serum by gas chromatography was used as a biochemical indicator of the smoking level because it provided an objective measure of nicotine intake that was not subject to reporting bias.[26,27] We used the base-10 logarithm of the average of the two cotinine measures (before and 28 days after challenge) as an indicator of the level of smoking. (The correlation between the two measures was 0.95 [P < 0.001], n = 348].) The correlation between $\log_{10}$ average cotinine level and the $\log_{10}$ number of cigarettes reported as smoked per day was 0.96 (P < 0.001, n = 372).

The remaining health practices were assessed by questionnaire before the viral challenge. The average number of alcoholic drinks per day was calculated on the basis of separate estimates of weekday and weekend drinking. A half-pint, bottle, or can of beer, a glass of wine, and a shot of whiskey contain approximately equal amounts of alcohol, and each was treated as a single drink. The exercise index included items on the frequency of walking, running, jogging, swimming, aerobic exercise, and work around the house. The quality-of-sleep index included items on feeling rested, difficulty falling asleep, and awakening early; and the dietary-habit index was made up of items designed to assess concern with a healthful diet and included the frequency of eating breakfast, fruits, and vegetables.

White-cell counts and total immunoglobulin levels

White-cell counts and total immunoglobulin levels were assessed as possible factors linking psychological stress and susceptibility to illness. Assays were performed in blood samples collected before the viral challenge. White cells were counted with an automatic cell counter, and differential counts (lymphocytes, monocytes, and neutrophils) were calculated from 200 cells in a stained film. Total serum and nasal-wash

IgA and IgE levels and total nasal-wash protein levels were assessed by enzyme-linked immunosorbent assay.[25] We used the base-10 logarithm of each differential count and immunoglobulin measurement.

Measures of personality

Because the degree of psychological stress might reflect stable personality styles rather than responses to environmental factors causing stress, two personality characteristics closely associated with stress – self-esteem and personal control (the expectation that one can control events) – were assessed before the viral challenge. Self-esteem was measured with the self-regard and social-confidence subscales of the Feelings of Inadequacy Scale[28] (reliability, $\alpha = 0.89$) and personal control with the personal-efficacy and inter-personal-control subscales of the Spheres of Control Scale[29] (reliability, $\alpha = 0.76$). A third personality characteristic, the degree of relative introversion or extraversion, was also assessed because some evidence had suggested that introverts were at higher risk for infection.[30,31] This characteristic was assessed with the Eysenck Personality Inventory[32] (reliability, $\alpha = 0.80$).

Statistical analysis

The primary analysis tested whether psychological stress was associated with a higher incidence of clinical colds. Secondary analyses assessed the importance of the two components of the definition of a clinical cold, documented infection and symptoms, in accounting for the association between stress and clinical colds. Specifically, we determined whether the relation between stress and colds was attributable to an increase in infection or to an increase in diagnosed colds among infected persons. The subjects who received saline were not included in these analyses.

Logistic regression was used to predict categorical outcomes.[33] We conducted a series of analyses. In the first stage, only the psychological-stress index was entered as a predictor. In the second, we entered the standard control variables in the initial step of the regression analysis and then tested whether there was a significant change in the log likelihood of a clinical cold when the stress index was added to the equation. Education, weight, the season, and the number of subjects sharing an apartment were entered as continuous variables, and the remainder of the standard controls as dummy (categorical) variables.[33] Because the predictor (the stress-index score) was a continuous variable, we have reported raw regression coefficients (b) and their standard errors.[33] To estimate the sizes of effects, we have also reported odds ratios and their 95 percent confidence intervals, derived from modified regression models in which the continuous stress-index score was replaced with a contrast between the subjects in the bottom and the top quartiles of the stress index. The odds ratio approximates how much more likely it was that the outcome (infection or clinical cold) would be present among those with the highest stress-index scores (top quartile group) than among those with the lowest scores (bottom quartile group).[33]

Additional analyses tested possible roles for immunity, health practices, and personality variables in mediating the relation between stress and clinical colds. In the first analysis, the possibility that white-cell counts, total antibody levels, or five different health practices operated as pathways through which psychological stress influenced the risk of having a clinical cold was assessed by entering these variables along with the standard control variables in the first step of the regression equation and then testing whether adding stress to the equation accounted for a significant change in the log likelihood of illness. In the second analysis, the possibility that the effects of stress might reflect differences in personality rather than reactions to environmental stress factors was assessed by adding first two personality variables associated with stress (self-esteem and personal control) and then another previously associated with susceptibility to infection (introversion–extraversion) to the set of control variables and testing for any additional contribution of stress. All the immune measures, health practices, and personality variables were entered as continuous variables.

Results

Preliminary analysis indicated that there were no statistically reliable interactions between the standard control variables and the stress index in predicting clinical colds (highest t = 1.62, P = 0.11).[33] The relations we report between the stress index and colds were thus similar for the five viruses and for groups defined by serologic status, age, sex, allergic status, education, weight, the number of subjects sharing an apartment, whether another subject in the same housing was infected, and the season.

There were, however, main effects of three standard control variables – serologic status (P < 0.001), the virus (P < 0.001), and whether another subject in the same apartment was infected (P < 0.02). The P value for the remaining variables was >0.20. Subjects who were seronegative at base line had more colds (49.3 percent) than those who were seropositive (22.2 percent). The incidence of colds was 61.1 percent for coronavirus, 42.4 percent for rhinovirus type 14, 37.5 percent for respiratory syncytial virus, 33.6 percent for rhinovirus type 9, and 23.3 percent for rhinovirus type 2. Finally, subjects sharing an apartment with an infected subject

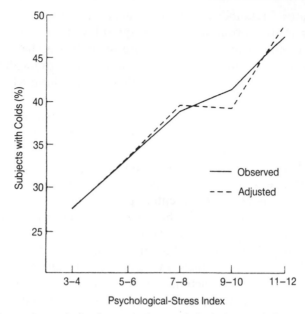

Figure 1. Observed association between the psychological-stress index and the rate of clinical colds and the association adjusted for standard control variables. For an explanation of the psychological-stress index, see the text. Only the 394 subjects who received virus are included.

had more colds (40.9 percent) than those without an infected apartment mate (26.4 percent). Although they were associated with the development of clinical colds, none of these three variables was reliably associated with the stress index (highest F = 1.44, P < 0.22).

As is apparent in Figure 1, the rate of clinical colds increased in a dose–response manner with increases in the stress-index score (b [±SE] = 0.01 ± 0.04, P < 0.02, n = 394; odds ratio for the comparison of the highest and lowest quartile groups = 1.98 [95 percent confidence interval, 1.10 to 3.56]). Moreover, entering the standard control variables into the equation before the stress index (adjusted rates are shown in Fig. 1) did not alter this association (b = 0.10 ± 0.05, P < 0.04, n = 394; odds ratio = 2.16 [95 percent confidence interval, 1.11 to 4.23]).

As is apparent in Figure 2, the rates of infection also increased with increases in the stress index (b = 0.15 ± 0.05, P < 0.005, n = 394; odds ratio for the comparison of the highest and lowest quartile groups = 3.45 [95 percent confidence interval, 1.51 to 7.87]). This relation was similarly unaltered by the inclusion of standard control variables in the equation (b = 0.17 ± 0.06, P < 0.004; odds ratio = 5.81 [95 percent confidence interval, 2.12 to 15.91]). The level of stress was not, however,

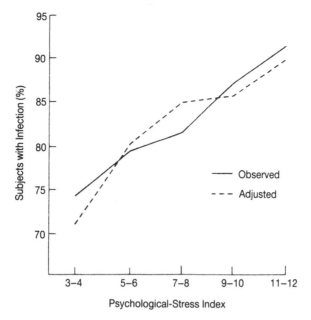

Figure 2. Observed association between the psychological-stress index and the rate of infection and the association adjusted for standard control variables. Only the 394 subjects who received virus are included.

reliably associated with the rate of clinical colds among infected persons ($b = 0.07 \pm 0.04$, $P = 0.13$; including the control variables; $b = 0.06 \pm 0.05$, $P = 0.24$, $n = 325$). Hence, the relation between stress and colds was primarily attributable to an increased rate of infections among subjects with higher stress-index scores, rather than to an increase in clinical colds among infected persons with higher stress scores.

The similar effect of stress at the various levels of each standard control variable (i.e., the lack of interaction between stress and each control variable) has already been mentioned. Of special importance in interpreting this study is the fact that stress had the same effects in all the challenge-virus groups regardless of the infectious status of apartment mates or prechallenge serologic status. The consistent effect of stress among the five viruses is illustrated in Figures 3 and 4, which present the rates of colds and infection (adjusted for standard control variables) according to challenge virus for subjects below the median value of the stress index (low stress) and above the median (high stress). That the effects of stress were similar for all viruses suggests the biologic generality of the effect. Table 1 presents similar data for base-line serologic status and the infectious status of subjects sharing the same apartment. The data on subjects housed together indicate that greater person-to-person

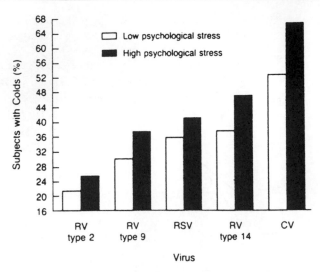

Figure 3. Subjects with low degrees of psychological stress (index values below the median) and high degrees of stress (values above the median) who had colds, according to challenge-virus group. The rates have been adjusted for the standard control variables. RV denotes rhinovirus, RSV respiratory syncytial virus, and CV coronavirus. Only the 394 subjects who received virus are included.

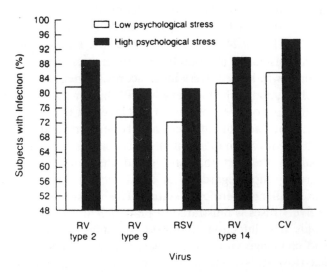

Figure 4. Subjects with low degrees of psychological stress (index values below the median) and high degrees of stress (values above the median) who were infected, according to challenge-virus group. The rates have been adjusted for the standard control variables. RV denotes rhinovirus, RSV respiratory syncytial virus, and CV coronavirus. Only the 394 subjects who received virus are included.

Table 1. *Rates of infection and colds among subjects with high and low stress-index scores, according to prechallenge serologic status and the infectious status of apartment mates**

	Infection		Colds	
	Low stress index	High stress index	Low stress index	High stress index
	incidence (%)			
Prechallenge serologic status				
Positive (n = 171)	67.2	79.8	18.7	25.5
Negative (n = 223)	86.2	92.4	43.7	55.2
Infectious status				
Not infectious (n = 91)	68.7	81.4	20.8	32.6
Infectious (n = 303)	81.2	88.3	37.2	44.6

*Rates of infection and clinical colds have been adjusted for standard control variables. The categorization of low and high degrees of stress is based on whether the subjects' stress-index scores fell below or above the median value. The infectious status of subjects sharing the same housing is considered "infectious" if any person housed with the subject was infected.

transmission among subjects with higher stress-index scores cannot explain the association between stress and colds (such transmission was possible only if the subject had an infected apartment mate). Finally, consistency among groups defined by prechallenge serologic status suggests that if an immune mechanism is the mediator of the relation between stress and colds, it is a primary and not a secondary (immune-memory) mechanism.

Additional analyses tested the possible roles of immunity, health practices, and personality variables in the relation between stress and clinical colds. In the first analysis, we assessed the possibility that measures of white-cell populations (differentials), total immunoglobulin levels, or health practices operate as pathways through which psychological stress is related to clinical illness. These variables were entered together, along with the standard controls, in the first step of a regression equation, with the stress index entered in the second step. The stress index continued to add to the predictive power of the equation even after the additional controls were entered ($b = 0.14 \pm 0.05$, $P < 0.01$). Hence, none of these variables were responsible for the association between stress and illness in this study.

In the second analysis, we assessed the possibility that effects of stress might actually reflect differences in personality rather than reactions to environmental stressors. Two personality variables associated with stress (self-esteem, $r = -0.52$, $P < 0.001$; and sense of personal control, $r = -0.25$, $P < 0.001$) and another previously associated with susceptibility to infection (introversion–extraversion, r with stress $= -0.04$, $P = 0.46$) were added to the first step of the regression (with standard controls, health practices, and immune controls), and the stress index was entered in the second step. The stress index continued to produce a unique contribution to the explanation of colds ($b = 0.13 \pm 0.06$, $P < 0.04$). Thus, none of the personality characteristics we studied could account for the relation between stress and illness.

Discussion

Psychological stress was associated with an increased risk of acute infectious respiratory illness in a dose–response manner; this risk was attributable to increased rates of infection. Although there was some person-to-person transmission of virus in this study, the effect of stress on colds was independent of whether such transmission was possible (i.e., whether a subject shared housing with another infected subject). Moreover, the relation between stress and colds was similar for those with and without infected apartment mates. In short, the stress index was associated with host resistance and not with differential exposure to virus.

The relation between stress and colds also proved to be independent of a variety of health practices. If the increased risk of illness for subjects with higher stress-index scores was not due to associations between stress and exposure to virus or between stress and health practices, what accounts for this relation? Evidence from both human and animal studies indicates that stress modulates immunity.[7–9] Although the immune measures assessed in this study (prechallenge white-cell counts and antibody levels) did not explain the relation between stress and colds, these are quantitative measures; qualitative (functional) measures of immunity were not assessed. Because the effects of stress were the same for both subjects who were seropositive at base line and those who were seronegative, an explanation of the association between stress and illness would need to focus on primary rather than secondary immune responses. Some examples of primary immune functions that could have a role in this association are endothelial or lymphocyte production of interferon, mucus production, and natural-killer-cell activity.[34]

The association between stress and clinical illness was limited (adjusted odds ratio $= 2.16$), and the detection of the effect required a large sample. The relation between stress and infection, however, is stronger (adjusted odds ratio $= 5.81$). Moreover, the consistency of the stress–illness relation among three very different viruses – rhinovirus, coronavirus, and respiratory syncytial virus (as well as among rhinovirus types) – was impressive. This observation suggests that stress is associated with the suppression of a general resistance process in the host, leaving persons susceptible to multiple infectious agents, or that stress is associated with the suppression of many different immune processes, with similar results.

Although psychological stress is conceptualized here as a response to environmental events, our measures may also reflect personality characteristics that are independent of environmental factors. However, self-esteem and personal control, two personality characteristics strongly associated with stress, did not account for the effect of stress in this study. Another personality characteristic previously found to predict susceptibility to infection, introversion–extraversion, similarly did not account for the effect of stress. Because the psychological stress index assesses negative cognitive and emotional states rather than environmental stress factors, however, it is possible that it reflects other, individual traits not controlled for in the current study.

The results of research on stress as a risk factor in verified infectious disease may have been inconsistent.[10] This inconsistency may be due to insensitive techniques for detecting a relatively small effect on clinical illness. Our data suggest that a relation between stress and susceptibility to illness may be best detected in studies that incorporate control for important demographic and biologic characteristics, reliable and broadly defined indexes of stress, controlled exposure to the infectious agent, and relatively large samples.

Acknowledgements

Supported by grants from the National Institute of Allergy and Infectious Diseases (A123072) and the Office of Naval Research (N00014-88-K0063), by a Research Scientist Development Award to Dr. Cohen from the National Institute of Mental Health (MH00721), and by the Medical Research Council's Common Cold Unit, Salisbury, United Kingdom.

We are indebted to S. Bull, J. Greenhouse, M. Jarvis, H. Parry, M. Russell, M. Sargent, J. Schlarb, S. Trickett, the medical, nursing, and technical staff of the Common Cold Unit, and the volunteers for their contributions to the research; and to J. Cunnick, R. Dawes, D. Klahr, K. Kotovsky, K. Matthews, B. Rabin, and M. Scheier for comments on an earlier draft of the manuscript.

References

1. Lazarus RS, Folkman S. Stress appraisal, and coping. New York: Springer, 1984.
2. Felten DL, Felten SY, Carlson SL, Olschowka JA, Livnat S. Noradrenergic sympathetic innervation of lymphoid tissue. J Immunol 1985; 135:Suppl 2:755S–765S.

3. Felten SY, Olschowka JA. Noradrenergic sympathetic innervation of the spleen. II. Tyrosine hydroxylase (TH)-positive nerve terminals from synaptic-like contacts on lymphocytes in the splenic white pulp. J Neurosci Res 1987; 18:37–48.

4. Shavit Y, Lewis JW, Terman GS, Gale RP, Liebeskind JC. Opioid peptides mediate the suppressive effect of stress on natural killer cell cytotoxicity. Science 1984; 223:188–90.

5. Rabin BS, Cohen S, Ganguli R, Lysle DT, Cunnick JE. Bidirectional interaction between the central nervous system and the immune system. Crit Rev Immunol 1989; 9:279–312.

6. Kiecolt-Glaser JK, Glaser R. Methodological issues in behavioral immunology research with humans. Brain Behav Immun 1988; 2:67–78.

7. Ader R, ed. Psychoneuroimmunology. New York: Academic Press, 1981.

8. Calabrese JR, Kling MA, Gold PW. Alterations in immunocompetence during stress, bereavement, and depression; focus on neuroendocrine regulation. Am J. Psychiatry 1987; 114:1123–34.

9. Kiecolt-Glaser JK, Glaser R. Psychosocial factors, stress, disease, and immunity. In: Ader R, Felten DL, Cohen N, eds. Psychoneuroimmunology. New York: Academic Press. 1991:849–67.

10. Cohen S, Williamson GM. Stress and infectious disease in humans. Psychol Bull 1991; 109:5–24.

11. Laudenslager ML. Psychosocial stress and susceptibility to infectious disease. In: Kurstak E, Lipowski AJ, Morozov PV, eds. Viruses, immunity and mental disorders. New York: Plenum Medical Books, 1987:391–402.

12. Graham NMH, Douglas RB, Ryan P. Stress and acute respiratory infection. Am J Epidemiol 1986; 124:389–401.

13. Boyce WT, Jensen EW, Cassel JC, Collior AM, Smith AH, Ramey CT. Influence of life events and family routines on childhood respiratory tract illness. Pediatrics 1977; 60:609–15.

14. Meyer RJ, Haggerty RJ. Streptococcal infections in families. Pediatrics 1962; 29:539–49.

15. Alexander R, Summerskill J. Factors affecting the incidence of upper respiratory complaints among college students. Student Med 1956; 4:61–73.

16. Cluff LE, Cantor A, Imboden JB. Asian influenza: infection, disease, and psychological factors. Arch Intern Med 1966; 117:159–63.

17. Beare AS, Reed SE. The study of antiviral compounds in volunteers. In: Oxford JS, ed. Chemoprophylaxis and virus infections. Vol. 2. Cleveland: CRC Press, 1977:27–55.

18. Henderson S, Byrne DG, Duncan-Jones P. Neurosis and the social environment. Sydney, Australia: Academic Press, 1981.

19. Cohen S, Williamson G. Perceived stress in a probability sample of the United States. In: Spacapan S, Oskamp S, eds. The social psychology of health. Newbury Park, Calif.: Sage, 1988:31–67.

20. Cronbach L. Coefficient alpha and the internal structure of tests. Psychometrika 1951; 16:297–334.

21. Zevon MA, Tellegen A. The structure of mood change: an idiographic/nomothetic analysis. J Pers Soc Psychol 1982; 43:111–22.

22. Afifi AA, Clark V. Computer-aided multivariate analysis. Belmont, Calif.: Lifetime Learning Publications, 1984.

23. Al Nakib W, Tyrrell DAJ. *Picornviridae*: rhinoviruses – common cold viruses. In: Lennette EM, Halonen P, Murphy FA, eds. Laboratory diagnosis of infectious diseases: principles and practice: Vol. 2. New York: Springer-Verlag, 1988:723–42.
24. Barclay WS, Al Nakib W. An ELISA for the detection of rhinovirus specific antibody in serum and nasal secretion. J Virol Methods 1987; 15:53–64.
25. Callow KA. Effect of specific humoral immunity and some non-specific factors on resistance of volunteers to respiratory coronavirus infection. J Hyg (Lond) 1985; 95:173–89.
26. Feyerabend C, Russell MAH. A rapid gas–liquid chromatographic method for the determination of cotinine and nicotine in biological fluids. J Pharm Pharmacol 1990; 42:450–2.
27. Jarvis MJ, Tunstall-Pedoe H, Feyerabend C, Vesey C, Saloojee Y. Comparison of tests used to distinguish smokers from nonsmokers. Am J Public Health 1987; 77:1435–8.
28. Fleming JS, Watts WA. The dimensionality of self-esteem: some results for a college sample. J Pers Soc Psychol 1980; 39:921–9.
29. Paulhus D. Sphere-specific measures of perceived control. J Pers Soc Psychol 1983; 44:1253–65.
30. Totman R, Kiff J, Reed SE, Craig JW. Predicting experimental colds in volunteers from different measures of recent life stress. J Psychosom Res 1980; 24:155–63.
31. Broadbent DE, Broadbent MHP, Phillpotts RJ, Wallace J. Some further studies on the prediction of experimental colds in volunteers by psychological factors. J Psychosom Res 1984; 28:511–23.
32. Eysenck HJ, Eysenck SBG. Manual of the Eysenck Personality Inventory. London: University of London Press, 1964.
33. Hosmer DW Jr, Lemeshow S. Applied logistic regression. New York: John Wiley, 1989.
34. Morahan PS, Murasko DM. Viral infections. In: Nelson DS, ed. Natural immunity in disease processes. New York: Academic Press, 1989:557–86.

Section 3

Personality, behaviour patterns and health

Readings

Coronary heart disease in the Western Collaborative Group Study: final follow-up experience of $8\frac{1}{2}$ years.
    R. H. Rosenman, R. J. Brand, C. D. Jenkins, M. Friedman, R. Straus and M. Wurm. *Journal of the American Medical Association*, **233**, 872–77, 1975.

Anger-coping types, blood pressure, and all-cause mortality: a follow-up in Tecumseh, Michigan (1971–1983).
    M. Julius, E. Harburg, E. M. Cottington and E. H. Johnson. *American Journal of Epidemiology*, **124**, 220–33, 1986.

Pessimistic explanatory style is a risk factor for physical illness: a thirty-five-year longitudinal study.
    C. Peterson, M. E. P. Seligman and G. E. Vaillant. *Journal of Personality and Social Psychology*, **55**, 23–7, 1988.

Effectiveness of hardiness, exercise and social support as resources against illness.
    S. C. Ouellette Kobasa, S. R. Maddi, M. C. Puccetti and M. A. Zola. *Journal of Psychosomatic Research*, **29**, 525–33, 1985.

Introduction

The theme underlying this set of readings is the role played by personality factors, behavior patterns and coping styles in vulnerability to illness. The idea that personality is relevant to disease aetiology has a long history in psychosomatic medicine, beginning with psychodynamic conceptualisations in which psychic conflicts or specific attitudes were thought to increase risk for particular disorders (Alexander, 1950; Grace and Graham, 1952). These formulations were based predominantly on retrospective assessments using poorly standardised measures, so doubts were raised about consistency, reliability and bias. More recently, hypotheses about specific personality types being linked with particular disorders, as in the 'cancer-prone personality' suggested by Temoshok (1987), have been developed using more systematic approaches. It has also been suggested by Friedman (Friedman and Booth-Kewley, 1987) that there might be a 'disease-prone personality', a constellation of negative affective traits such as anxiety, depression and hostility that increase disease risk in a general fashion across different medical problems.

Biomedical scientists have remained sceptical of these hypotheses, and this is perhaps not surprising given the inconsistencies in the literature and the failure to link personality and behaviour patterns with credible psychobiological mechanisms. One of the major difficulties has been teasing out cause and effect relationships, since many studies of psychological factors have been carried out on diagnosed groups of patients. The presence of a serious medical condition may lead to changes in psychological factors as the individual faces threats to his or her well-being and the prospect of a curtailed lifespan. Diagnostic labelling can itself have adverse psychological and psychophysiological consequences (Rostrup and Ekeberg, 1992). These factors limit the inferences that can be drawn from cross-sectional studies. Another factor bedevilling the interpretation of studies is negative affectivity, a pervasive tendency to dysphoric mood (Watson and Pennebaker, 1989). Negative affectivity is associated with subjective complaints about health, increased symptom perception and use of health services, and may also lead to spurious reporting of negative life events and poor social supports (Schroeder and Costa, 1984). Added to these considerations is the dispute over the consistency of personality traits, with modern theorists favouring interactionist views in which situational and dispositional factors are both influential on the behaviour that is displayed (see Carver and Scheier, 1992).

There is a clear need for standardised assessments of personality factors, the application of multivariate techniques to control for the influence of potentially confounding variables, and the use of longitudinal designs that track the impact of personal factors on health prospectively. The selection of readings for Section 3 reflects these concerns for methodological rigour. The readings illustrate some of the themes that have been prominent in research on personality and behaviour pattern in disease risk, including Type A coronary prone behaviour (*Rosenman et al.*), suppression of anger (*Julius et al.*), pessimism/optimism (*Peterson et al.*) and hardiness (*Kobasa et al.*). These characteristics are perhaps best seen within an interactionist perspective as factors influencing the ways in which people cope with adverse events. Potentially damaging psychobiological stress responses of the type illustrated in Section 2 will arise when external demands are not adequately matched by personal and social resources (Steptoe, 1991). The personal characteristics described in these readings may influence coping effectiveness, either increasing risk (as in the case of Type A behaviour, suppressed anger and pessimism), or acting as stress buffers (hardiness and optimism).

Type A behaviour and coronary heart disease

The Type A behaviour pattern has been one of the most influential constructs in studies of psychosocial factors in disease aetiology. The 'action–emotion' complex first described by Friedman and Rosenman in 1959 is characterised by hostility and aggression, competitiveness, vocational ambition and a sense of time urgency. The reading from *Rosenman and colleagues* describes the results of the study that established Type A behaviour as an independent risk factor for coronary heart disease. Their Western Collaborative Group Study used all the techniques of rigorous epidemiological research available at the time. A prospective design was used, studying the evolution of heart disease in Type A and Type B middle-aged men over an eight-and-a-half year period. Clinical examination eliminated those with pre-existing disease in order to rule out the possibility that Type A behaviour might have arisen after disease onset, producing a spurious association. Type A behaviour was assessed using the Structured Interview, considered to be the best method of measurement (Matthews and Haynes, 1986). Regular clinical examinations, assessments of outcome by clinicians who were blind to behavioural classification, and a fairly complete follow-up further ensured against bias.

The study showed that coronary heart disease rates were predicted by conventional risk factors such as age, education, body weight, smoking, blood pressure level, cholesterol concentration, diabetes and physical activity level. In addition, men classified as Type A had a higher risk. Multivariate analyses were performed to show that the difference between Type A and Type B men was not accounted for by other risk factors, either individually or in combination. In the multivariate analysis, the relative risk of coronary heart disease in Type A over Type B men was somewhat reduced but remained highly significant. These results have been replicated in the Framingham Heart Study and in other prospective investigations (Matthews and Haynes, 1986). Studies of mechanism have suggested that Type A men show greater cardiovascular and neuroendocrine responses to challenging situations than do Type B individuals (e.g. Friedman *et al.*, 1975). The evidence appeared so convincing in the late 1970s that a review panel convened by the National Heart, Lung and Blood Institute in the USA endorsed Type A behaviour as an independent risk factor for coronary heart disease (Review Panel, 1981).

Since this time, the concept of Type A behaviour has experienced changing fortunes. A number of studies failing to document any association between coronary heart disease and Type A behaviour have been reported (Shekelle *et al.*, 1985; Appels *et al.*, 1987). A longer-term follow-up of the Western Collaborative Group Study itself found no relationship between Type A behaviour and coronary mortality (Ragland and Brand, 1988), while in the Framingham Study, Type A was related to incidence of angina pectoris but not to myocardial infarction or fatal cardiac events (Eaker *et al.*, 1989). Several explanations for these discrepancies have been put forward (Miller *et al.*, 1991). Changes in the behaviour pattern over time are probably not responsible, since relatively consistent results have been reported from reassessments of the same individuals after 25 years (Carmelli *et al.*, 1991). One possibility is that the measurement technique is at fault and that questionnaire measures are less sensitive than the Structured Interview. However, negative results have arisen from investigations using the interview, while Type A questionnaires did predict coronary heart disease in the Western Collaborative Group and Framingham studies, but not in other investigations. Another possibility is that the cultural context of Type A behaviour has changed. The pattern was first identified in middle-aged men working in corporations in California in the 1960s, and it may be that other cultural settings do not elicit this aggressive competitive response pattern in the same fashion. A further explanation is that the global Type A construct is too broad, and that only specific components may be pathogenic. Attention has focused particularly on hostility, since this is the element that has been found to predict coronary heart disease most strongly (Dembroski *et al.*, 1989). Whatever the explanation, the association between Type A behaviour and coronary heart disease that emerges from the behavioural epidemiological literature has to be viewed with more caution than it was a decade ago. On the other hand, the impact of Type A modification on recurrence of coronary events described in Section 6 (*Friedman et al.*) lends weight to the arguments in favour of the concept.

Suppressed anger and health

The reading from *Julius, Harburg, Cottington and Johnson* is another study that uses epidemiological methods to evaluate the role of psychological characteristics in health risk. The investigation took place in the context of a well-established longitudinal study of the population of Tecumseh, Michigan, USA. This small and stable community is accustomed to clinical research, and follow-up rates were high despite the 12-year period over which deaths were monitored.

The study concerns the influence of suppressed anger on mortality and its relationship with high blood pressure. The relevance of suppressed anger to high blood pressure has been implicated in a number of studies (see Johnson *et al.*, 1992). In this reading, suppressed anger was not construed as a personality trait so much as coping response to harassing situations. Thus, measurement was not conducted using a questionnaire, but rather by assessing reactions to hypothetical scenarios in which respondents were confronted with arbitrary and unwarranted verbal attacks. The construct identified by the investigators involved failure to express anger or to protest when provoked, coupled with feeling guilty or sorry afterwards. This pattern of coping was not related to high blood pressure. Nonetheless, suppressed anger did predict future mortality, with premature death being more common among men and women who reported high levels of suppressed anger. The effect was independent of conventional risk factors such as age, sex, smoking, education, body weight and the presence of coronary heart disease. However, an interaction was seen with blood pressure, such that suppressed anger predicated increased mortality among subjects with high blood pressure, but not in those with normal blood pressure. The results were most striking when analysed in terms of subjects' responses to hypothetical unprovoked attacks from their spouses rather than from policemen; it may be that this scenario was particularly vivid and immediately relevant to respondents.

This study relates suppressed anger to all-cause mortality rather than death from any specific illness. It is probable that in this middle-aged sample, coronary heart disease would have figured prominently as a cause of premature death, but precise causes of death were not established. It might appear surprising that suppressed anger is pathogenic, since it could be seen as antithetical to the overt hostility component of Type A behaviour. It may be that both excessive expression and suppression of hostile emotions are problematic, and that the healthy path lies in situationally appropriate responses. Moreover, as *Julius and colleagues* pointed out, data from the Framingham study have indicated that both Type A behaviour and suppressed hostility are related to future coronary heart disease.

If suppressed anger is conceptualised as a coping response to harassing social interactions, it might be predicted that its relevance would depend on exposure to these situations. Thus, some participants who responded with high suppressed anger scores might experience no adverse effects because they rarely encountered provocative situations. No data concerning exposure were recorded in this study.

However, other studies have suggested that anger inhibition may have adverse effects when combined with chronic stressors such as dissatisfaction with co-workers (Cottington *et al.*, 1986). *Julius et al.* did not observe any association between suppressed anger and high blood pressure, but elsewhere researchers have identified direct relationships between suppressed anger or inhibited expression and blood pressure levels (Gold and Johnston, 1990). The mechanisms underlying these processes are not clear and there may be a range of processes involved in linking suppressed anger with health. One possibility is that when people cope with aggravating circumstances by inhibiting anger, they show heightened cardiovascular and neuroendocrine stress responses of the type described in Section 2 that in turn promote health risk. For example, Vögele and Steptoe (1993) found that adolescents at risk for cardiovascular disease who inhibited anger were more responsive physiologically to challenging tasks than were those who did not suppress anger. It is interesting that failure to express feelings has also been linked with poor immune function (Pennebaker *et al.*, 1988). Another intriguing possibility is that emotional inhibition may be an obstacle to effective doctor–patient communication. Roter and Ewart (1992) found that patients with essential hypertension tended to give a false impression to their physicians that they were in a good psychological state, and this may militate against appropriate aid being mobilised when necessary.

Pessimism and illness

The reading from *Peterson, Seligman and Vaillant* concerns the role of pessimism in health. These investigators construed pessimism as an explanatory or attributional style, a way of accounting for negative events in one's life, and pessimists as people who explain negative events as being due to stable, enduring and global factors in themselves, rather than as incidents resulting from chance or external causes. Pessimistic explanatory style can be seen as a method of cognitive coping with adverse events. This theory developed from research on the effects of uncontrollable aversive stimulation (see Section 2), with the notion that not just events themselves but the internal explanations people make for events might be damaging (Abramson *et al.*, 1978). It has been applied principally to studies of depression, but this reading shows the relevance of pessimism to general physical health.

The study took advantage of a longitudinal survey of men originally recruited in the 1940s. The sample was highly selected: not only were all the participants Harvard graduates, but they were selected as being the most healthy psychologically and physically and among the academically most able. One might expect such a group to enjoy good health in later life, so the influence of pessimistic coping is all the more striking. Modern techniques for assessing explanatory style such as the Attributional Style Questionnaire had not been formulated at the time this study began (Peterson *et al.*, 1982). The investigators took advantage of methods that have been developed for assessing cognitive coping through the analysis of written texts. This method, which is described in the reading, shows high correlations with qeustionnaire measures (Schulman *et al.*, 1989). Health outcome was based on periodic physician assessments and not on self-report, and attrition was low. *Peterson and his colleagues* found that a pessimistic explanatory style predicted later poor health in this population. The pattern evolved as subjects grew older. Importantly, the association remained significant after controlling statistically for initial psychological and physical health status, so was not due to the influence of a sub-group of participants who were vulnerable from the beginning. The physicians' ratings of health were confined to problems of non-psychiatric illness, suggesting an influence of pessimistic style on general health status.

Peterson et al. were not able to assess life experiences over the years since the study began. The presumption is, however, that pessimists coped less effectively with stressful life events and difficulties. The results are consistent with shorter-term findings relating self-reported health and pessimism (Peterson, 1988). Several possible pathways through which pessimism might influence health are proposed in the reading. Pessimists may fail to seek medical advice at the appropriate time, may experience more negative life events due to a relative inability to maintain relationships, or may display poorer health-related behaviours of the type described in Section 4 (Lin and Peterson, 1990). Kamen-Siegel *et al.* (1991) have shown that a pessimistic explanatory style is associated with poor immune function in elderly men and women, suggesting that resistance to infection may be compromised.

People who are low on pessimistic explanatory style tend to be optimistic in their outlook, and a related literature on the construct of optimism has developed over recent years. Scheier and Carver (1992) have defined optimism as the disposition to believe in favourable rather than unfavourable outcomes to problems. Optimism has been associated with coping responses such as problem-solving as opposed to avoidance, with faster recovery following surgery, and with more positive outlooks in chronic illness (Taylor *et al.*, 1992). As such, it is relevant not only to health risk, but also to the patterns of coping with illness and disability discussed in Section 5. Optimists also engage in higher levels of positive health practices (Steptoe *et al.*, 1994). Consequently, it would appear from this literature that characteristic forms of coping with life experience do have an impact on physical health. This theme is taken up in the next reading.

Multiple personal resources against illness

The perspective adopted in this Section is that personality and behaviour patterns are resources that modulate people's responses to the potentially traumatic experiences they have in life. However, comparatively few studies have assessed the role of personal resources longitudinally in relation to illness, while also measuring life stress in an objective fashion. The reading from *Kobasa, Maddi, Puccetti and Zola* is notable for taking a multidimensional approach to the investigation of resources against illness. They studied the combined effects of hardiness, exercise and social support on ill-health among participants reporting high levels of negative life events.

The reading is important in introducing the influential concept of hardiness. Hardiness is the name given by Kobasa (1979) to a constellation of personality constructs presumed to be relevant to coping with stressful events. It includes dimensions of commitment versus alienation, sense of control as opposed to powerlessness, and challenge rather than threat. The hardy individual is one who becomes actively involved in what he or she is doing, who believes in personal ability to influence events, and who perceives changes in life as challenges rather than as threats. Hardy people cope effectively because they transform potentially stressful situations into more benign events by appraising them positively. *Kobasa et al.* studied a group of male business executives who had reported high levels of stressful life events over the previous year. They found that rates of self-reported illness over the subsequent year were lower among hardy individuals, in men who exercised regularly, and in those reporting high levels of social support. The three resources against illness acted in concert. Thus, men who scored high on all three resources had substantially reduced illness rates compared with those who scored low. In multiple regression analysis, the three resources predicted illness independently of one another, with hardiness accounting for most of the variance.

The concept of hardiness is attractive, since it implies that certain global ways of coping with life are more adaptive. It shows some similarity to other descriptions such as the 'sense of coherence' formulated by Antonovsky (1987). The results of the reading confirm data from a previous longitudinal study of managers (Kobasa *et al.*, 1982) and are consistent with the research on social support discussed in Section 1. The concept of hardiness has, however, come in for a variety of criticisms concerning the unitary nature of the construct and its independence from neuroticism (Funk, 1992; Williams *et al.*, 1992). It appears that the 'challenge' component of hardiness is somewhat independent of the other two. At least some of the explanation for why hardy individuals appear healthier is that they are also low in neuroticism. The fact that objective measures of illness status were not collected in the study raises the possibility that hardiness may affect the way people appraise health problems and report illness, rather than having a direct impact on the development of disease *per se*.

The role of exercise in moderating reactions to stressful events has, however, been endorsed in other investigations. Longitudinal studies randomising sedentary individuals to exercise training or control conditions have documented improvements in psychological well-being coupled with reports of improved coping ability (Steptoe, 1992). Psychophysiological studies have shown associations between fitness, exercise and reduced responsivity to experimental stressors, and to some extent these relationships have been confirmed in ecological studies. For example, Brown (1991) showed that fitness buffered the impact of negative life events on self-reported health and clinic visits in a cohort of students.

These readings therefore suggest that many aspects of people's habitual way of coping with life stress may be relevant to disease risk. It remains to be resolved whether particular personality or behaviour patterns have specific relationships with single disorders, or whether the associations relate to general vulnerability. The role of coping is taken up again in Section 5, where its relevance to adjustment to illness and disability is discussed.

References

Abramson, L. Y., Seligman, M. E. P. and Teasdale, J. D. (1978). Learned helplessness in people: critique and reformulation. *Journal of Abnormal Psychology*, **87**, 49–74.

Alexander, F. (1950). *Psychosomatic Medicine.* New York: Naughton.

Antonovsky, A. (1987). *Unravelling the Mystery of Health.* San Francisco: Jossey-Bass.

Appels, A., Mulder, P., Van't Hof, M., Jenkins, C. D., van Houten, J. and Tan, F. (1987). A prospective study of the Jenkins Activity Survey as a risk indicator for coronary heart disease in the Netherlands. *Journal of Chronic Disease*, **40**, 959–65.

Brown, J. D. (1991). Staying fit and staying well: physical fitness as a moderator of life stress. *Journal of Personality and Social Psychology*, **60**, 555–61.

Carmelli, D., Dane, A., Swan, G. and Rosenman, R. (1991). Long-term changes in Type A behavior: a 27 year follow-up of the Western Collaborative Group Study. *Journal of Behavioral Medicine*, **14**, 593–606.

Carver, C. S. and Scheier, M. F. (1992). *Perspectives on Personality*, Second edition. Boston: Allyn and Bacon.

Cottington, E. M., Matthews, K. A., Talbott, D. and Kuller, L. H. (1986). Occupational stress, suppressed anger, and hypertension. *Psychosomatic Medicine*, **48**, 249–60.

Dembroski, T. M., MacDougall, J. M., Costa, P. T. and Grandits, G. A. (1989). Components of hostility as predictors of sudden death and myocardial infarction in the Multiple Risk Factor Intervention Trial. *Psychosomatic Medicine*, **51**, 514–22.

Eaker, E. D., Abbott, R. D. and Kannel, W. B. (1989). Frequency of uncomplicated angina pectoris in Type A compared with Type B persons (The Framingham Study). *American Journal of Cardiology*, **63**, 1042–5.

Friedman, H. S. and Booth-Kewley, S. (1987). The 'disease-prone personality': a meta-analytic view of the construct. *American Psychologist*, **42**, 539–55.

Friedman, M., Byers, S., Diamant, J. and Rosenman, R. H. (1975). Plasma catecholamine response of coronary-prone subjects (Type A) to a specific challenge. *Metabolism*, **24**, 205–10.

Funk, S. C. (1992). Hardiness: a review of theory and research. *Health Psychology*, **11**, 335–45.

Gold, A. and Johnston, D. W. (1990). Does anger relate to hypertension and heart disease? In: *Current Developments in Health Psychology*, pp. 105–27. P. Bennett, D. Spurgeon and J. Weinman (eds.). London: Harwood.

Grace, W. J. and Graham, D. T. (1952). Relationship of specific attitudes and emotions to certain bodily diseases. *Psychosomatic Medicine*, **14**, 243–51.

Johnson, E. H., Gentry, W. D. and Julius, S. (eds.) (1992). *Personality, Elevated Blood Pressure and Essential Hypertension*. Washington: Hemisphere.

Kamen-Siegel, L., Rodin, J., Seligman, M. E. P. and Dwyer, J. (1991). Explanatory style and cell-mediated immunity in elderly men and women. *Health Psychology*, **10**, 229–35.

Kobasa, S. C. (1979). Stressful life events, personality and health: an enquiry into hardiness. *Journal of Personality and Social Psychology*, **37**, 1–11.

Kobasa, S. C., Maddi, S. R. and Kahn, S. (1982). Hardiness and health: a prospective study. *Journal of Personality and Social Psychology*, **42**, 168–77.

Lin, E. H. and Peterson, C. (1990). Pessimistic explanatory style and response to illness. *Behaviour Research and Therapy*, **28**, 243–8.

Matthews, K. A. and Haynes, S. G. (1986). Type A behavior pattern and coronary disease risk: update and critical evaluation. *American Journal of Epidemiology*, **123**, 923–60.

Miller, T. Q., Turner, C. W., Tindale, R. S., Posavac, E. J. and Dugoni, B. L. (1991). Reasons for the trend toward null findings in research on Type A behavior. *Psychological Bulletin*, **110**, 469–85.

Pennebaker, J. W., Kiecolt-Glaser, J. K. and Glaser, R. (1988). Disclosure of traumas and immune function: health implications for psychotherapy. *Journal of Consulting and Clinical Psychology*, **56**, 239–45.

Peterson, C. (1988). Explanatory style as a risk factor for illness. *Cognitive Therapy and Research*, **12**, 119–32.

Peterson, C., Semmel, A., Von Bayer, C., Abramson, L. Y., Metalsky, G. I. and Seligman, M. E. P. (1982). The Attributional Style Questionnaire. *Cognitive Therapy and Research*, **6**, 287–99.

Ragland, D. R. and Brand, R. J. (1988). Coronary heart disease mortality in the Western Collaborative Group Study: follow-up experience of 22 years. *American Journal of Epidemiology*, **127**, 462–75.

Review Panel (1981). Coronary-prone behavior and coronary heart disease: a critical review. *Circulation*, **63**, 1199–215.

Rostrup, M. and Ekeberg, O. (1992). Awareness of high blood pressure influences on psychological and sympathetic responses. *Journal of Psychosomatic Research*, **36**, 117–23.

Roter, D. L. and Ewart, C. K. (1992). Emotional inhibition in essential hypertension: obstacle to communication during medical visits? *Health Psychology*, **11**, 163–69.

Scheier, M. F. and Carver, C. S. (1992). Effects of optimism on psychological and physical well-being: theoretical overview and empirical update. *Cognitive Therapy and Research*, **16**, 201–28.

Schroeder, D. H. and Costa, P. T. (1984). Influence of life events stress on physical illness: substantive effects or methodological flaws? *Journal of Personality and Social Psychology*, **46**, 853–63.

Schulman, P., Castellan, C. and Seligman, M. E. P. (1989). Assessing explanatory style: the content analysis of verbatim explanations and the Atrributional Style Questionnaire. *Behaviour Research and Therpay*, **27**, 505–12.

Shekelle, R. B., Hulley, S. B., Neaton, J. D., Billings, J. H., Borhani, N. O., Gerace, T. A., Jacobs, D. R., Lasser, N. L., Mittlemark, M. B. and Stamler, J. (1985). The MRFIT behavior pattern study. II. Type A behavior and incidence of coronary heart disease. *American Journal of Epidemiology*, **122**, 559–70.

Steptoe, A. (1991). The links between stress and illness. *Journal of Psychosomatic Research*, **35**, 633–44.

Steptoe, A. (1992). Physical activity and psychological well-being. In: *Physical Activity and Mental Health*, pp. 207–29. N. G. Norgan (ed.). Cambridge: Cambridge University Press.

Steptoe, A., Wardle, J., Vinck, J., Tuomisto, M., Holte, A. and Wichstrøm, L. (1994). Personality and attitudinal correlates of healthy and unhealthy lifestyles in young adults. *Psychology and Health*, in press.

Taylor, S. E., Kemeny, M. E., Aspinwall, L., Schnieder, S. G., Rodriguez, R. and Herbert, M. (1992). Optimism, coping, psychological distress, and high-risk sexual behaviour among men at risk for Acquired Immunodeficiency Syndrome (AIDS). *Journal of Personality and Social Psychology*, **63**, 460–73.

Temoshok, L. (1987). Personality, coping style, emotion, and cancer: towards an integrative model. *Cancer Surveys*, **6**, 545–67.

Vögele, C. and Steptoe, A. (1993). Anger inhibition and family history as modulators of cardiovascular responses to mental stress in adolescent boys. *Journal of Psychosomatic Research*, **37**, 503–14.

Watson, B. and Pennebaker, J. W. (1989). Health complaints, stress, and distress: exploring the central role of negative affectivity. *Psychological Review*, **96**, 234–54.

Williams, P. G., Wiebe, D. J. and Smith, T. W. (1992). Coping processes as mediators of the relationship between hardiness and health. *Journal of Behavioral Medicine*, **15**, 237–55.

Coronary heart disease in the Western Collaborative Group Study: final follow-up experience of $8\frac{1}{2}$ years

Ray H. Rosenman, MD, Richard J. Brand, PhD,
C. David Jenkins, PhD, Meyer Friedman, MD,
Reuben Straus, MD, and Moses Wurm, MD

From the Harold Brunn Institute, Mount Zion Hospital and Medical Center, San Francisco, USA (Drs. Rosenman and Friedman), the School of Public Health, University of California, Berkeley, USA (Dr. Brand), the Department of Behavioral Epidemiology, Boston School of Medicine, Boston, USA (Dr. Jenkins), the Research Laboratories, St. Joseph Hospital, Burbank, Calif, USA (Drs. Straus and Wurm)

Abstract

Clinical coronary heart disease (CHD) occurred in 257 subjects during eight to nine years of follow-up (average, $8\frac{1}{2}$ years) in a prospective study of 39- to 59-year-old employed men. Incidence of CHD was significantly associated with parental CHD history, reported diabetes, schooling, smoking habits, overt behavior pattern, blood pressure, and serum levels of cholesterol, triglyceride, and β-lipoproteins. The type A behavior pattern was strongly related to the CHD incidence, and this association could not be explained by association of behavior pattern with any single predictive risk factor or with any combination of them.
   (*JAMA* 233:872–877, 1975)

Our earlier studies indicated a significant association between the type A behavior pattern and both the prevalence[1-3] and incidence[4] of clinical coronary heart disease (CHD). Pattern A is characterized by enhanced aggressiveness, ambitiousness, competitive drive, and chronic sense of time urgency.[1,2] The converse, more relaxed, type B subject exhibited substantially lower CHD incidence[4] and less basic atherosclerosis.[5] The association of various facets of pattern A with increased levels of CHD risk factors and higher CHD prevalence has been confirmed by other investigators.[6–10]

Keys[11] recently observed that the classical risk factors account for only about half of the CHD incidence in middle-aged American men and that other variables contribute significantly to the incidence. The present findings indicate that the behavior pattern is one such important factor.

Methods and materials

The Western Collaborative Group Study (WCGS)[3] was initiated in 1960–1961 as a prospective epidemiological investigation of CHD incidence in 3,524 men, aged 39 to 59 years at intake, and employed in ten California companies. The methodology had been described in previous reports.[3,4] Comprehensive data were obtained at intake and annually until the study was terminated, providing eight to nine years of follow-up, at which time a sufficient incidence of CHD had occurred as to make it unlikely that further follow-up would provide additional significant information. The intake studies were accomplished over an 18-month period from June 1960 to December 1961. Annual resurveys were done during the calendar 12-month period, ending in December 1969, during which time the subjects were studied in order of intake, with minor exceptions. Excluded from longitudinal analyses were 78 men under or over specified intake ages, 141 subjects with CHD manifest at intake, 106 employees of one firm that excluded itself from follow-up, and 45 subjects who were lost to the study because of early relocation, non-CHD death, or self-exclusion prior to the first follow-up. This left 3,154 initially well subjects at risk for CHD. Manifest CHD occurred in 257 subjects during the follow-up period, and death occurred in 140 subjects: 31 of their initial CHD event, 19 of a recurring CHD event, and 90 of non-CHD causes, including seven subjects who had developed manifest CHD. The remaining subjects were considered to be non-CHD cases, including 2,391 subjects who were examined throughout the entire period of follow-up and 423 subjects who were variously lost to follow-up. The death rate per 1,000 person-years was 2.10 from CHD events and 3.78 from non-CHD causes.

The behavior pattern was classified at intake from the tape-recorded, structured interview developed for this purpose[3] and administered by trained interviewers. The final rating was made after audition of the tape-recorded interview and without knowledge of other intake-history or measurement. This was done to avoid possible bias introduced by knowledge of subjects' other attributes. The 3,154 subjects at risk included 1,589 assessed as exhibiting type A behavior patterns and 1,565 assessed as exhibiting type B behavior patterns. Death from CHD events occurred in 34 type A and 16 type B subjects and from non-CHD causes in 51 type A and 39 type B subjects, including five type A and two type B subjects with manifest CHD. The death rate per 1,000 person-years was 2.92 for type A and 1.32 for type B subjects for CHD causes, and 4.38 for type A and 3.21 for type B subjects for non-CHD causes. The 2,391 subjects without manifest CHD included 1,129 type A and 1,262 type B subjects. The 506 men who were lost on or before final follow-up are also considered to be non-CHD cases and include 282 type A and 224 type B subjects. The total number of person-years of follow-up was 11,642 for type A and 12,148 for type B subjects. Thus, there was a slightly greater loss to follow-up of type A than of type B men, proportionately speaking. The excess of type A men in the CHD-incidence group, accordingly, is not a function of a greater loss of type B subjects from the initial populations at risk. Association between behavior pattern and CHD is slightly underestimated by using CHD rates based on number at risk at intake rather than on person-years of exposure to risk. Nevertheless, in what follows, rates based on number at risk at intake are required by the multivariate adjustment method to be described here that plays a major role in data analysis.

All electrocardiograms were screened by a cardiologist while those considered definitely or probably indicative of myocardial infarction were referred to an independent medical referee who was solely responsible for all diagnosis of manifest CHD, and this selection was made in the absence of any knowledge of the variables under investigation.[3]

The category termed "symptomatic myocardial infarction (MI)" includes 135 subjects, of whom 31 died in association with their initial CHD event. The diagnosis of acute MI in 104 surviving subjects was based on the occurrence of a symptomatic CHD event accompanied by definitive electrocardiographic and serum enzyme changes. Postmortem examination was performed on 24 of the 31 deceased subjects and demonstrated the presence of acute coronary thrombosis or acute MI in 23 instances and of severe, diffuse, coronary atheroclerosis in one subject, who was found dead in bed. No other anatomic or toxicological findings were noted to controvert inclusion of this subject as a case of sudden CHD death. The diagnosis of acute MI was confirmed by antemortem hospital findings in four of the seven deceased subjects who were not autopsied. Three other deceased subjects who were not autopsied were included because of sudden death. One subject died suddenly while driving his car, and the other two subjects died suddenly. None of the three had any other acute or chronic illness that might controvert including them as cases of sudden CHD death.

The category termed "unrecognized MI" is herein used to designate 71 subjects whose interval ECG during annual resurvey was adjudged by the independent electrocardiographer and medical referee to show definite evidence of the occurrence of MI that, however, was either "silent" or clinically unrecognized. The category of "angina pectoris (without MI)" was devised for 51 subjects by the medical referee, on the basis of the development of classical Heberden disease, and excluded subjects whose symptoms were atypical or doubtful.

The analyses are based on intake data, except for fasting scrum triglyceride levels, which were determined at the first annual resurvey examination. Among the 578 subjects with a history of parental CHD, 481 (83.2%) reported this at intake and the remaining 97 (16.8%) reported this during the first five years of follow-up. The statistical significance of categorical data was analyzed by the x^2-test, and of continuous variables by Student t-test. For behavior pattern, a multivariate adjustment using the Mantel-Haenszel x^2 method of analysis was utilized.[12] The association between behavior pattern and CHD incidence was adjusted one at a time and then in combination with other risk factors that were associated with the behavior pattern.

Results

Single predictive factors and CHD incidence

There were 3,154 intake subjects at risk for initial occurrence of CHD, 2,249 of whom were aged 39 to 49 years, and 905 aged 50 to 59 years. Clinical CHD was observed in 257 subjects during the mean $8\frac{1}{2}$ years of follow-up, an average annual incidence of 9.6/1,000 subjects at risk. (Relevant intake findings in the 257 CHD subjects are compared with those of all subjects in Tables 1 and 2.) Descriptive results, in the form of CHD rates and means, are provided for assessing the magnitude of association between each risk factor and CHD to indicate clinical significance of findings. Measures of statistical significance are provided to show the extent to which chance can be eliminted as an explanation of observed associations.

The educational level was inversely related to CHD incidence in both age groups, although annual income was not related to CHD rates. Subjects with a history of parental CHD and those with reported diabetes each exhibited higher CHD incidence of about the same proportion in both age groups, but statistical significance was not reached in the older group because of the smaller number of subjects. This exemplifies the difficulty in interpreting the possible difference between clinical and statistical significance. For example, the rate of CHD in older subjects with parental history of CHD was 5.4% higher than in those without such

Table 1. *Prospective history*

	Intake Age 39–49 yr				Intake Age 50–59 yr			
	Total Subjects	Subjects With CHD*	CHD Rate†	Significance‡ (P)	Total Subjects	Subjects With CHD	CHD Rate†	Significance‡ (P)
No of Subjects	2,249	145	7.6		905	112	14.6	
Schooling								
High school or less	961	77	9.4	.05	463	66	16.8	.01
Some college	300	17	6.7		131	22	19.8	
College graduate	987	50	6.0		311	24	9.1	
Annual income								
<$10,000	1,023	65	7.5	NS	368	41	13.1	NS
$10,000–$14,999	904	59	7.7		307	47	18.0	
≥$15,000	320	21	7.7		228	24	12.4	
Medical history								
Parental CHD	411	38	10.9	.025	167	27	19.0	NS
No parental CHD	1,838	107	6.9		738	85	13.6	
Diabetes history	74	9	14.3	.05	56	11	23.1	NS
No diabetes history	2,175	136	7.4		849	101	14.0	
Physical activity at work								
Sedentary and light	2,048	133	7.6	NS	800	96	14.1	NS
Moderate and heavy	200	12	7.1		103	15	17.1	
Exercise habits								
None or occasional	1,689	118	8.2	NS	649	90	16.3	.05
Regular	560	27	5.7		256	22	10.1	
Smoking habits								
Never smoked	536	19	4.2	.001	179	15	9.9	NS
Pipe or cigar only	407	17	4.9		159	19	14.1	
Former cigarette	239	16	7.9		132	12	10.7	
			10.?		435	66	17.9	

	No. at risk	CHD*	Rate†	P‡	No. at risk	CHD*	Rate†	P‡
None	1,182	52	5.2		470	46	11.5	
Yes	1,067	93	10.3	.03	435	66	17.9	.02
1–15/day	214	11	6.0		108	9	9.8	
16–25/day	433	36	9.8		164	26	18.7	
26+/day	420	46	12.9	.001	163	31	22.4	.01
Systolic blood pressure, mm Hg								
<120	592	21	4.2		175	11	7.4	
120–159	1,597	112	8.2		664	85	15.1	
≥160	60	12	23.5	.001	66	16	28.5	.001
Diastolic blood pressure, mm Hg								
<95	2,070	126	7.2		792	89	13.2	
≥95	179	19	12.5	.05	113	23	23.9	.01
Serum total cholesterol, mg/100 ml								
<220	1,093	35	3.8		359	26	8.5	
220–259	728	52	8.4		321	46	16.9	
≥260	421	58	16.2	.001	220	40	21.4	.001
Fasting serum triglycerides, mg/100 ml								
<100	600	19	3.7		250	21	9.9	
100–176	1,038	70	7.9		408	48	13.8	
≥177	496	50	11.9	.001	212	35	19.4	.05
Serum β-/α-lipoprotein ratio								
<2.01	1,291	59	5.4		487	45	10.9	
2.01–2.35	278	22	9.3		99	16	19.0	
≥2.36	674	64	11.2	.001	313	50	18.8	.01
Behavior pattern								
Type A	1,067	95	10.5		522	83	18.7	
Type B	1,182	50	5.0	.001	383	29	8.9	.001

*Coronary heart disease.

†Average annual rate/1,000 subjects at risk.

‡Analyzed by χ^2 test. NS indicates not significant at $P < .05$.

Table 2. *Mean values*

	Intake Age 39–49 yr			Intake Age 50–59 yr		
	Total Subjects	Subjects With CHD*	Significance† (P)	Total Subjects	Subjects With CHD	Significance† (P)
No. of Subjects	2,249	145	⋯	905	112	⋯
Age, yr:						
All subjects	43.3 ± 3.1‡	44.3 ± 3.5	.01	53.6 ± 2.7	54.0 ± 2.8	.05
Type A subjects	43.4 ± 3.1	44.4 ± 3.5	NS	53.7 ± 2.7	54.0 ± 2.8	NS
Type B subjects	43.3 ± 3.1	43.9 ± 3.4	NS	53.5 ± 2.7	53.8 ± 3.0	NS
No. of cigarettes/day (current smokers)	24.5 ± 11.3	27.5 ± 10.8	.03	24.0 ± 11.9	26.2 ± 11.0	.02
Height, cm	178 ± 6	178 ± 6	NS	176 ± 6	176 ± 6	NS
Weight, kg	77.2 ± 9.6	79.3 ± 9.9	.01	76.5 ± 9.4	78.7 ± 9.6	.01
Weight gain, kg§	5.7 ± 6.9	6.1 ± 7.2	NS	6.7 ± 8.3	6.7 ± 8.6	NS
Blood pressure, mm/Hg						
Systolic	127.4 ± 14.2	132.9 ± 15.5	.01	131.8 ± 16.7	138.6 ± 19.2	.01
Diastolic	81.4 ± 9.6	83.8 ± 9.9	.01	83.7 ± 9.9	87.3 ± 10.5	.01
Serum lipids						
Cholesterol, mg/100 ml	224.2 ± 43.8	253.1 ± 56.0	.01	231.9 ± 41.9	246.1 ± 39.0	.01
Triglycerides, mg/100 ml	146.2 ± 84.0	166.9 ± 77.0	.01	150.3 ± 103.4	164.8 ± 95.6	.01
β-/α-lipoprotein ratio	1.99 ± 1.05	2.44 ± 1.33	.01	2.08 ± 1.10	2.34 ± 1.00	.01

*Coronary heart disease.

†Analyzed by Student *t*-test. NS indicates not significant at $P < .05$.

‡Mean value ± standard deviation.

§Mean weight gain from age 25 yr to intake.

history, while the corresponding increment in the younger group was only 4.0% (Table 1). Nevertheless, because of the respective differences in the numbers of subjects involved, the observed findings reached statistical significance only in the younger group. However, the magnitude of the observed differences suggests clinical significance in both age groups.

Reported occupational-physical activity was not associated with differences in CHD rates. However, men reporting regular exercise habits (daily, purposeful calisthenics, walking, or hobby exercise) had lower CHD rates than those reporting only occasional avocational exercise, and differences were significant in the older group. Smoking habits were related to CHD incidence in both decades—with higher rates for current cigarette smokers—and rates of CHD were significantly related to reported daily amount smoked at intake.

There was no significant difference in the average weight gain between age 25 years and intake for subjects with or without CHD. However, subjects suffering CHD exhibited higher mean weights at intake. Average systolic and diastolic blood pressures, and serum levels of cholesterol and triglycerides, and β-/α-lipoprotein ratios were significantly higher in subjects of both age groups who later had CHD, compared to the non-CHD population, and the CHD rate was proportional to the degree of measured level of each factor. Significantly higher rates of CHD were observed in subjects of both age groups classified at intake as type A compared to those with the type B behavior pattern.

Different initial manifestations of CHD and predictive factors

Among the 257 subjects suffering clinical CHD during follow-up, the initial manifestation in 135 men was symptomatic myocardial infarction (including 19 subjects who died of sudden CHD death, as adjudged by history and postmortem findings), "silent" and clinically unrecognized myocardial infarction in 71, and classical angina pectoris without infarction in 51.

The incidence of symptomatic CHD events in the total population, including fatal and nonfatal infarction and sudden CHD death, as found at earlier follow-up[4] was significantly associated with parental history of CHD, cigarette smoking and the number smoked per day, the type A behavior pattern, both systolic and diastolic blood pressure, serum levels of cholesterol and triglycerides, and the β-/α-lipoprotein ratio. The incidence of "silent" and clinically unrecognized myocardial infarction and of angina pectoris was also associated with each of these factors in a similar direction, but the differences did not reach statistical significance in every instance. Thus, the incidence of unrecognized infarction was significantly associated (probability $[P] < .05$) with cigarette smoking and the number smoked daily, with systolic blood pressure, and with behavior pattern type A. The incidence of angina pectoris was significantly associated with parental history of CHD, reported diabetes, systolic and diastolic blood pressure, serum cholesterol level, and behavior pattern type A.

Postmortem findings in most of the subjects who died of initial or recurring CHD events, as well as of all causes, have been carefully collected. The relationship of the prospectively studied variables to the degree of coronary atherosclerosis and to the mechanism of CHD death will be separately reported, since the findings are too extensive for inclusion in the present discussion. Data regarding fatal cases, accordingly, are not reported herein.

CHD incidence and behavior pattern

Table 3 shows CHD incidence in the two age groups by type of initial manifestation in subjects with type A and type B behavior. In the younger group, type A behavior was significantly associated with incidence of both symptomatic and unrecognized infarction. The twofold higher incidence of angina pectoris in type A compared to type B subjects was not statistically significant because of the relatively small number of subjects in this category. In the older group, type A subjects had significantly more symptomatic infarction and angina pectoris. The observed relationship of the behavior pattern to the incidence of unrecognized infarction in the two age groups emphasizes again the difference between clinical and statistical significance. Thus, a 2% difference in the incidence of unrecognized infarction between type A and type B subjects in the older group did not reach statistical significance, while a 1.6% difference in the younger group was statistically significant (Table 3). The magnitude of the observed differences suggests that they are both clinically important, even though the differences did not reach statistical significance in both age groups.

In view of the association of type A with other risk factors for CHD, it was important to reexamine the incidence of CHD in type A and type B subjects stratified against all factors found to be significantly related to the CHD incidence.[4] The results of this survey are shown in Table 4. The higher CHD incidence in type A subjects prevailed when subjects were stratified by each of the predictive risk factors. The type A and type B subjects exhibited no significant differences of mean age, height, or weight. These results were corrected for each single risk factor in studying the association between the behavior pattern and the CHD incidence. No single risk factor had a substantial impact on the degree of association.

The possibility that the combination of effects of all risk factors may

Table 3. CHD* by type of manifestation and behavior pattern

	Intake Age 39–49 yr				Intake Age 50–59 yr				Intake All Ages			
	All Subjects	Type A	Type B	Significance‡	All Subjects	Type A	Type B	Significance‡	All Subjects	Type A	Type B	Significance‡
No. of subjects at risk	2,249	1,067	1,182	...	905	522	383	...	3,154	1,589	1,565	...
Subjects with CHD												
No.	145	95	50		112	83	29		257	178	79	
Incidence†	7.6	10.5	5.0	.001	14.5	18.7	8.9	.001	9.6	13.2	5.9	.001
Subjects with myocardial infarction												
No.	120	79	41		86	62	24		206	141	65	
Incidence†	6.3	8.7	4.1	.001	11.1	14.0	7.3	.01	7.7	10.4	4.9	.001
Symptomatic												
No.	79	52	27		56	41	15		135	93	42	
Incidence†	4.1	5.7	2.7	.005	7.2	9.2	4.5	.025	5.0	6.9	3.2	.001
Unrecognized												
No.	41	27	14		3.0	21	9		71	48	28	
Incidence†	2.1	3.0	1.4	.05	3.9	4.7	2.7	NS	2.6	3.6	1.7	.01
Subjects with angina pectoris												
No.	25	16	9		26	21	5		51	37	14	
Incidence†	1.3	1.8	0.9	NS	3.4	4.7	1.5	.05	1.9	2.7	1.1	.005

*Coronary heart disease.

†Average annual rate per 1,000 subjects at risk.

‡Probabilities are based on χ^2 test of significance. NS indicates not significant at $P < .05$.

Table 4. *Prospective history and findings by behavior pattern*

	Age 39–49 yr						Age 50–59 yr					
	Subjects at Risk		Subjects With CHD*		Rate of CHD†		Subjects at Risk		Subjects With CHD		Rate of CHD†	
	Type A	Type B	Type A	Type B	Type A	Type B	Type A	Type B	Type A	Type B	Type A	Type B
No. of subjects	1,067	1,182	95	50	10.5	5.0	522	383	83	29	18.7	8.9
Parental history of CHD												
Yes	214	197	23	15	12.6	9.0	103	64	20	7	22.8	12.9
No	853	985	72	35	9.9	4.2	419	319	63	22	17.7	8.1
Smoking habits												
Never smoked	221	315	11	8	5.9	3.0	90	89	10	5	13.1	6.6
Pipe or cigar	191	216	11	6	6.8	3.3	81	78	17	2	24.7	3.0
Former cigarette	110	129	11	5	11.8	4.6	91	41	10	2	12.9	5.7
Current cigarette	545	522	62	31	13.4	7.0	260	175	46	20	20.8	13.4
Current cigarette usage												
None	522	660	33	19	7.4	3.4	262	208	37	9	16.6	5.1
1–15 day	95	119	3	8	3.7	7.9	65	43	8	1	14.5	2.7
≥16/day	450	403	59	23	15.4	11.4	195	132	38	19	22.9	16.9

Systolic blood pressure, mm Hg											
<120	264	328	17	4	7.6	1.4	95	80	7	4	8.7	5.9
120–159	771	826	69	43	10.5	6.1	381	283	64	21	19.8	8.7
≥160	32	28	9	3	33.1	12.6	46	20	12	4	30.7	23.5
Diastolic blood pressure, mm Hg											
<95	970	1,100	81	45	9.8	4.8	448	344	64	25	16.8	8.5
≥95	97	82	14	5	17.0	7.2	74	39	19	4	30.2	12.1
Serum cholesterol, mg/100 ml											
<220	486	607	24	11	5.8	2.1	211	148	20	6	11.2	4.8
220–259	352	376	32	20	10.7	6.3	179	142	36	10	23.7	8.3
≥260	226	195	39	19	20.3	11.5	130	90	27	13	24.4	17.0
Fasting serum triglycerides, mg/100 ml											
<100	252	348	12	7	5.6	2.4	151	99	16	5	12.5	5.9
100–176	500	538	48	22	11.3	4.8	238	170	37	11	18.3	7.6
≥177	247	249	30	20	14.3	9.6	114	98	26	9	26.8	10.8
Serum β-/α-lipoprotein ratio											
<2.36	733	836	57	24	9.1	3.4	323	263	43	18	15.7	8.1
≥2.36	331	343	38	26	13.5	8.9	196	117	39	11	23.4	11.1

*Coronary heart disease.

†Average annual rate/1,000 subjects at risk. Difference of rates between type A and type B subjects are tested for significance by Mental–Haenszel χ^2, with adjustment for factors indicated. For each factor the adjusted association between behavior pattern and CHD incidence is significant at $P < .001$.

explain a substantial part of the behavior pattern-CHD association then was studied by the Mantel-Haenszel procedure[12] in each age group. This method of analysis, in addition to providing a test of statistical significance, gives a summary measure of association, which is computed in a way that is analogous to direct adjustment of rates. The resulting measure can be interpreted, in this case, as an approximate relative risk that gives the ratio of the CHD rate in type A subjects divided by the CHD rate in type B subjects.

In this analysis, the behavior pattern-CHD relationship was viewed when simultaneous adjustment was made for parental history of CHD, current cigarette usage, systolic and diastolic blood pressure, serum levels of cholesterol and triglyceride, and β-/α-lipoprotein ratios, all treated as categorical variables as indicated in Table 4. Simultaneous adjustment eliminates any apparent increase of CHD risk in type A subjects that stems from the tendency of these subjects to have a relatively higher occurrence of any of these other risk factors. In the younger age group, the approximate relative risk (odds ratio[13]), which assesses the association between behavior pattern and CHD incidence is 2.21 $(P < .0001)$ before adjustment and 1.87 $(P < .003)$ after adjustment for the other risk factors. In the older group, the ratio is 2.31 $(P < .0002)$ before adjustment and 1.98 $(P < .019)$ after adjustment. The results of these analyses thus incidated that the predictive relationship of the behavior pattern to the CHD incidence could not be "explained away" by other risk factors, a finding similar to that at the $4\frac{1}{2}$-year follow-up in which the same issue was studied by means of both bivariate and multivariate analyses.[4]

Comment

Epidemiological studies have confirmed a relationship between the incidence of clinical CHD and prospective risk factors, including age, parental history of premature CHD, elevated systolic and diastolic blood pressures, cigarette smoking, and higher serum concentrations of cholesterol, triglycerides, and β-lipoproteins. These findings are again confirmed in the present $8\frac{1}{2}$-year follow-up of a large population. However, the predictive relationship of any single risk factor with the incidence of CHD may be a reflection of its association with other risk factors. Accordingly, any attempts at causal interpretation of the data observed in these univariate analyses requires caution. It is beyond the scope of the present report to investigate the multivariate relationships of all of the risk factors studied herein, as was done for the behavior pattern. Although these factors are important in prediction of relative risk of CHD, even the combination of such risk factors cannot definitively predict CHD in prospective studies of middle-aged American men, indicating that other variables must play an important pathogenetic role in the CHD incidence.[11]

The present findings reaffirm earlier follow-up studies[4] and indicate that the overt behavior pattern is prominent among variables in the list of major risk factors. The results also confirm that this relationship is not the artifact of the association of the behavior pattern with other risk factors and suggest that the pathogenetic force of type A behavior on the CHD incidence is due primarily to factors other than the classical risk factors, perhaps operating through various neurohormonal pathways. However, it seems clear that behavior pattern A indicates a pathogenetic force operating in addition to, as well as in conjunction with, the classical risk factors.

The findings would appear to have important clinical implications for the primary prevention of CHD. Moreover, evaluating patients with CHD for presence of the coronary-prone behavior pattern may well improve the prognostic prediction of the course of the disease. It has not yet been shown whether altering facets of the behavior pattern in surviving type A CHD patients reduces their risk of reinfarction, but research along these lines is strongly indicated.

Acknowledgements

This study was supported by the National Heart and Lung Institute, research grant HL-03429.

Herman N. Uhley, MD, screened all the ECGs; Harold Rosenblum, MD, served as independent medical referee; and Robert I. Sholtz, MS, assisted in the analysis of the data.

References

1. Friedman M, Rosenman RH: Association of specific overt behavior pattern with blood and cardiovascular findings: Blood cholesterol level, blood clotting time, incidence of arcus senilis and clinical coronary artery disease. *JAMA* 169:1286–1296, 1959.

2. Rosenman RH, Friedman M: Association of specific behavior pattern in women with blood and cardiovascular findings. *Circulation* 24:1173–1184, 1961.

3. Rosenman RH, Friedman M, Straus R, et al: A predictive study of coronary heart disease: The Western Collaborative Group Study. *JAMA* 189:15–26, 1964.

4. Rosenman RH, Friedman M, Straus R, et al: Coronary heart disease in the western collaborative group study: A follow-up experience of $4\frac{1}{2}$ years. *J Chronic Dis* 23:173–190, 1970.

5. Friedman M, Rosenman RH, Straus R, et al: The relationship of behavior pattern A to the state of the coronary vasculature: A study of 51 autopsy subjects. *Am J Med* 44:525–537, 1968.

6. Brozek J, Keys A, Blackburn H: Personality differences between potential coronary and non-coronary subjects. *Ann NY Acad Sci* 134:1057–1063, 1966.

7. Caffrey B: Behavior patterns and personality characteristics related to prevalence rates of coronary heart disease in American monks. *J Chronic Dis* 22:93–103, 1969.

8. Liljefors I, Rahe RH: An identical twin study of psychosocial factors in coronary heart disease in Sweden. *Psychosom Med* 32:523–542, 1970.

9. Jenkins CD: Psychologic and social precursors of coronary disease. *N Engl J Med* 284:244–255, 307–317, 1971.

10. Ganelina IE, Kraevskij JM: Premorbid personality traits in patients with cardiac ischemia. *Cardiologia* 2:40–45, 1971.

11. Keys A: The epidemiology of coronary heart disease. *CVD Epidemiology Newsletter*, 1972, pp 2–5.

12. Mantel N, Haenszel W: Statistical aspects of the analysis of data from retrospective studies of disease. *J Natl Cancer Inst* 22:719–748, 1959.

13. Fleiss JL: *Statistical Methods for Rates and Proportions*. New York, John Wiley & Sons, Inc, 1973, pp 43–46.

Anger-coping types, blood pressure, and all-cause mortality: a follow-up in Tecumseh, Michigan (1971–1983)

Mara Julius, Ernest Harburg, Eric M. Cottington, and
Ernest H. Johnson

*The University of Michigan, School of Public Health, Department of
Epidemiology, Ann Arbor, MI 48109-2029, USA; The University of
Michigan, College of Literature, Science, and the Arts, Department of
Psychology, Ann Arbor, MI, USA; Allegheny-Singer Research Institute,
Pittsburgh, PA, USA; The University of Michigan, Medical School,
Division of Hypertension, Ann Arbor, MI, USA.*

Abstract

Julius, M. (U. of Michigan, School of Public Health, Ann Arbor, MI 48109-
2029), E. Harburg, E. M. Cottington, and E. H. Johnson. Anger-coping types,
blood pressure, and all-cause mortality: a follow-up in Tecumseh, Michigan
(1971–1983). *Am J Epidemiol* 1986; 124:220–33.

This study examined prospectively (1971–1983) the relationship between
anger-coping types, blood pressure, and all-cause mortality in a sample of men
and women aged 30–69 ($n = 696$) of the Tecumseh Community Health Study.
Subjects who indicated that they were likely to suppress their anger in response to
two hypothetical anger-provoking situations had 1.7 times the mortality risk of
those who expressed their anger (95% confidence interval (CI) = 1.03–3.05).
Subjects who suppressed their anger when unjustifiably confronted by their
spouse had twice the mortality risk of those who expressed their anger (95%
CI = 1.13–3.38). For high vs. low suppressed anger towards a policeman, the
mortality risk was 1.24 (95% CI = 0.72–2.14). These relationships were invariant
across age, sex, and education groups, even when medical risk factors were
adjusted for, i.e., smoking, relative weight, blood pressure, coronary heart
disease status, forced expiratory volume at one second (FEV_1), and chronic
bronchitis. However, suppressed anger measures significantly interacted with

Abbreviation: FEV_1, forced expiratory volume at one second.

Reprinted from Julius, M., Harburg, E., Cottington, E. M. and Johnson, E. H.
Anger-coping types, blood pressure and all-cause mortality: a follow-up in
Tecumseh, Michigan (1971–1983). *American Journal of Epidemiology*, **124**,
220 33, 1986.

elevated blood pressure to predict the highest mortality risk. These results suggest that persons with high mortality risk can be identified in part by how they cope with anger, and by the joint effect of anger-coping type (a behavioral trait) and elevated blood pressure (a biological trait).

anger; blood pressure; follow-up studies; mortality

The association between anger-hostility and health status has long been emphasized by researchers, with particular attention given to cardiovascular disorders such as coronary heart disease and hypertension (1–6), as well as to coronary heart disease complications of hypertension (7). Recent investigations have also indicated that anger-hostility may be the most important "coronary prone behavior" that underlies the confirmed relationship between the Type A behavior pattern and both the incidence of coronary heart disease in prospective studies (8) and the severity of basic coronary artherosclerosis (9, 10).

The purpose of the present study was to examine the relationships between anger-coping types, blood pressure, and all-cause mortality. These anger types, namely keeping "anger in" or letting "anger out" were first suggested by Funkenstein et al. (3), by classifying behaviors to laboratory-induced provocation; later, a self-report measure was developed by Harburg et al. (4) for assessing these specific components for anger-coping behavior in their social expression. The Harburg et al. model from which this measure is derived, is based on the thesis that psychophysiologic responses of anger are induced in those social situations whereby the person perceives 1) a loss or threat of loss of 2) something felt to be possessed (rights, or physical objects, etc.) through 3) perceived arbitrary (unfair) acts by others (person, group or society). When the loss is felt to be sudden, and is perceived to be highly arbitrary involving a matter strongly valued, then anger behavior will be more intense. Responses to the hypothetical situations, which compose the measure using these model elements, even though "subjective," appear to be related to other self-reported measures of "anger expression" (11) and blood pressure in a variety of studies (4, 12–15) and in recent unpublished observations (16). A recent study of 674 men and women whose survey responses in 1965–1967 were related to coronary heart disease events eight years later in Framingham, Massachusetts, showed results pertinent to the issue of anger behavior and cardiovascular events (15, 17, 18). Briefly, women (aged 45–64) who developed coronary heart disease scored significantly higher on measures of Type A behavior, suppressed hostility (not showing or discussing anger), tension, and anxiety symptoms than women free of coronary heart disease signs. Men exhibiting Type A behavior, work overload, suppressed hostility (not showing anger), and frequent job promotions were at increased risk of developing coronary heart disease (especially in the 55–64-year-old group). Type A behavior and not discussing anger were independent predictors of coronary heart disease incidence when controlling for standard risk factors (cholesterol, weight, cigarette smoking, glucose intolerance, and blood pressure). The measures of suppressed anger-hostility in this study were constructed ex post facto and allowed discovery of these interesting relationships.

Recently, prospective studies (19, 20) have found a strong association between hostility, as measured by the Minnesota Multiphasic Personality Inventory items derived by Cook and Medley (21), and subsequent coronary heart disease morbidity and all-cause mortality over follow-up periods of 20–25 years. One major problem is whether this Minnesota Multiphasic Personality Inventory subscale is actually appropriate for assessing the various dimensions of anger and hostility (6, 10, 22). Moreover, it has been recently pointed out (11) that this psychometric measure probably assesses either the quality and quantity of social support or "cynicism" rather than a specific dimension of anger-hostility. There is, therefore, conceptual confusion regarding the underlying trait measured by the Cook and Medley Hostility Inventory. Thus, to test the important hypothesis linking anger-hostility to disease states and mortality rates, appropriate measures of suppressed anger, based on a specific conceptual model such as the one used in the present study, are necessary.

The specific aims of the present analysis, formulated in 1971–1972, were to test for 1) the association between suppressed anger and blood pressure; 2) the relationship of suppressed anger and mortality; and 3) the joint relationship of suppressed anger, blood pressure, and mortality (when mortality data were available in adequate numbers in follow-ups through the Tecumseh Project). The original statements of these hypotheses were directional and specific to expectations derived from prior research and theory.

Materials and methods

The present analyses are based on data collected from a subsample of the Tecumseh Community Health Study, a longitudinal epidemiologic study of acute and chronic diseases in a whole community in Michigan. The study started in 1957 and has collected data on several occasions since 1959. Objectives and methods of the overall study design have been described elsewhere (23).

Sample

During the fourth Medical Tests Series in 1971–1972 a psychosocial study of life change events, anger-coping types, and psychologic well-being was conducted (24). Participants in the Medical Tests Series eligible for the Life Change Event Study were residents of a 20 per cent stratified sample of dwelling units in the study area, men and women aged 30 through 69 years, who were also examined in the Third Series of examinations in 1967–1969. The overall response rate in the Medical Tests Series was 88 per cent. Of the 736 respondents eligible for the Life Change Event Study, 696 or 95 per cent agreed to participate, 324 men and 372 women.

The demographic characteristics of this subsample are similar to the Tecumseh Study cohort, as well as to the population of the community. Tecumseh, a community of about 10,000 people, has a predominantly white, Anglo-Saxon, middle-class population. In 1971, over 98 per cent of the Life Change Event Study sample was white, with an average age of 47 years. The majority of the sample were married (95 per cent) and less than 1 per cent had never married. The median education level achieved was high school graduation. The median family income level was between $10,000 and $12,000 per year in 1967–1969, with 7 per cent receiving less than $5,000 annually. Sixty-four per cent of the study population were in the labor force during the 1967–1969 examination. Of those in the labor force, the majority (71 per cent) were lower white- and blue-collar workers (e.g., clerical, sales, operatives, laborers), while 29 per cent were in the three top professional categories according to the census classification of occupations. The demographic characteristics of Tecumseh remain relatively stable and there has been little relative change since these statistics were compiled.

Data collection

All medical and psychologic data were collected in the Tecumseh Community Health Study clinic in 1971–1972. The medical data included blood pressure and weight measured at the beginning of the examination. Demographic and health-related information was obtained by a standard Tecumseh Community Health Study questionnaire. All subjects also completed the psychosocial questionnaire for the Life Change Event Study.

Mortality status was determined in 1978–1979 for virtually everyone who was ever examined in the Tecumseh Study. After 1979, mortality status was updated by screening daily reports in local newspapers. Persons not positively identified as deceased were assumed to be living. Thus, for the cohort analyzed here, a less complete ascertainment of mortality status occurred after 1979. To evaluate the extent to which estimates of the effects of anger on mortality are biased by using mortality status information after 1979, separate analyses were performed with mortality status as of 1979 *and* mortality status as of 1983 as the dependent variables. The point estimates produced by these analyses were very similar, although those based on the smaller number of deaths as of 1979 ($n = 28$) were generally nonsignificant. For example, the spouse-specific expression of anger item (anger in/anger out) had an adjusted relative risk of 1.93 (95 per cent confidence interval (CI) = 0.93–4.01) with mortality as of 1979 as the dependent variable and an adjusted relative risk of 1.98 (95 per cent CI = 1.13–3.38) with mortality as of 1983 as the dependent variable. Given that the incomplete ascertainment after 1979 does not appear to severely bias the estimates and that a larger number of deaths had accumulated by 1983, all analyses presented in this report use mortality status as of 1983 as the dependent variable.

Measures

Blood pressure was measured with a standard sphygmomanometer. All readings were taken with the subject seated and using his/her right arm. Both systolic pressure and diastolic (fifth phase) pressure were recorded.

Anger-coping types were assessed using a format developed by Harburg et al. (4). All subjects responded to two hypothetical anger-provoking situations involving injustices perpetrated by a power figure (termed an unjustified attack throughout the paper). In one situation, the power figure was a policeman; in the other, one's spouse or "sweetheart." The anger-provoking situation involving the spouse is as follows: "Imagine that your (husband/wife/sweetheart) yelled in anger or blew up at you for something that wasn't your fault." For each situation, three items were measured. These include whether anger would be expressed or not, what level of guilt would result later if there was a display of anger in response, and would the subject just leave or protest the unjustified attack.

The possible responses used to assess whether anger would be expressed were 1) "I'd get angry or mad and show it; 2) I'd get annoyed and show it; 3) I'd get annoyed, but would keep it in; 4) I'd get angry or mad, but would keep it in; 5) I wouldn't feel angry or annoyed." The responses used to assess the level of guilt associated with a hypothetical display of anger by the subject in response to the attack were 1) "I'd feel very guilty or sorry; 2) I'd feel somewhat guilty or sorry; 3) I'd feel a little guilty or sorry; 4) I wouldn't feel at all guilty or sorry." Finally, the possible responses used to assess how much the subject would protest the attack were 1) "I'd just remain quiet; 2) I'd just leave; 3) I'd protest a little; 4) I'd protest strongly" (to the policeman/spouse directly either by doing or saying something).

For each situation, separate anger, guilt, and protest scores were constructed by recoding items as "anger out" (codes 1, 2), "anger in" (codes 3–5), "guilt" (codes 1–3), "no guilt" (code 4), "no protest" (codes 1, 2) and "protest" (codes 3, 4). It is assumed that each recoded item is an indicator of a suppressive anger process. Scoring was arranged such that high scores represent a more suppressed response. Therefore, anger-out, no guilt, and protest were each coded "0" and anger-in, guilt, and no protest were each coded "1".

Finally, cumulative anger-guilt protest indices of suppressed anger were also developed for each situation separately and combined. These measures were constructed by summing the recoded responses described above. Thus, those persons with a high score (2+ out of three items) on an anger-guilt-protest index in each role situation are more likely to not express their anger, to feel guilty, and to not protest an unjustified attack. We will label these anger-guilt-protest indices as "suppressed anger" and designate the specific role situation as suppressed anger/spouse or suppressed anger/policeman. The score which combines six items from both role situations (high score is 3+) was labeled as the "total suppressed anger index." If more role situations are used, one can detect a consistent response set by an individual across many situations, creating a measure of a "personality trait" (13, 25). It is well to remember that using only two role situations restricts the measures of suppressed anger as a *trait*; yet in this study, using the spouse situation approximates a trait measure, since 95 per cent of the sample were married and 4 per cent widowed, and the marital relationship constitutes a chronic social condition with intense interaction. On the other hand, the policeman situation represents an infrequent but highly severe stress experience, as the attacker is a formal sanctioning authority figure, and the coping response should be salient to the respondent.

A number of variables were considered to have potential confounding effects. Those ascertained during the Medical Tests Series interviews and medical tests, in 1971–1972, included sex, age in years, education in years, relative weight, cigarette smoking, and blood pressure. Certain indicators of physical status and morbidity obtained at the Third Series of examinations in 1967–1969 were also included as possible confounding variables. They are 1) a diagnosis of suspect or probable coronary heart disease, defined as a probable history of myocardial infarction or angina or electrocardiographic evidence of myocardial infarction (Minnesota codes 1–1 or 1–2); 2) chronic bronchitis or persistent cough or phlegm; and 3) FEV_1 score, forced expiratory volume at one second adjusted for sex, age, and height using the FEV_1 values of nonsmoking respondents without respiratory disease or symptoms. The results of multivariate analyses presented in this report are adjusted for all of these nine risk variables.

As previously described, mortality from all causes as of 1983 was selected as the dependent variable. Analyses for separate causes of death were not possible for two reasons. First, death certificate information was only available for a subset of the population (i.e., persons who died before 1980). Second, the small number of deaths for any single cause precluded reliable cause-specific risk estimates.

Table 1. *Relative mortality risk for the traditional risk factors based on multiple logistic analyses: Tecumseh, Michigan, 1971–1983*

Health risk variable	Relative risk estimate†	95% confidence interval
Sex (male/female)	2.25***	1.30–3.91
Age (≥45/<45)	10.28***	3.77–28.04
Cigarette smoking (yes/no)	1.34	0.75–2.41
Relative weight (≥110/<110)	1.02	0.54–1.92
Systolic pressure (≥140/<140)	2.65***	1.55–4.54
Education (<high school/≥high school)	1.52*	0.89–2.58
Chronic bronchitis status (suspect or probable/ negative)	1.43	0.79–2.61
FEV$_1$ score (<10/≥10)	1.41	0.81 2.45
Coronary heart disease status (suspect or probable/ negative)	2.54**	1.14–5.66

*$p < 0.10$ (one-tail); **$p < 0.05$ (one-tail); ***$p < 0.01$ (one-tail).
†Each relative risk estimate is based on a logistic model with all the other variables included as main effects.

To test the expected relationships between the measures of available health risk factors (i.e., sex, age, education, relative weight, smoking, blood pressure, coronary heart disease status, bronchitis and FEV$_1$) and mortality and to partially test the external validity of our sample, relative risk estimates were computed (table 1). Results confirm that all nine risk factors, except relative weight, had mortality risks greater than 1.00 and most were significant at the $p = 0.05$ level or marginally significant, $p \leq 0.10$. Results of a multiple logistic regression of these risk factors considered as continuous variables (except sex and coronary heart disease status) on all-cause mortality (data not shown) revealed that sex (males more than females), older age, higher systolic and diastolic blood pressures, lower forced expiratory capacity FEV$_1$, and fewer number of years in school were significantly and independently ($p < 0.05$) related to the all-cause mortality status. Furthermore, similar predictors of death were reported for the entire Tecumseh Study cohort (26).

In the present analysis both systolic and diastolic measures were examined separately. Each yielded the same results. The two variables were highly correlated and the inclusion of both in multiple adjustment equations is confounding. Therefore, in this paper, only results for systolic pressure are presented.

The statistical approach was to first examine univariate associations, then test for statistical significance using multivariate analyses allowing for adjustments of confounding variables. A total of 53 persons (7.6 per cent) died during the 12-year follow-up period; 36 (11.1 per cent) were men and 17 (4.6 per cent) were women. To determine the univariate associations (unadjusted) between the measures of anger-coping types and mortality, the per cent deceased were compared among persons grouped according to their anger-coping responses. This crude analysis allowed an initial evaluation of the presence and magnitude of the suppressed anger-mortality association. For the situation-specific and total suppressed anger indices, the distribution of scores was divided into thirds. The significance of each association was determined by the chi-square statistic. In all multivariate analyses presented in this paper, testing for the relationships between anger-coping measures and mortality, the possible confounding effects of the nine available health risk factors were adjusted for. Because of the small number of deaths, the unit of analyses was the entire sample rather than age/sex-specific groups. Finally, all statistical tests are one-tailed; this usage allows for specific directional hypotheses.

Results

The hypothesis that suppressed anger would be directly related to higher blood pressure was not supported. None of the suppressed anger indices were significantly correlated with systolic pressure or diastolic pressure controlling for age and relative weight. Moreover, a comparison of adjusted mean blood pressure across levels of the separate anger, guilt, and protest items did not reveal any significant trends in this sample.

An item analysis (figure 1) revealed that no significant associations with mortality were observed for any of the separate anger-coping items to an unjustified attack by a policeman. However, two out of three anger-coping items to an unjustified attack by one's spouse did predict mortality risk. Persons who would hold in their anger to their spouse were 2.4 times as likely to die over the follow-up period compared with those who would express their anger to their rate ($p = 0.001$). Moreover, this mortality rate was found to be greater than the mortality rates for persons classified by any of the other items. Although experiencing guilt in response to becoming angry at one's spouse did not significantly predict mortality, the results were in the predicted direction. Finally, those respondents who did not protest an unjustified attack by their spouse were 1.7 times as likely to have died during the follow-up period compared with those who protested the attack ($p = 0.023$).

Indices of suppressed anger (figure 2) were also associated with mortality. Persons who scored high on suppressed anger (anger-in, feeling

Table 2. *Multiple logistic regression of all-cause mortality on anger-coping types: Tecumseh, Michigan, 1971–1983*

Anger-coping variable	Logistic coefficient†	Standard error
Total suppressed anger index	0.134*	0.097
Suppressed anger/spouse index	0.317**	0.168
Anger (in)	0.687**	0.331
Guilt (yes)	0.043	0.331
Protest (no)	0.561**	0.339
Suppressed anger/policeman index	0.079	0.160
Anger (in)	0.190	0.331
Guilt (yes)	−0.130	0.336
Protest (no)	0.310	0.349

$*p < 0.10$ (one-tail); $**p < 0.05$ (one-tail).

†Based on models with the following covariates included: age, sex, cigarette smoking, systolic pressure, education, relative weight, chronic bronchitis, coronary heart disease status, FEV_1 score.

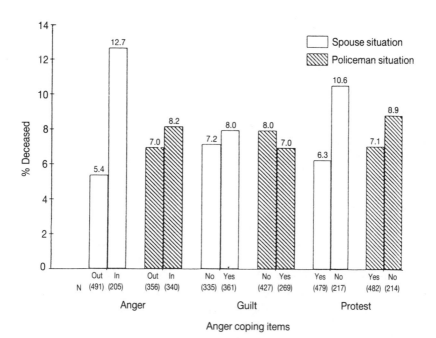

Figure 1. Per cent deceased (unadjusted all-cause mortality rates) by response categories to individual anger items in two hypothetical anger-provoking stituations, i.e., unjustified attack by spouse and by policeman: Tecumseh, Michigan, 1971–1983.

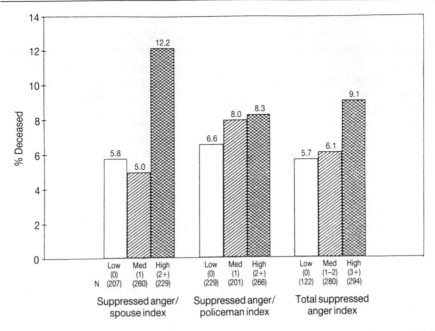

Figure 2. Per cent deceased (unadjusted all-cause mortality rates) by low, medium, and high suppressed anger index categories to hypothetical anger-provoking situations for spouse, policeman, and total suppressed anger (spouse and policeman): Tecumseh, Michigan, 1971–1983.

guilty, not protesting) in response to an unjustified attack by their spouse were 2.1 times as likely ($p = 0.005$) to have died during the follow-up period compared with those who scored low in suppressed anger (express their anger, not feel guilty, and protest). No significant association was observed between the suppressed anger/policeman index and mortality, but the linear pattern is consistent with the expected trend. Finally, those respondents who scored high on the total suppressed anger index were 1.6 times as likely to have died during the follow-up period compared with those with moderate or low scores ($p = 0.03$).

Results based on multiple logistic regression analyses controlling for the potential confounding effects of age, sex, education, relative weight, cigarette smoking, systolic pressure, chronic bronchitis status, coronary heart disease status, and FEV_1 score were obtained (table 2). The suppressed anger indices were treated as continuous variables in these analyses. The logistic coefficients for the associations between the anger-coping variables and mortality indicate that anger-in towards one's spouse, not protesting an unjustified attack by spouse, and the suppressed anger/spouse and total suppressed anger index were all significantly associated with increased mortality risk.

Table 3. *Relative mortality risk for the anger-coping variables based on multiple logistic analyses: Tecumseh, Michigan, 1971–1983*

Anger-coping variable	Relative risk estimate†	95% confidence interval
Total suppressed anger index		
High/medium + low	1.77**	1.03–3.05
High/low	1.38	0.60–3.05
Suppressed anger/spouse index		
High/medium + low	1.95**	1.13–3.38
High/low	1.83*	0.93–3.60
Items		
Anger (in/out)	1.99**	1.15–3.43
Guilt (yes/no)	1.04	0.61–1.80
Protest (no/yes)	1.75**	1.01–3.06
Suppressed anger/policeman index		
High/medium + low	1.24	0.72–2.14
High/low	1.36	0.70–2.64
Items		
Anger (in/out)	1.21	0.70–2.08
Guilt (yes/no)	0.87	0.51–1.52
Protest (no/yes)	1.36	0.77–2.42

$*p < 0.10$ (one-tail), $**p < 0.05$ (one-tail).

†Relative risk estimates are based on logistic models with the following variables included as covariates: age, sex, cigarette smoking, relative weight, systolic pressure, education, chronic bronchitis, coronary heart disease status, FEV_1 score.

Given that each of the suppressed anger indices, and the anger, guilt, and protest items making up each index could be treated as dichotomous variables, relative risk estimates were also calculated (table 3). The adjusted relative risk estimate for persons with high scores on the total suppressed anger index was 1.77 ($p < 0.05$) in comparison with 1.95 ($p < 0.05$) for the spouse and 1.24 for the policeman (not significant). For the spouse-specific anger, guilt, and protest items, the adjusted relative risk estimate ranged from 1.04 for guilt to 1.99 for anger-in. The relative risk estimates for the anger and protest items were significant, $p < 0.05$. The adjusted relative risk estimates for the policeman-specific anger, guilt, and protest items ranged from 0.87 for the guilt item to 1.36 for the protest item; these estimates were not significant.

We next tested for interaction effects among specific predictors of mortality. Multiple logistic regression was used to test whether the associations between mortality and the various measures of anger-coping

Table 4. *Multiple logistic regression of all-cause mortality: test for interaction effects between anger-coping variables and systolic pressure: Tecumseh, Michigan, 1971–1983*

Anger-coping variable	Interaction term with systolic pressure†		Logistic coefficient‡
Total suppressed anger index	×	Systolic pressure	0.012**
Suppressed anger/spouse index	×	Systolic pressure	0.017**
Anger (in)	×	Systolic pressure	0.028**
Guilt (yes)	×	Systolic pressure	0.029**
Protest (no)	×	Systolic pressure	0.010
Suppressed anger/policeman index	×	Systolic pressure	0.017**
Anger (in)	×	Systolic pressure	0.006
Guilt (yes)	×	Systolic pressure	0.053***
Protest (no)	×	Systolic pressure	0.018

$**p < 0.05$ (one-tail); $***p < 0.01$ (one-tail).

†The pattern of results is the same for diastolic blood pressure.

‡All coefficients are based on models with the following covariates included: age, sex, cigarette smoking, systolic pressure, education, relative weight, chronic bronchitis status, coronary heart disease status, FEV_1 score, and the appropriate anger variable.

responses were significantly modified by other risk factors. There was no evidence beyond chance levels that the relationships between anger-coping types and mortality were significantly different across age, sex, or education status. However, data show that significant interactions were found between the anger-coping variables and systolic pressure (table 4). Given the high correlation between systolic pressure and diastolic pressure, only the interactions involving systolic pressure are presented here. In these analyses the suppressed anger indices and systolic pressure were treated as continuous variables. Systolic pressure modified the relationships between several anger-coping variables and mortality. It interacted with the total suppressed anger index and the spouse- and policeman-specific indices, and with certain items: namely, anger-in toward one's spouse, and both of the situation-specific guilt items. Similar interaction terms involving diastolic pressure and these same anger-coping variables were found to be statistically significant or in the predicted direction.

Results from stratified contingency table analyses using unadjusted mortality rates are presented to give the reader a sense of the magnitude and direction of the significant modifying effects of systolic pressure (figure 3). The spouse and policeman suppressed anger indices significant-

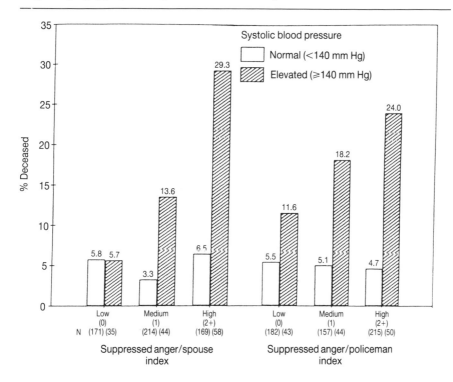

Figure 3. Per cent deceased (unadjusted all-cause mortality rates) by low, medium, and high suppressed anger response categories for suppressed anger/spouse and policeman indices, and normal and elevated blood pressure scores: Tecumseh, Michigan, 1971–1983.

ly predict higher mortality only for those respondents with systolic pressure greater than or equal to 140 mmHg. Individuals with elevated systolic pressure who scored high on the suppressed anger/spouse index were about five times as likely to have died during the follow-up period compared with those hypertensives who expressed their anger ($p < 0.002$). The results for the suppressed anger/policeman index also show about twice the mortality among persons who had elevated systolic pressure and suppressed their anger compared with those with elevated blood pressure but who scored low on suppressed anger.

In addition to the spouse- and policeman-specific suppressed anger indices, persons who had elevated systolic pressure and scored high on the total suppressed anger index (figure 4) were, on the average, five times as likely to have died during the follow-up period compared with hypertensives who expressed their anger (low scores), $p = 0.04$.

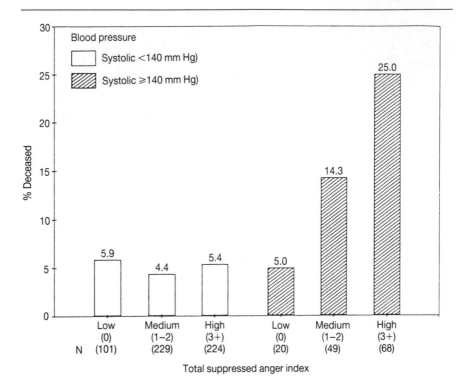

Figure 4. Per cent deceased (unadjusted all-cause mortality rates) by low, medium, and high suppressed anger response categories for the total suppressed anger index (spouse and policeman), and normal and elevated blood pressure scores: Tecumseh, Michigan, 1971–1983.

Discussion

Measures of suppressed anger were found to be significantly related to high all-cause mortality in a 12-year follow-up study (1971–1983) of 696 persons sampled from the town of Tecumseh, Michigan. While the number of deaths was low ($n = 53$), a similar pattern of relationships held both for items as well as index measures even when adjusted for standard health risk factors. Although the suppressed anger measures have been related to higher blood pressure levels in other studies, they were not directly related in this sample. However, suppressed anger did statistically interact with elevated blood pressure levels to predict significantly higher per cent mortality, even with adjustments. These findings urge the importance of considering both psychosocial and physiologic risk factors when identifying individuals at increased mortality risk.

Several limitations of the study design that may influence the results deserve mention. While the study had complete ascertainment of deaths through 1978–1979, there was less complete ascertainment after 1979. If persons who suppressed anger were more likely to have died during the follow-up period, then the observed estimates of effect using mortality status as of 1983 may be biased away from the null value. While this is possible, it seems unlikely, and the relative risk estimates based on follow-up through 1979 and follow-up through 1983 were similar. Nevertheless, only a complete ascertainment of deaths after 1979 can eliminate the potential for this kind of bias. Such an ascertainment of deaths through 1985 is currently being planned.

There was a two- to five-year lag time between classification of disease status (e.g., coronary heart disease, chronic bronchitis) in 1967–1969 and the assessment of psychologic characteristics in 1971–1972. Thus, an unknown number of people were falsely classified as nondiseased in multivariate analyses controlling for these conditions. Greenland (27) has demonstrated that controlling for a misclassified confounding variable can retain confounding in the estimate of effect. Little can be done in the present study to address this potential problem, given that clinical examination data were not collected in 1971–1972. Nevertheless, it is likely that not controlling for the misclassified confounding variables would have produced more severely distorted risk estimates, particularly since suppressed anger has been linked to coronary heart disease (15, 17, 18).

Finally, the small number of deaths, especially among females, precluded reliable sex-specific analyses. However, there is reason to believe that the effect of suppressed anger may be different for men and women. While the modifying effects of sex were examined by entering the appropriate interaction term into logistic models, the sample size may not have been large enough to detect statistically significant interactive effects. Further follow-up of this cohort should provide a more powerful test of the potential modifying effects of sex.

The model of suppressed anger on which the measures in this study are based assumes that anger is induced by perceived unjust deprivation of a felt possession, such as one's rights. One of many coping responses to the experience of an angry attack is what is here termed suppressed anger. If this response is consistent across many social situations and the attacks are chronic (as from a spouse), then a state of resentment will arise. In this state, angry feelings and their biologic processes are aroused by internal hostile attitudes as a chronic condition. When this psycho-physiologic anger process interacts with elevated blood pressure, then a morbid condition and mortality may result.

Early research by Funkenstein et al. (3) identified "anger-in" and "anger-out" coping responses to angry attack. Both of these coping types were significantly associated with blood pressure reactions to laboratory stress. They also reported "anger without physiologic" responses to the same stress situations by a subset of subjects; they termed this coping response "mastery of stress." Systematic research on this particular anger-coping response is lacking in the psychosomatic research literature.

Further research by Harburg et al. (28), however, has revealed another common response to attack, namely "reflective." Here the subject attempts to constrain anger and solve the problem which the angry attacker provokes. Thus a typical response may be "let's talk about this later" or "what's bothering you" even when feeling angry. This response type was found to be more prevalent among women than men, middle rather than working class, and showed no differences between blacks and whites. Of most interest was the finding which indicated that reflective responses were related to lower blood pressure levels for black males who resided in high-stress urban areas. Since the present survey did not include chances to respond in the reflective response mode, further study of this coping mode is important. For example, some "reflective" persons may easily constrain their anger and solve problems related to their experience of anger. Other reflective persons may impede problem resolutions by "keeping anger in," feeling "guilt about anger," *and* "brooding" about unjust attacks—all parts of a process we have termed suppressed anger.

More recent investigations (6, 10, 11) have determined that anger-hostility is one of the important "coronary-prone behaviors," if not the most important, that underlie the confirmed relationship between the Type A behavior pattern and heart disease. Paradoxically, but psychologically prevalent among Type A persons, those who chronically suppress anger may also at times be more overtly explosive as a result of an increase in the intensity of their angry feelings, when problems are not being resolved or they sense they are not controlling the means to resolve problems. This suggests that persons who are either excessive "anger-in" or "anger-out" responders may exhibit higher levels of blood pressure. Thus, as found in the Detroit Project (28), both "anger-in" and "anger-out" responses to provocation had an influence on the level of blood pressure. Similarly, in a study of breast cancer (29), the only significant differences in psychologic attributes between women with benign lumps and those with malignant tumors was in how they handled their emotions, particularly anger. Both "extreme suppressors" (those who had not openly shown anger more than once or twice in their lives) and "exploders" (who had frequent outbursts of temper and very rarely concealed their feelings) had higher rates of diagnosed breast cancer than women with "normal" emotional response patterns. There are few investigations of the association between the paradoxical response types who exhibit both "anger-in" and "anger-out" and health outcomes. Many studies do show that suppressing emotional expression is related to disease states. In one study of tumor formation, the "denial" and "repression" of emotional discharge was the most significant difference between lung cancer patients and controls (30). Suppressed anger has also been related to diagnosed rheumatoid arthritis with measures similar to those in the present study (31). In sum, these findings suggest that the health consequences of anger-response behaviors are broad and are consistent with the present observation that suppressed anger significantly predicts all-cause mortality.

Although there appears to be a consistency in findings relating anger-hostility to a variety of disease states, there are a number of problems measuring coping responses to anger. Measures of anger-hostility have been related to coronary heart disease (15, 17, 18), but the measures used were constructed ex post facto by a panel of experts who selected items judged to measure suppressed anger. Similarly, other studies (19, 20) relating coronary heart disease morbidity and mortality to anger-hostility selected items from the Minnesota Multiphasic Personality Inventory (21) also on an ex post facto basis. Thus, to date, there are no standardized tests of anger-coping types and suppressed anger that have been validated across different populations and disease states. Measures to observe and classify various categories of anger-coping responses must now be specifically constructed and tested to investigate the relationship between suppressed anger, disease states and mortality. The strategy of reinterpreting personality inventories, for example the Minnesota Multiphasic Personality Inventory (22, pp. 53–54) or the Cattell 16 Personality Factor Inventory (10, pp. 180–181), is not efficient for this task. Even if certain combinations of items appear as factors and are related to morbidity and mortality, it is not clear which dimension of anger is being measured (e.g., experience of anger – frequency, intensity, and duration, or expression of anger – anger in, anger out). In sum, there are conceptual and methodological problems concerning anger behavior in the social and psychologic areas which require new measures based on explicit models.

In terms of therapy, these measurement problems also apply to designs aimed at changing medical and behavioral risk factors for disease states. For example, a recent study by Friedman et al. (32) used a sample ($n = 862$) of postmyocardial infarction patients who volunteered to participate in an experiment aimed at reducing Type A behavior. Control groups received group cardiological counseling ($n = 270$) while the experimental group ($n = 592$) received group Type A behavior counseling in addition to cardiological counseling. The experiment, which lasted three years, suggests that the degree of Type A behavior reduction was significantly greater in the experimental group than in the control group. Even more important, the cumulative cardiac recurrence rate was 7.2 per cent for the experimental group, which was significantly less ($p < 0.005$) than the 13 per cent observed for the controls. The design and intervention aims of the study by Friedman et al. are novel and the results are intriguing; nevertheless, it is unclear what components of Type A behavior are being reduced. Moreover, anger-hostility has been pointed out to be one of the most important coronary prone behaviors of Type A, and it is unclear in the study by Friedman et al. what dimensions of anger behavior are being modified.

It might well be that a counseling program aimed at discussing and/or modifying response behavior to handling emotions in general and anger in particular, could have beneficial effects on more than one health outcome for those identified as having "disruptive anger-coping responses," e.g., extreme suppressors, or exploders. These disruptive anger-coping responses can be viewed as specific stressors which in turn disrupt the body's biochemical balance which then precipitates diseases, e.g., tumors, lung and breast cancer, arthritis, and heart disease (33). For example, in a two-year follow-up study of 160 women examined bioscopically for breast turmor, tests of anger expression were given before diagnosis; the findings strongly suggest that "release or suppression of anger influences the serum IgA [Immunoglobulin type A] levels in everyone. The study has demonstrated that altered expression of anger is much more frequent in cancer patients ... and that serum IgA levels may correlate to some extent with tumour mass ..." (34, pp. 398–399). Conversely "benign anger-coping responses." e.g., reflective or the as yet unknown anger-specific behaviors of Type B, may be part of a psychosocial immunity to morbid and lethal health outcomes. Our future research efforts are aimed at continuing the present investigation prospectively to ascertain cause-specific mortality and relate these to suppressed anger, separately and in interaction with other medical risk factors.

Acknowledgements

This work was supported in part by the National Institutes of Health grant nos. HL09814-03, MH25279, and 5 T32 MH16806, and the Michigan Heart Association.

The authors thank M. Higgins and A. Schork for their comments on earlier drafts; T. Karunas for processing 1971/1972 data, and S. McCallum for preparation of the manuscript.

References

1. Alexander FG. Emotional factors in essential hypertension: presentation of a tentative hypothesis. Psychosom Med 1939;1:173–9.
2. Dunbar E. Emotions and bodily changes: a survey of literature on psychosomatic interrelationships, 1910–1945. New York: Columbia University Press, 1947.
3. Funkenstein DH, King SH, Drolette ME. The direction of anger during a laboratory stress-inducing situation. Psychosom Med 1954;16:404–13.
4. Harburg E, Erfurt JC, Hauenstein LS, et al. Socioecological stress, suppressed hostility, skin color, and black-white male blood pressure: Detroit. Psychosom Med 1973;35:276–96.
5. Schwartz GE, Weinberger DA, Singer JB, Cardiovascular differentiation of happiness, sorrow, anger, and fear following imagery and exercise. Psychosom Med 1981;43:343–67.
6. Rosenman RH. Health consequences of anger and implications for treatment. In: Chesney MA, Rosenman RH, eds. Anger and hostility in cardiovascular and behavioral disorders. Washington: Hemisphere Publishing Corp., 1985.
7. Diamond EL. The role of anger and hostility in essential hypertension and coronary heart disease. Psych Bull 1982;92:410–33.
8. Matthews KA, Glass DC, Rosenman RH, et al. Competitive drive, Pattern A, and coronary heart disease: a further analysis of some data from the Western Collaborative Group Study. J Chronic Dis 1977;30:489–98.
9. Dembroski TM, MacDougall JM, Williams RB, et al. Components of Type A, hostility, and anger-in: relationship to angiographic findings. Psychosom Med 1984;47:219–33.
10. Williams RB Jr, Barefoot JC, Shekelle RB. The health consequences of hostility. In: Chesney MA, Rosenman RH, eds. Anger and hostility in cardiovascular and behavioral disorders. Washington: Hemisphere Publishing Corp., 1985.
11. Spielberger CD, Johnson EH, Russell SF, et al. The experience and expression of anger: construction and validation of an anger expression scale. In: Chesney MA, Rosenman RH, eds. Anger and hostility in cardiovascular and behavioral disorders. Washington: Hemisphere Publishing Corp., 1985.
12. Esler M, Julius S. Zweifler A, et al. Mild high-renin essential hypertension: neurogenic human hypertension? N Engl J Med 1977;296:405–11.
13. Gentry WD, Chesney AP, Gary HE, et al. Habitual anger-coping styles. I. Effect on mean blood pressure and risk for essential hypertension. Psychosom Med 1982;44:195–202.
14. Chesney AP, Gentry WD, Gary HE, et al. Life strain as a conditional variable in the anger expression-blood pressure relationship. (Unpublished manuscript.)
15. Haynes SG, Lewis S, Scotch N, et al. The relationship of psychosocial factors to coronary heart disease in the Framingham Study: I. Methods and risk factors. Am J Epidemiol 1978;107:362–83.
16. Johnson EH. Anger and anxiety as determinants of elevated blood pressure in adolescents: The Tampa Study. PhD dissertation. University of South Florida, Tampa, 1984.
17. Haynes SG, Feinlicb M, Levine S, et al. The relationship of psychosocial

factors to coronary heart disease in the Framingham Study. II. Prevalence of coronary heart disease. Am J Epidemiol 1978;107:384–402.

18. Haynes SG, Feinlieb M, Kannel WB. The relationship of psychosocial factors to coronary heart disease in the Framingham Study. III. Eight-year incidence of coronary heart disease. Am J Epidemiol 1980;111:37–58.

19. Shekelle RB, Gale M, Ostfeld AM, et al. Hostility, risk of CHD, and mortality. Psychosom Med 1983;45:109–14.

20. Barefoot JC, Dahlstrom WG, Williams RB Jr. Hostility, CHD incidence and total mortality: a 25-year follow-up study of 255 physicians. Psychosom Med 1983;45:59–63.

21. Cook WW, Medley DM. Proposed hostility and pharisaic-virtue scales for the MMPI. J Appl Psych 1954;38:414–18.

22. Megargee EI. The dynamics of aggressions and their application to cardiovascular disorders. In: Chesney MA, Rosenman RH, eds. Anger and hostility in cardiovascular and behavioral disorders. Washington: Hemisphere Publishing Corp., 1985.

23. Napier JA, Johnson BC, Epstein FH. The Tecumseh Community Health Study. In: Kessler II, Levin ML, eds. The community as an epidemiologic laboratory: a casebook of community studies. Baltimore: Johns Hopkins Press, 1970.

24. Julius M. Psychosocial factors of stress and their influence on mental and physical health. ScD dissertation. University of Zagreb, Yugoslavia, 1978.

25. Newcomb TM. Social psychology. New York: The Dryden Press, 1950:452–7.

26. Higgins M, Keller J, Landis R. Causes and predictors of death in the population of Tecumseh, Michigan. Presented at the 9th International Scientific Meeting of the International Epidemiological Association, Edinburgh, England, 1981.

27. Greenland S. The effect of misclassification in the presence of covariates. Am J Epidemiol 1980;112:564–9.

28. Harburg E, Blakelock EH Jr, Roeper PJ. Resentful and reflective coping with arbitrary authority and blood pressure: Detroit. Psychosom Med 1979;41:189–202.

29. Greer S, Morris T. Psychological attitudes of women who develop breast cancer: a controlled study. J Psychosom Res 1975;19:147–53.

30. Kissen DM. Psychosocial factors, personality and lung cancer in men aged 55–64. Br J Med Psychol 1967;40:29–43.

31. Harburg E, Kasl SV, Tabor J, et al. The intrafamilial transmission of rheumatoid arthritis. IV. Recalled parent–child relations by rheumatoid arthritics and controls. J Chronic Dis 1969;22:223–39.

32. Friedman M, Thorensen CE, Gill JJ, et al. Alteration of Type A behavior and reduction in cardiac recurrences in postmyocardial infarction patients. Am Heart J 1984;108:237–48.

33. Jemmott JB III, Locke SE. Psychosocial factors, immunologic mediation, and human susceptibility to infectious diseases: How much do we know? Psych Bull 1984;95:78–108.

34. Pettingale KW, Greer S, Tee DEH. Serum IgA and emotional expression in breast cancer patients. J Psychosom Res 1977;21:395–9.

Pessimistic explanatory style is a risk factor for physical illness: a thirty-five-year longitudinal study

Christopher Peterson, Martin E. P. Seligman and
George E. Vaillant

University of Michigan, University of Pennsylvania, Dartmouth Medical School, USA

Abstract

Explanatory style, the habitual ways in which individuals explain bad events, was extracted from open-ended questionnaires filled out by 99 graduates of the Harvard University classes of 1942–1944 at age 25. Physical health from ages 30 to 60 as measured by physician examination was related to earlier explanatory style. Pessimistic explanatory style (the belief that bad events are caused by stable, global, and internal factors) predicted poor health at ages 45 through 60, even when physical and mental health at age 25 were controlled. Pessimism in early adulthood appears to be a risk factor for poor health in middle and late adulthood.

Do our habits of explaining bad events when we are young predict our physical health in later life? Several lines of evidence imply that such explanatory styles might predict subsequent ill health. For example, research with animals suggests that uncontrollable bad events make poor immune functioning and illness more likely (Laudenslager, Ryan, Drugan, Hyson, & Maier, 1983; Sklar & Anisman, 1979; Visintainer, Volpicelli, & Seligman, 1982). And research with humans suggests that individuals who explain such bad events pessimistically have lowered immune function (Kamen, Rodin, & Seligman, 1987) and, over a 1-year span, make more doctor visits than do individuals who explain bad events optimistically (Peterson, 1988). We set out to investigate whether

Peterson, C., Seligman, M. E. P. and Vaillant, G. E. Pessimistic explanatory style is a risk factor for physical illness: a thirty-five-year longitudinal study. *Journal of Personality and Social Psychology*, **55**, 23–7. Copyright (1988) by the American Psychological Association. Reprinted by permission.

individuals who explain bad events pessimistically in early adulthood have more illness in middle and late adulthood.

We believe that an adequate investigation of early psychological precursors of illness and death should meet several stringent methodological requirements:

1. The research design must be longitudinal and span enough time for change in illness status to occur; this may require several years or even decades. Our study covers a 35-year period.
2. The initial health status of research participants must be known when the investigation begins. We began with certifiably healthy members of the Harvard University classes of 1942–1944.
3. An adequate number of research participants must be studied because links between psychology factors and illness—if they exist—are probably modest. We used 99 subjects.
4. Objective measures of health and illness that go beyond self-report must be available at the time the investigation begins, during the study, and at the time at which it ends. We used physician examinations numerically rated by an internist who was blind to other data.
5. There must be minimal attrition over the course of the investigation. We had less than 5% attrition.

Our study met these criteria and found that a cognitive personality variable, explanatory style, predicts health two and three decades later in life.

Explanatory style is the habitual way in which people explain the bad events that befall them (Peterson & Seligman, 1984a). Three dimensions of these explanations are of interest: stability versus instability, globality versus specificity, and internality versus externality. A stable cause invokes a long-lasting factor ("it's never going to go away"), whereas an unstable cause is transient ("it was a one-time thing"). A global cause is one that affects a wide-domain of activities ("it's going to ruin everything I do"), whereas a specific cause is circumscribed ("it has no bearing on my life"). Finally, an internal cause points to something about the self ("it's me"), whereas an external cause points to other people or circumstances ("it's the heat in this place").

Explanatory style emerged from the reformulation of the learned helplessness model as a way of accounting for the diversity of people's responses to uncontrollable bad events (Abramson, Seligman, & Teasdale, 1978). A person who explains such events with stable, global, and internal causes shows more severe helplessness deficits than a person who explains them with unstable, specific, and external causes. These deficits include passivity, depression, poor problem solving, low self-esteem, poor immune function, and higher morbidity (Kamen et al., 1987; Maier &

Seligman, 1976; Peterson, 1988; Seligman, 1975). Explanatory style is a prime candidate as a psychological precursor of good or bad health because it affects the severity of deficits following uncontrollable aversive events (Peterson & Seligman, 1984a).

Researchers usually use a questionnaire to measure explanatory style (Peterson et al., 1982), but also suitable and validated is a procedure that content analyzes natural speech for explanations (e.g., Peterson, Bettes, & Seligman, 1985; Peterson, Luborsky, & Seligman, 1983). It is called the CAVE technique (Content Analysis of Verbatim Explanations). Causal explanations are frequent in written and spoken material when bad events are on focus (cf. Weiner, 1985). Judges extract and rate causal explanations according to their stability, globality, and internality. Explanatory style assessed in this way is blind and reliable, with accumulating validity (Peterson & Seligman, 1984b). It is also stable: Explanations for bad events correlate .55 over 52 years (Burns & Seligman, 1987). Most important for the present purposes, the CAVE technique allows explanatory style to be measured using verbatim statements from the distant past.

We used the CAVE procedure to analyze open-ended questionnaires completed in 1946 (at approximately age 25) by participants in the well-known Study of Adult Development at the Harvard University Health Sciences. This project is an ongoing longitudinal investigation initiated by Clark Heath and Arlie Bock in 1937 to study "the kinds of people who are well and do well" (Vaillant, 1977, p. 3). Our major hypothesis was that the men who explain bad events pessimistically, with stable, global, and internal causes, will show worse health outcomes later in life than men who explain bad events with unstable, specific, and external causes. Furthermore, this relation should hold above and beyond their initial health status.

Method

Subjects and procedure

The Study of Adult Development began with mentally and physically healthy and successful members of the classes of 1942 through 1944 at Harvard University. Potential subjects were first screened on the basis of academic success (40% of the entire student body was excluded), then on the basis of physical and psychological health (another 30% was excluded), and finally on the basis of nominations by college deans of the most independent and healthy individuals. In all, 268 young men were included in the study. See Vaillant (1977, pp. 30–49) for details of the selection procedure.

Each subject, while an undergraduate, took an extensive physical examination and completed a battery of personality and intelligence tests. After graduation, the subjects completed annual questionnaires about employment, family, health, and so on. The results of periodic physical examinations of each subject, conducted by his own doctor, are also available. A total of 10 men withdrew from the study during college, and 2 more men withdrew after graduation.

For the present investigation, we studied 99 of these subjects, chosen arbitrarily according to the first letter of their last names. We used this sample size because previous investigations of explanatory style have consistently found significant correlations in samples of this size (see Peterson, Villanova, & Raps, 1985; Sweeney, Anderson, & Bailey, 1986).

Assessment of explanatory style

Using the CAVE technique, we analyzed the responses of these 99 men to open-ended questionnaires completed in 1946 that asked about difficult wartime experiences:

What difficult personal situations did you encounter (we want details), were they in combat or not, or did they occur in relations with superiors or men under you? Were these battles you had to fight within yourself? How successful or unsuccessful in your own opinion were you in these situations? How were they related to your work or health? What physical or mental symptoms did you experience at such times?

When a bad event involving the subject was described, along with a causal explanation, both were extracted and written on index cards. The index cards were shown to four independent judges, blind to the source of the quotes, the health of the individual, and the other statements he had made. Judges rated each cause on 7-point scales according to its stability, globality, and internality.

The ratings were averaged into a composite (across judges, across events, and across dimensions) so that each research participant had an explanatory style score ranging from relatively unstable, specific, and external to relatively stable, global, and internal. For the 99 men, a total of 1,102 bad events and causal explanations were identified (average = 11.1). Rating reliability, estimated by alpha coefficients, was highly satisfactory: .85 for stability, .77 for globality, .90 for internality, and .89 for the composite of stability + globality + internality. To make the procedure more concrete, we present in Table 1 some of the explanations made by those participants at age 25 who were among the least and the most healthy at age 55.

Subject consistency (the tendency for an individual to explain different

Table 1. *Examples of explanations of men who were least and most healthy at age 55*

Subject	Health (age 55)	Representative explanation (age 25)
314	Deceased (=5)	"I cannot seem to decide firmly on a career . . . this may be an unwillingness to face reality." (rating = 5.75)
316	Deceased (=5)	"What I feel is characterized more by confusion than by sense." (rating = 5.67)
327	Deceased (=5)	"(I dislike work because I have) . . . fear of getting in a rut, doing the same thing day after day, year after year." (rating = 5.42)
347	Deceased (=5)	"I have symptoms of fear and nervousness . . . similar to those my mother has had. She is still very nervous." (rating = 4.67)
301	Healthy (=1)	"My career in the Army has been checkered, but on the whole characteristic of the Army." (rating = 3.92)
315	Healthy (=1)	"I occasionally feel lazy . . . (due to) . . . lack of physical exercise." (rating = 3.75)
305	Healthy (=1)	"I tried to bluff my way through a situation . . . I didn't know the facts, a situation common to all green junior officers when they are first put in charge of men." (rating = 2.75)
320	Healthy (=1)	"Accused of violating a confidence . . . because the officer had not bothered to get all the facts." (rating = 1.83)

Note: Explanation ratings range from *optimistic* (1) to *pessimistic* (7).

events in the same way) was assessed by looking at the 59 men who made 10 or more causal explanations. As estimated by alpha coefficients, the consistencies of their first 10 explanations was .40 for stability, .46 for globablity, .48 for internality, and .61 for the composite. These figures seem notable in that explanations measured with the CAVE procedure reflect not only individual differences in explanatory style but also variation produced by the reality of the actual events explained (see Peterson & Seligman, 1984a).

Assessment of physical health

Health status at eight ages was scored from serial physical exams by the men's personal physicians and rated by a research internist in the following way. 1 = good health, normal; 2 = multiple minor complaints, mild back trouble, prostatitis, gout, kidney stones, single joint problems, chronic ear problems, and so on; 3 = probably irreversible chronic illness without disability, illness that will not fully remit and will probably progress, for example, treated hypertension, emphysema with cor pulmonale, and diabetes; 4 = probably irreversible chronic illness with disability, for example, myocardial infarction with angina, disabling back trouble, hypertension and extreme obesity, diabetes and severe arthritis, and multiple sclerosis; and 5 = deceased. Health scores were available for each subject at ages 25 (approximately the time of completion of the open-ended questionnaire from which causal explanations were extracted), 30, 35, 40, 45, 50, 55, and 60. From age 50 on, the research internist also had available blood and urine tests, an electrocardiogram, and a chest X-ray for most subjects. Again, see Vaillant (1977) for details of these procedures.

In 1945, a global measure of college soundness was made for each subject by an examining psychiatrist using a 3-point scale estimating the participant's likelihood of encountering emotional difficulties in the future. Although recognizing the limitations of this rating, we used it in subsequent analyses to control for the initial emotional well-being of the subjects (cf. Schleifer, Keller, Siris, Davis, & Stein, 1985).

Results

Overall, men who explained bad events with stable, global, and internal causes at age 25 were less healthy later in life than men who made unstable, specific, and external explanations. This correlation held even when initial physical and emotional health were held constant.

Table 2 presents the means and standard deviations of our major variables. As one would expect, overall health status gradually worsened with age, and variability in health across subjects increased. Also included in this table is the number of deceased subjects at each age.

We correlated composite explanatory style scores with the measures of objective health status available at various ages, partialing out health status at age 25. We partialed out the rating of college soundness as well. Results are shown in Table 3. As can be seen, explanatory style is initially unrelated to physical illness, but as time passes, the hypothesized correlation emerges. Its most robust level was reached at age 45, approximately 20 years after the time that explanatory style was assessed. After this time, the correlation between explanatory style and illness somewhat falls off.

A particularly stringent way to investigate our hypothesis is to correlate explanatory style with health at a particular age, partialing out health status not at age 25 but at the immediately preceding age. These analyses

Table 2. *Means and standard deviations of overall health status and number of deceased subjects*

Variable	M	SD	No. deceased
Composite explanatory style	3.60	0.45	—
College soundness	1.80	0.71	—
Physical health			
Age 25	1.16	0.66	0
Age 30	1.20	0.71	0
Age 35	1.30	0.84	0
Age 40	1.41	0.94	2
Age 45	1.60	1.05	4
Age 50	1.91	1.14	5
Age 55	2.21	1.24	9
Age 60	2.67	1.83	13

Note: N = 99.

test whether explanatory style (at age 25) predicts *changes* in health at later ages. So, at age 40, the partial correlation (controlling for health at age 35) was .19 ($p < .06$), and at age 45, the partial correlation (controlling for health at age 40) was .42 ($p < .001$). The other partial correlations (at ages 30, 50, 55, and 60) did not attain significance, although all were positive.

We conducted several additional analyses, with the following results. First, when examined separately, the individual dimensions of explanatory style (stability, globality, and internality) showed the same relations with health. Second, the relation between explanatory style and health was linear and did not depend simply on including deceased subjects in the analyses. Third, explanatory style was not related to the number of explanations offered by a subject, nor to Thematic Apperception Test measures of motives and clinical ratings of defense mechanisms made by other researchers (cf. Vaillant, 1977). Fourth, the number of explanations offered by a subject tended to predict subsequent health but independently of explanatory style.

Discussion

What have we accomplished in the present study? We believe that we have shown unambiguously that a psychological variable—pessimistic explanatory style—predicts physical illness two and three decades later. Prediction is successful even when possible third variables like initial physical health and initial emotional health are controlled. Whether psychological states influence health and illness is hotly debated. This debate is typically characterized more by opinions than evidence. The present study is an empirical foray into this controversy, one that sides with the claim that psychological factors can predispose physical health and illness.

Explanatory style did not predict immediate health status. This is not surprising because there was little variation. But in early middle age (35–50), health becomes more variable, and psychological factors come to play a role, perhaps by contributing to lifestyle, self-care, and social support. In late middle age (50–60), the relation between explanatory style and health falls off a bit, and we have no good explanation why. Perhaps constitutional factors or alcoholism, or both, dominate the health picture, and psychological factors from youth thus play a smaller role.

According to the learned helplessness reformulation, explanatory style influences the generality of deficits following bad events (Peterson & Seligman, 1984a). This proposal has been contested, but the present results extend and clarify its empirical support in several ways. First, our study goes beyond questionnaire approaches to explanatory style and its consequences. We found that people indeed offer spontaneous causal explanations for events they encounter. We found that different explanations by the same person are consistent with respect to their stability, globality, and internality. We found that explanatory style predicts an objectively measured health outcome decades later.

Second, although most investigations of the helplessness reformulation focus on depression, explanatory style pertains to a much wider range of outcomes. The present study links illness to explanatory style, just as other recent studies show that explanatory style predicts good or bad performance in academic, athletic, and work domains (cf. Kamen & Seligman, 1985; Nolen-Hoeksema, Girgus, & Seligman, 1986; Peterson & Barrett, 1987; Peterson & Seligman, 1984b; Seligman & Schulman, 1986). Explanatory style influences helplessness, and because helplessness is involved in many important failures of human adaptation, one should expect explanatory style to be broadly relevant. A difficult question thus arises: Granted that someone explains bad events with stable, global, and internal causes, what dictates the particular consequence he may suffer— depression, illness, job failure, and so on? Future studies are needed that simultaneously look at these different outcomes of pessimistic explanatory style.

Qualifications of the present research should be made clear. Our sample was originally chosen to be nonrepresentative, so generalization is of course a problem. All of the subjects began the study as healthy, and the present results might not have been obtained had the subjects been ill to start. Also, the study did not test the whole of helplessness theory,

Table 3. *Partial correlations between explanatory style and poor physical health*

Poor health: Age	Partial *r*
30	.04
35	.03
40	.13
45	.37****
50	.18*
55	.22**
60	.25***

Note: $N = 99$. Partialed out are initial physical and mental health.
$*p < .10.$ $**p < .05.$ $***p < .02.$ $****p < .001.$

which is a diathesis-stress model. Explanatory style (the diathesis) predicted subsequent illness, but we do not know if this is because particular bad events (the stress) were processed through the style. Some of our measures were less than ideal, particularly that of college soundness. Finally, the various correlations in Table 3 are not independent of each other, because a subject's prior health constrained his later health.

These qualifications aside, what have we not accomplished in the present study? Basically, we do not know the mechanism by which pessimistic explanatory style puts one at risk for eventual poor health. Explanatory style could influence illness in several ways (cf. Peterson & Seligman, 1987). Perhaps individuals who offer stable, global, and internal explanations become passive in the face of illness. Not seeking medical advice or not following medical advice are two helpless behaviors that might exacerbate illness (Seligman, 1975). Similarly, individuals with a negative explanatory style might neglect the basics of health care in the first place, either because they see no connection between anything they might do and the onset or offset of illness or because they feel that behaviors that promote health are useless (Becker, 1974; O'Leary, 1985; Wallston & Wallston, 1982).

People who offer stable, global, and internal explanations for bad events tend to be poor problem solvers (Alloy, Peterson, Abramson, & Seligman, 1984). They may experience more numerous and severe bad life events because they never nip a crisis in the bud. Increased illness may be a consequence of these accumulated life changes (Rabkin & Struening, 1976). Yet another possible mechanism is loneliness and lack of social support. The person who makes negative explanations for bad events is socially withdrawn (Anderson, Horowitz, & French, 1983).

Supportive social contacts with others may buffer one against illness (Cobb, 1976), and perhaps explanatory style affects long-term health through an interpersonal pathway.

Finally, a negative explanatory style may affect immune function, making morbidity and mortality more likely. By analogy to animal studies, helpless people may have less competent immune systems (Jemmott & Locke, 1984). Data from our research group suggest that people who make stable, global, and internal explanations for bad events show increased immunosuppression (Kamen et al., 1987).

Peterson (1988) conducted a preliminary investigation of what mediates the correlation between explanatory style and illness and found that pessimistic explanatory style predicted stressful life events, unhealthy habits, and low self-efficacy to change these habits for the better. These in turn predicted reports of poor health. However, this investigation is limited because it was cross-sectional. Longitudinal studies are obviously needed to map out the process by which pessimistic individuals eventually become ill. So, in a longitudinal study, Peterson and Lin (1987) found that pessimistic college students who developed colds or flus were less likely than their optimistic counterparts to take mundane steps to combat their illness, like sleeping more, increasing fluid intake, and curtailing activities.

Bidirectional influence among each of these variables, health, and explanatory style is perhaps to be expected. We regard explanatory style as traitlike because it is stable across time and situation (Peterson & Seligman, 1984a). We hasten to add that we do not regard traits as rigidly fixed. To date, we know little about the origins of explanatory style. Early socialization and early experience with loss may mold explanatory style. And experiences later in life, like illness or therapy, may encourage someone to be more versus less pessimistic.

In conclusion, we doubt that any single mechanism will prove responsible for the risk that pessimism creates for a nonspecific variable like poor health. Although mechanisms remain to be investigated, it is clear that the person who habitually explains bad events by stable, global, and internal causes in early adulthood is at risk for poor health in middle age. It may be important that training programs exist that reliably change this explanatory style for the better (Beck, Rush, Shaw, & Emery, 1979).

Acknowledgements

This research was supported by a Virginia Tech Travel Grant to Christopher Peterson, by Public Health Service Grant MH-19604 and the MacArthur Foundation Research Network on Determinants and Consequences of Health-Promoting and Health-Damaging Behavior to Martin E. P. Seligman and

Christopher Peterson, and by Public Health Service Grants MH-39799 and KO MH-00364 to George E. Vaillant.

We thank Linda Blumenthal, Vicki Gluhoski, Margaret Hahn, Susan Hilderley, Sara Koury, Tara Mitchell, and Peter Schulman for their assistance with data collection and analysis and Lisa Bossio for her editorial help in preparing this article.

References

Abramson, L. Y., Seligman, M. E. P., & Teasdale, J. D. (1978). Learned helplessness in people. Critique and reformulation. *Journal of Abnormal Psychology, 87*, 49–74.

Alloy, L. B., Peterson, C., Abramson, L. Y., & Seligman, M. E. P. (1984). Attributional style and generality of learned helplessness. *Journal of Personality and Social Psychology, 46*, 681–687.

Anderson, C. A., Horowitz, L. M., & French, R. deS. (1983). Atrributional style of lonely and depressed people. *Journal of Personality and Social Psychology, 45*, 127–136.

Beck, A. T., Rush, A. J., Shaw, B. F., & Emery, G. (1979). *Cognitive therapy of depression.* New York: Guilford.

Becker, M. H. (1974). *The health belief model and personal health behavior.* Thorofare, NJ: Slack.

Burns, M., & Seligman, M. E. P. (1987). Unpublished raw data.

Cobb, S. (1976). Social support as a moderator of life stress. *Psychosomatic Medicine, 38*, 300–314.

Jemmott, J. B., & Locke, S. E. (1984). Psychosocial factors, immunologic mediation, and human susceptibility to infectious disease: How much do we know? *Psychological Bulletin, 95*, 78–108.

Kamen, L. P., Rodin, J., & Seligman, M. E. P. (1987). *Explanatory style and immune functioning.* Unpublished manuscript, University of Pennsylvania, Philadelphia.

Kamen, L. P., Seligman, M. E. P. (1985). *Explanatory style predicts college grade point average.* Unpublished manuscript, University of Pennsylvania, Philadelphia.

Laudenslager, M. L., Ryan, S. M., Drugan, R. C., Hyson, R. L., & Maier, S. F. (1983). Coping and immunosuppression: Inescapable but not escapable shock suppresses lymphocyte proliferation. *Science, 221*, 568–570.

Maier, S. F., & Seligman, M. E. P. (1976). Learned helplessness: Theory and evidence. *Journal of Experimental Psychology, 105*, 3–46.

Nolen-Hoeksema, S., Girgus, J. S., & Seligman, M. E. P. (1986). Learned helplessness in children: A longitudinal study of depression, achievement, and explanatory style. *Journal of Personality and Social Psychology, 51*, 435–442.

O'Leary, A. (1985). Self-efficacy and health. *Behaviour Research and Therapy, 23*, 437–451.

Peterson, C. (1988). Explanatory style as a risk factor for illness. *Cognitive Therapy and Research, 12*, 117–130.

Peterson, C., & Barrett, L. C. (1987). Explanatory style and academic performance among university freshmen. *Journal of Personality and Social Psychology*, *53*, 603–607.

Peterson, C., Bettes, B. A., & Seligman, M. E. P. (1985). Depressive symptoms and unprompted causal attributions: Content analysis. *Behaviour Research and Therapy*, *23*, 379–382.

Peterson, C., & Lin, E. (1987). *Pessimistic explanatory style and response to illness*. Unpublished manuscript, University of Michigan, Ann Arbor.

Peterson, C., Luborsky, L., & Seligman, M. E. P. (1983). Attributions and depressive mood shifts: A case study using the symptom–context method. *Journal of Abnormal Psychology*, *92*, 96–103.

Peterson, C., & Seligman, M. E. P. (1984a). Causal explanations as a risk factor for depression: Theory and evidence. *Psychological Review*, *91*, 347–374.

Peterson, C., & Seligman, M. E. P. (1984b). *Content analysis of verbatim explanations*. Unpublished manuscript, University of Pennsylvania, Philadelphia.

Peterson, C., & Seligman, M. E. P. (1987). Explanatory style and illness. *Journal of Personality*, *55*, 237–265.

Peterson, C., Semmel, A., von Bayer, C., Abramson, L. Y., Metalsky, G. I., & Seligman, M. E. P. (1982). The Attributional Style Questionnaire. *Cognitive Therapy and Research*, *6*, 287–299.

Peterson, C., Villanova, P., & Raps, C. S. (1985). Depression and attributions: Factors responsible for inconsistent results in the published literature. *Journal of Abnormal Psychology*, *94*, 165–168.

Rabkin, J. G., & Struening, E. H. (1976). Life events, stress, and illness. *Science*, *194*, 1013–1020.

Schleifer, S. J., Keller, S. E., Siris, S. G., Davis, K. L., & Stein, M. (1985). Depression and immunity. *Archives of General Psychiatry*, *42*, 129–133.

Seligman, M. E. P. (1975). *Helplessness: On depression, development, and death*. San Francisco: Freeman.

Seligman, M. E. P., & Schulman, P. (1986). Explanatory style as a predictor of productivity and quitting among life insurance agents. *Journal of Personality and Social Psychology*, *50*, 832–838.

Sklar, L. S., & Anisman, H. (1979). Stress and coping factors influence tumor growth. *Science*, *205*, 513–515.

Sweeney, P. D., Anderson, K., & Bailey, S. (1986). Attributional style in depression: A meta-analytic review. *Journal of Personality and Social Psychology*, *50*, 974–991.

Vaillant, G. E. (1977). *Adaptation to life*. Boston: Little, Brown.

Visintainer, M. A., Volpicelli, J. R., & Seligman, M. E. P. (1982). Tumor rejection in rats after inescapable versus escapable shock. *Science*, *216*, 437–439.

Wallston, K. A., & Wallston, B. S. (1982). Who is responsible for your health? The construct of health locus of control. In G. S. Sanders & J. Suls (Eds.), *Social psychology of health and illness* (pp. 65–95). Hillsdale, NJ: Erlbaum.

Weiner, B. (1975). "Spontaneous" causal thinking. *Psychological Bulletin*, *97*, 74–84.

Effectiveness of hardiness, exercise and social support as resources against illness

Suzanne C. Ouellette Kobasa, Salvatore R. Maddi,
Mark C. Puccetti and Marc A. Zola

*Department of Behavioral Sciences, The University of Chicago,
5848 S. University Avenue, Chicago, IL 60637, USA*

Abstract

The effects of the resistance resources of personality hardiness, exercise, and social support, taken singly and in combination, on concurrent and prospective levels, and probability of illness were studied. In 1980, 85 male business executives identified as high in stressful events were tested for the three resistance resources. Predicting their illness scores in 1980 formed the concurrent aspect of the study. For the prospective aspect, illness scores in 1981 were available on 70 of the subjects. With regard to resistance resources, when there are none, one, two or three, the level and probability of both concurrent and prospective illness drop in a regular and marked fashion. These results highlight the importance of multiple resistance resources. Estimates of relative effectiveness indicate that hardiness is the most important of the resistance resources studied.

Recently, a shift has occurred in research on the relationship between stressful events and illness symptoms toward identifying moderating variables. The list of moderators, called resistance resources by Antonovsky [1], is growing. Now that research has suggested the importance of various individual resistance resources, it is time to consider their joint effects on the stress–illness relationship. The present study makes a start on this endeavor. The three resistance resources considered here are personality hardiness [2], exercise [3], and social support [4]. All three have received considerable attention lately.

Introduced by Kobasa [2], hardiness is considered a personality style consisting of the interrelated orientations of commitment (vs alienation),

Reprinted from *Journal of Psychosomatic Research*, **29**, Kobasa, S. C. O., Maddi, S. R., Puccetti, M. C. and Zola, M. A., Effectiveness of hardiness, exercise and social support as resources against illness, 525–33. Copyright (1985), with kind permission from Pergamon Press Ltd, Headington Hill Hall, Oxford OX3 0BW, UK.

control (vs powerlessness), and challenge (vs threat). Persons high in commitment find it easy to involve themselves actively in whatever they are doing, being generally curious about and interested in activities, things and people [5]. Persons high in control believe and act as if they can influence the events taking place around them through what they imagine, say and do [6]. Challenge involves the expectation that life will change and that the changes will be a stimulus to personal development.

These various beliefs and tendencies are considered very useful in coping with stressful events [7]. Optimistic cognitive appraisals are likely, in which the events will tend to be perceived as natural changes, meaningful and interesting despite their stressfulness. In that sense, the stressful events will be held in perspective. Decisive coping actions will also be taken to find out more about the changes constituting the event, with emphasis on incorporating them into an ongoing life plan and on learning from them whatever may be of value for the future. In these ways, hardy persons will transform stressful events into less stressful forms.

In contrast, persons low in hardiness tend to find themselves and the environment boring, meaningless and threatening. They feel powerless in the face of overwhelming forces, believing that life is best when it involves no disruptive changes. As such, they have little conviction that development is either possible or important, and tend to be passive in their interactions with the environment. When stressful events occur, these persons will have little basis for optimistic appraisal or decisive actions that could transform the events. As their personalities provide little or no buffer, the stressful events are free to have a debilitating effect on health.

The initial retrospective empirical demonstration that executives high in hardiness are freer of illness in the face of mounting stressful events [1] has since been replicated with a prospective design and data analysis [7]. Further, hardiness appears independent of other potential resistance resources, such as exercise [8] and constitutional strengths [9], and of various demographic factors, such as age, education, income and job level [1, 9]. Although there is some relationship between hardiness and perceived social support [8], it is far from large enough to suggest that they are the same thing.

Exercise has been widely considered to protect health. The evidence is most complete regarding cardiovascular disorders. Generally, the studies are longitudinal, obtaining self-report measures of exercise first and then checking periodically for evidence of heart symptoms. The consensus of these studies [3, 10], appears to be that exercise decreases the likelihood of heart attacks. Even among subjects showing constitutional risk factors, those who exercised had fewer heart attacks than those who were sedentary. Apparently, the beneficial effect of exercise is not restricted to sports, but includes physical labor as well [3].

Explanations of these results [3, 10, 11] assume that vigorous exercise increases the efficiency of cardiac action, slowing the heart, and regulating rhythm. Further, levels of energy expenditure probably increase fibromolytic activity, and finally increase collateral circulation of the luminal area of coronary arteries. In this fashion, exercise can protect health by decreasing organismic strain resulting from stressful events. These assumptions are based on some evidence [12, 13] that inactivity is associated with cardiac arrhythmia and other signs of circulatory impairment.

The evidence that exercise protects against other illnesses is less clear, though it has been implicated in this fashion [14, 15]. Recently, Kobasa *et al.* [8] reported finding that exercise was associated with lower overall illness scores in executives under stress, and that this buffering effect was distinct from that attributable to hardiness. Whereas hardiness leads to decreasing the stressfulness of events, thereby decreasing their ability to produce sympathetic arousal (or organismic strain), exercise may have its general buffering effect by relieving the organismic strain directly, without altering the precipitating events [8]*.

Social support has long been regarded as an important basis for resisting debilitation by stressful events [16, 17]. The early emphasis on possession of social resources, such as education, wealth and majority status in society has shifted to perceived support from others [4]. Despite definitional and measurement controversies surrounding this apparently heterogeneous construct, there is evidence that perceived support aids in maintaining health. Some studies report this as a main effect whereas others find instead the interaction with stressful events that is most consistent with social support as a buffer [18].

The general presumption about how social support protects health emphasizes both the resources and the encouragement it provides the person. When experiencing stressful events, it is buffering for the person to have others to turn to who can provide either the knowledge and information that helps in determining what to do, or the basic appreciation and encouragement that can soothe the pain, or both. Thus, social support may be similar to hardiness in aiding transformation of events into a less stressful form and similar to exercise in decreasing the strain resulting from experience of the stressful events.

Not very much is known about the buffering effects of combinations of hardiness, exercise, and social support. In one relevant study, Kobasa, Maddi and Puccetti [8] did find that subjects who are high in both

*Supported in whole by NIMH grant No. 28839-05 to Kobasa and Maddi.

hardiness and exercise are more resistant in the face of stressful events than are those high in one but not the other. Another study [19] found a similar additive effect of hardiness and social support at work. These findings suggested the present study, in which an attempt is made to determine the effects on illness score of resistance resources present. In addition, estimates of the relative effectiveness of each resistance resource will be obtained. These buffering effects should be apparent on illness symptoms not only concurrent with the stressful event and resistance resource measurements, but subsequent to that time as well.

Method

Overview of procedure

The subjects for this study were those of the male business executives in the longitudinal sample of the Chicago Stress Project who were above the median on stressfu! life events scores in 1980. In September of that year, all subjects in the longitudinal sample completed a questionnaire sent and returned in the mail as part of the annual testing program of the Project. The stressful life events and illness symptom portions of the questionnaire were to be filled out for the immediately preceding one-year period. Also included were measures of hardiness, exercise, and social support. In September of 1981, the annual testing included of relevance to this study a repeat of the illness symptom measure, to be filled out for the immediately preceding year.

The number of subjects who, in 1980, completed all measures and were above the sample median in stressful life events, numbered 85. By 1981, this group had dwindled to 70. The reasons for sample attrition were retirement, job transfer, and failure to complete the questionnaire sent in 1981.

Measure of stressful life events

An adapted, revised version of the Schedule of Recent Life Events [20] was used. The original scale lists numerous events, and provides for each a stressfulness weight that has been determined through the consensus of a large sample of judges. This measure has consistently shown a low, positive correlation with measures of illness. For purposes of this study, certain modification was made in the scale along the lines of suggestions made by veteran stress researchers [21]. Specifically, items emerging from a pilot study as distinctive to the population of business executives were added [1]. Also, ambiguous items, (e.g., 'change in financial condition') were clarified (e.g., 'improvement in financial condition' and 'worsening of financial condition').

Measure of hardiness

The multifaceted style of hardiness has come to be measured by five scales [7, 9]. Employed as negative indicators of commitment were the Alienation from Work and Alienation from Self scales of the Alienation Test [5]. High scores on Alienation from Self reflect a lack of involvement with one's particular skills and sentiments, with a passive attitude toward decision-making and goal setting. Sample items include 'the attempt to know yourself is a waste of effort,' and 'I long for a simple life in which body needs are the most important things and decisions don't have to be made.' High scores on Alienation from Work indicate a lack of personal investment in that area of life involving socially-productive activity. To the extent that these items depict work as linking the individual to society, they portray a general sense of meaninglessness, apathy and detachment. Sample items are, 'I find it difficult to imagine enthusiasm concerning work,' and 'I find it hard to believe people who actually feel that the work they perform is of value to society.' Across various adult samples, the Alienation from Self and Alienation from Work scales have shown an average internal consistency (Coefficient Alpha) of 0.85 and 0.79, respectively, and stability correlations of 0.77 and 0.70, over a three-week period [5].

Consistent with their roots in existential psychology, these scales show construct validity in negative relationships with such variables as empathy, endurance, achievement motivation, purpose-in-life, and role consistency [5]. Also, there are positive relationships between Alienation from Work and amount of leisure activities and between Alienation from Self and TV watching [22].

The challenge component of hardiness was measured negatively by the Security Scale of the California Life Goals Evaluation Schedule [23]. Examples of items are 'From each according to his ability; to each according to his needs,' and 'To achieve freedom from what is a large enough goal for anyone.' This true–false scale has been used widely with normal adult samples and has established reliability and validity [23]. It measures the degree to which safety, stability and predictability is deemed important. Persons high on this scale are unlikely to perceive changes as stimulating challenges to growth.

An emphasis on control was measured negatively by the External Locus of Control Scale [24] and the Powerlessness Scale of the Alienation Test [5]. The first of these scales consists of pairs of items in a forced-choice format. Examples of item-pair members showing an internal locus are 'People's misfortunes result from the mistakes they make,' and 'Capable people who fail to become leaders have not taken advantage of their opportunities.' Considerable research has shown this scale to be a reliable and valid index of the belief that one is controlled by external forces [6]. Although newer, the Powerlessness Scale shows an average internal consistency (Coefficient Alpha) of 0.88 over several adult samples, and a stability correlation of 0.71 over a three-week period [5]. Sample items are 'Most of my activities are determined by what society demands,' and 'It doesn't matter if people work hard at their jobs; only a few bosses profit.' Relevant to construct validation are a negative correlation with dominance and positive correlations with trait anxiety, external locus of control, and conformism [5].

The five scales of this composite have shown moderately high intercorrelations and jointly define the first and only large factor in a principal components factor analysis [7]. In addition, this hardiness composite has shown a stability correlation of 0.61 over a five-year period [23]. Following these precedents, subjects' scores on the five scales were standardized and added to obtain a measure of hardiness.

Measure of exercise

Following epidemiological procedures [3], subjects were asked (1) 'Do you engage in organized sports (e.g., jogging, tennis, softball) regularly?', (2) 'Do you engage in non-sports exercise (e.g., gardening, home repair) regularly?', (3) 'How many hours per week do you spend in sports and non-sports exercise?', and (4) 'On the average, how strenuous is the sports and non-sports exercise you engage in?' The last question was scored 0 (mild), 1 (moderate), or 2 (strenuous). The distribution of hours given in response to the third question was divided into thirds, yielding scores of 0, 1, and 2. The first two questions were scored simply 0 (no) or 1 (yes). Adding a subject's score on all four questions yielded his composite exercise score.

Measure of social support

Perceived social support at work was assessed by the Staff Support subscale of the Work Environment Scale [25]. This subscale, consisting of nine True–False items, was designed to measure the extent to which employees perceive their superiors in the organization as supportive. The original instrument was modified slightly to insure that subjects at the upper job levels would be able to answer the questions with reference to a superior. Sample items from this subscale are 'Superiors really stand up for their people,' and 'Those at the top give full credit to ideas contributed by others.' Moos [25] has used this subscale with a variety of occupational groups, and found it reliable and valid.

Measure of illness

Symptomatology was measured through the Seriousness of Illness Survey [26], a self-report checklist of 126 commonly recognized physical and mental symptoms and illnesses. In the development of this checklist, a severity weight for each disorder was obtained by asking a large sample of physicians and lay persons to rate each of them in terms of prognosis, duration, threat to life, degree of disability and degree of discomfort. The resulting scale of seriousness of illness has served as a frequent tool in stress and illness studies [27]. For present purposes, several symptoms of obvious irrelevance to the male sample were deleted.

Results

Relationship among resistance resources

As in previous years, hardiness and exercise were unrelated in 1980 ($r = 0.009$), rendering it unlikely that one exercises out of a sense of hardiness or feels hardy merely because of exercising. In 1980, hardiness did show a correlation of 0.23 ($p < 0.05$) with social support, which is not large enough, however, to suggest identity. Exercise and social support are also uncorrelated ($r = -0.02$), raising no question concerning their independence as buffers.

Number of resistance resources and illness

Table I shows the likelihood that illness score will be above the median of all subjects in the relevant year for various numbers of resistance resources. Concerning resistance resources, a score above the median for all subjects in 1980 was regarded as evidence that a resistance resource was strongly present. In addition, the mean illness scores for the various combinations of resistance resources is also shown. The 1980 and 1981 columns indicate illness means and likelihoods that are, respectively, concurrent with and following after estimates of stressful life events and resistance resources.

As shown in Table I, the probability that a subject will be above the median in illness increases as the number of resistance resources decreases. This relationship is summarized by Kendall's Tau$_C$ statistic, a

Table I. *Illness as a function of number of resistance resources among subjects high in stressful life events*

Resistance resources, 1980	n		Mean illness		Illness probability*	
	1980	1981	1980†	1981‡	1980§	1981‖
All three high	13	13	357.04	601.46	7.69	23.11
Two high	26	22	2049.27	1702.13	57.69	50.00
One high	32	24	3336.18	2715.58	71.87	62.50
None high	14	11	6474.35	5635.91	92.85	81.80

*The entries indicate the percentage of subjects in the various resistance resource categories falling above the illness median for all 71 subjects.
†For entries in this column, $F = 8.38$ ($p < 0.0001$).
‡For entries in this column, $F = 4.94$ ($p < 0.003$).
§For entries in this column, Kendall's $Tau_C = 0.52$ ($p < 0.0001$).
‖For entries in this column, Kendall's $Tau_C = 0.39$ ($p < 0.001$).

measure of association between two ordinal-level variables. The larger the statistic, the more likely a person in a 'higher' category in one variable will be so in the other. For purposes of analysis, subjects with three resistance resources were coded '1', those with two '2', those with one '3', and those with no resources '4'. Subjects below the median in illness were coded '1' and those above '2'.

Given this initial suggestive finding, attention was next turned to actual illness scores. Table I also shows that among highly stressed subjects, strength in all three resistance resources is associated with the lowest illness in both 1980 and 1981. High scores on two out of the three resistance resources yields the next lowest illness scores in both years. When subjects are high in only one resistance resource, illness scores are further elevated in both years. Finally, the highest illness scores in both years occur when subjects are low in all three resistance resources. Given the central question of the differential effects of the individual combinations of resistance resources, a planned comparison test was carried out in conjunction with a regular analysis of variance. The latter provides a general summary of the relationship between all groups of means being examined, but the nature of this investigation poses questions concerning the relationship between separate pairs of means.

With 4 degrees of freedom for the four categories of resistance resources, 3 orthogonal planned comparisons are permitted. Since the effects of each group combination are of central interest, the three

Table II. *Planned comparisons between resistance resource combinations*

Contrast	Mean difference	T value*	df	Sig. of T
1980 Illness				
3 Resources vs 2 Resources	−1692	−4.28	31.5	<0.001
2 Resources vs 1 Resource	−1287	−1.89	51.2	<0.030
1 Resource vs 0 Resources	−3138	−1.78	16.1	<0.050
1981 Illness				
3 Resources vs 2 Resources	−1101	−1.89	31.1	<0.40
2 Resources vs 1 Resource	−1013	−1.13	39.3	0.134
1 Resource vs 0 Resources	−2920	−1.56	13.9	<0.070

*For these analyses, a separate rather than pooled variance estimate was employed. The former is deemed more appropriate when there is some question concerning the homogeneity of variance assumption.

comparisons selected examined the groups pairwise as resistance sources decreased. The three specific hypotheses would then be:

1. Subjects with three resistance resources are healthier than those with two.
2. Subjects with two resistance resources are healthier than those with one.
3. Subjects with one resistance resource are healthier than those with none.

These comparisons are of course among the most stringent, but at the same time provide the clearest picture of the relationship between the groups. The results of the planned comparison analysis are presented in Table II. For both 1980 and 1981 illness, the overall ANOVA F's shown in Table I were highly significant: 1980 illness $F(3,81) = 8.38$, $p < 0.001$; 1981 illness $F(3,66) = 4.94$, $p < 0.003$. These overall statistics justify the subsequent planned comparisons.

Table II indicates that for the most part the hypotheses concerning the differential effects of the separate resistance resource groups were confirmed. For concurrent illness, the addition of one resource led to a significant decrease in illness in every instance. For prospective illness, the results were only slightly less positive. Three resources provided significantly more protection than two, and the difference between one and no resources was of borderline significance. Only the two versus one resource comparison failed to reach significance, and that result was none the less in the predicted direction. The strength of the above findings led to a final analysis, one that

Table III. *Multiple regression of illness with hardiness, social support, and exercise*

Variable	Multiple R	Cumulative R square	B^*	Beta*	F	Sig. of F
1980 Illness						
Hardiness	0.47	0.22	354.3	0.352	12.83	<0.01
Exercise	0.56	0.32	−980.2	−0.314	11.89	<0.01
Social support	0.59	0.35	−305.5	−0.194	3.72	<0.05
1981 Illness						
Hardiness	0.58	0.33	415.1	0.453	18.97	<0.01
Exercise	0.62	0.39	−357.4	−0.232	5.26	<0.01
Social support	0.65	0.43	−615.7	−0.213	4.73	<0.01

*The sign for hardiness is positive rather than negative because hardiness has been measured as a negative indicator. That is, the hardiness scale is constructed and scored in such a way that the higher a subject's score, the lower that subject's hardiness.

attempted to compare the buffering effectiveness of particular resistance resources. This seemed a logical refinement of the finding that a combination of resources in any pattern proved to buffer illness to a greater degree than any combination of fewer resources. To investigate the independent role of particular resistance resources, a multiple regression analysis was performed. Table III summarizes these results.

When the dependent variable is 1980 (or concurrent) illness, regression estimates show hardiness to be the most effective buffer, though exercise is also strong, leaving the smallest role for social support. As Table III shows, all three resources contribute significantly to the variance of 1980 illness. But hardiness alone explains almost one quarter of the variance of concurrent illness, and over 60% of all the variance accounted for in the analysis. The addition of exercise to the equation substantially increases the R^2 (by 10%), but the addition of social support adds little to the model (an additional 3%). These data seem to suggest that hardiness was the major force in the previously discussed grouping of resistance resources.

When the dependent variable is 1981 (or subsequent) illness, the estimates shown in Table III indicate that hardiness shows an even more pronounced buffering effect, and that exercise is now a slightly weaker moderator than social support. Here hardiness alone accounts for fully one third of the variance of 1981 illness and over three quarters of all variance explained. Social support and exercise, while again producing significant parameters, explain roughly 6 and 4% of the variance in subsequent illness. Again, hardiness appears to have been the most important resistance resource in the various combinations already analyzed.

Discussion

A combination of the three resistance resources of hardiness, social support and exercise appears to decrease illness likelihood in the face of highly stressful conditions to less than 10% concurrently and less than 24% subsequently. The trend toward lowered illness scores as the number of resistance resources increases is regular both concurrently and prospectively. In pinpointing the relative effectiveness of resistance resources, hardiness emerges as a more important buffer than are exercise and social support. Hardiness provides substantial protection against both concurrent and future illness. Social support and exercise appear to provide some protection both concurrently and prospectively, but their effects are relatively small compared to the contribution of hardiness.

The results of this study are understandable if certain implications of the manner in which the three resistance resources enact their buffering effect are considered. Because hardiness leads to transformation of events into less stressful forms, this resistance resource should have a strong buffering effect not only concurrently, but in the long run as well. In contrast, if exercise buffers by reducing the organismic strain produced by stressful events without altering them, they should last longer and thereby retain their ability to induce strain each time they are re-encountered. Thus, an executive experiencing a destructive relationship with his boss may, through hardiness, transform the situation by open discussion of differences, resolve to change, etc. He is thereby protected against strain in the future by the new accord with his superior. In contrast, the strain produced by the destructive relationship may be reduced by jogging, but the untransformed relationship retains its ability to reinduce strain. This is not to say, however, that exercise has no prospective value. Indeed, one might argue that the person who exercises regularly develops some degree of continued constitutional protection against strain. But, this is still a palliative effect. The role of exercise would remain one of warding off the effects of strain that have already manifested themselves. Thus, hardiness remains the most important prospective buffer of the deleterious effects of stress. Exercise levels in 1980 buffer 1981 illness, but the effects are relatively small.

Social support appears to emerge as a less critical buffer. But some indices in this study give it a role, and other studies have found it to be important (though they generally have not also measured hardiness and exercise). At the outset, it should be noted that many investigators [17] have recognized the heterogeneous quality of the social support construct.

The obtained correlation of hardiness and social support suggests that some meanings of the latter may overlap with the former. Hardiness has an active emphasis in that it predisposes persons to interact more intensely with stressful events in order to transform them into less stressful forms. When hardiness is controlled statistically (as in the regression analyses of this study), perhaps all that is left are the more passive implications of social support, namely, the reassurance about self and distraction from troubles that can be provided by affectionate others. This study suggests that these passive implications of social support have an only modest buffering effect. This is understandable in that they would not encourage transformational coping. In this regard, Kobasa and Puccetti [19] have reported that as stressful events at work mounted, social support from the family (perhaps likely to emphasize reassurance and distraction) was actually associated with increased illness when hardiness was low. It may be that the important place given to social support in previous conceptualizations of stress resistance is based on the undetected overlap of this admittedly heterogeneous construct with such personality constructs as hardiness.

This study provokes curiosity about how many resistance resources it is useful to have in the attempt to remain healthy despite stressful circumstances. Concurrently and prospectively, it appears that the more resources one possesses, the less likely one is to be at risk for serious illness. With respect to the differential effects of the separate sources, hardiness clearly emerges as the most powerful buffer both concurrently and prospectively. Social support and exercise also provide assistance in both temporal dimensions. These effects, however, are less marked than that of hardiness. If you could have only one resistance resource, hardiness would be the best. There are, of course, other putative resources [7], and their contribution to reduction of illness singly and in combination with the buffers of this study should be investigated.

Acknowledgement
We wish to thank Christine Hinze for help in this work.

References
1. ANTONOVSKY A. *Health, Stress and Coping*. Washington: Jossey-Bass, 1979.
2. KOBASA SC. Stressful life events, personality and health: An inquiry into hardiness. *J Person Soc Psychol* 1979; **37**: 1–11.
3. PAFFENBARGER RJ, HALE WE. Work activity and coronary heart mortality. *New Engl J Med* 1975; **292**: 545.

4. COBB S. Social support as a moderator of life stress. *Psychosom Med* 1976; **38**: 300–314.
5. MADDI SR, HOOVER M, KOBASA SC. Alienation and exploratory behavior. *J Person Soc Psychol* 1982; **42**: 884–890.
6. PHARES EJ. *Locus of Control in Personality*. Morristown, NJ: Central Learning Press, 1976.
7. KOBASA SC, MADDI SR, KAHN S. Hardiness and health: A prospective study. *J Personal Soc Psychol* 1982; **42**: 168–177.
8. KOBASA SC, MADDI SR, PUCCETTI MC. Personality and exercise as buffers in the stress–illness relationship. *J Behav Med* 1982; **5**: 391–403.
9. KOBASA SC, MADDI SR, COURINGTON S. Personality and constitution as mediators in the stress–illness relationship. *J Hlth Soc Behav* 1981; **22**: 368–378.
10. EPSTEIN L, MILLER GJ, STITT FW, MORRIS JN. Vigorous exercise in leisure time, coronary risk factors, and resting electrocardiogram in middle-aged civil servants. *Br Heart J* 1976; **38**: 403.
11. BOYER JM. Effects of chronic exercise on cardiovascular function. *Phys Fitness Res Digest* 1972; **2**: 1.
12. KARKOVEN MJ, RAUTAHARJU PM, ORMA E, PENSAR S, TAAKUNEN J. Heart disease and employment: Cardiovascular studies in lumberjacks. *J Occupational Med* 1961; **3**: 49.
13. SAMUELSON R. Effects of severe systemic hypoxia on myocardial excitation. *Acta Physiol Scand* 1973; **88**: 267.
14. INSULL W, editor. *Coronary Risk Handbook*. New York: American Heart Association, 1973.
15. WEINER H. *Psychobiology and Human Disease*. New York: Elsevier, 1977.
16. RABKIN JG, STRUENING EL. Life Events, stress, and illness. *Science* 1976; **194**: 1013–1020.
17. HOUSE JS. *Work Stress and Social Support*. Reading, Mass.: Addison–Wesley, 1981.
18. GORE S. The effect of social support in moderating the health consequences of unemployment. *J Hlth Soc Behav* 1978; **19**: 157–165.
19. KOBASA SC, PUCCETTI MC. Personality and social resources in stress-resistance. *J Personal Soc Psychol* 1983; **45**: 839–850.
20. HOLMES TH, RAHE RH. The Social Readjustment Rating Scale. *J Psychosom Res* 1967; **11**: 213–218.
21. DOHRENWEND BS, KRASNOFF L, ASKENASY AR, DOHRENWEND BP. Exemplification of a method for scaling life events: The PERI Life-Events Scale. *J Hlth Soc Behav* 1978; **19**: 205–229.
22. CSIKSZENTMIHALYI M. *Beyond Boredom and Anxiety*. San Francisco: Jossey-Bass, 1975.
23. HAHN NE. *California Life Goals Evaluation Schedule*. Palo Alto: Western Psychological Services, 1966.
24. ROTTER JB, SEEMAN M, LIVERANT S. Internal vs external locus of control of reinforcement: A major variable in behavior theory. In *Decisions, Values and Groups* (Edited by WASHBURNE NF). London: Pergamon Press, 1962.
25. MOOS RH. *The Human Context: Environmental Determinants of Behavior*. New York: Wiley, 1976.

26. WYLER AR, MASUDA M, HOLMES TH. Magnitude of life events and seriousness of illness. *Psychosom Med* 1971; **33**: 115–122.
27. DOHRENWEND BS, DOHRENWEND BP, editors. *Stressful Life Events: Their Nature and Effects*. New York: Wiley, 1974.

Section 4

Health practices and the modification of health risk behaviour

---

Readings

A multivariate analysis of health-related practices: a nine-year mortality follow-up of the Alameda County Study.
    D. L. Wingard, L. F. Berkman and R. J. Brand. *American Journal of Epidemiology*, **116**, 765–75, 1982.

The Health Belief Model and participation in programmes for the early detection of breast cancer: a comparative analysis.
    M. Calnan. *Social Science and Medicine*, **19**, 823–30, 1984.

Health promotion and the compression of morbidity.
    J. F. Fries, L. W. Green and S. Levine. *Lancet*, **i**, 481–3, 1989.

Community education for cardiovascular health.
    J. W. Farquhar, N. Maccoby, P. D. Wood, J. K. Alexander,
    H. Breitrose, B. W. Brown, W. L. Haskell, A. L. McAlister,
    A. J. Meyer, J. D. Nash and M. P. Stern. *Lancet*, **i**, 1192–5, 1977.

Primary prevention of cancer among children: changes in cigarette smoking and diet after six years of intervention.
    H. J. Walter, R. D. Vaughan and E. L. Wynder. *Journal of the National Cancer Institute*, **81**, 995–9, 1989.

Introduction

The acknowledgement of the role of lifestyle in the aetiology of many major diseases has been one of the most profound shifts in medical thinking in the twentieth century. In both the developed and the developing world, practices such as smoking and drinking are now believed to make a substantial contribution to premature mortality. The fervour with which lifestyle change has been promoted by governments world-wide reflects the seriousness with which these findings are regarded (US Department of Health and Human Services, 1990; Department of Health, 1992) and the wealth of research and polemic on this topic makes the choice of literature very difficult. The readings that have been selected in this section represent a number of important themes, including the initial observations that behaviour and health are related (*Wingard et al.*), the predictors of health behaviour (*Calnan*), the determination of appropriate endpoints in health promotion research (*Fries et al.*), and the evaluation of the efficacy of intervention strategies (*Farquhar et al., Walter et al.*).

The basic epidemiological work in this field has been concerned with the links between common behaviours such as smoking, exercise and dietary choice, and a variety of endpoints from general health status, through morbidity from specific diseases, to mortality. Many studies focus on a single behaviour; studies on smoking and mortality in British doctors (Doll and Bradford-Hill, 1954), dietary fat and cardiovascular disease (Keys, 1970), fruit intake and lung cancer (Fontham, 1990) and sexual behaviour and HIV infection (van Griensven *et al.*, 1989) exemplify this approach. Other research has taken the perspective of a behavioural profile across a range of health practices, and has evaluated outcome in relation to the extent of compliance with current guidelines (Belloc and Breslow, 1972). There are drawbacks and benefits to each strategy. The single behaviour approach may overstate the adverse impact of any individual behaviour, since one damaging behaviour is likely to be correlated with other equally damaging behavioural patterns. The use of summary methods, where a range of behaviours are combined in a *health practices index*, gives a better reflection of the lifestyle concept, but requires care in identifying the appropriate weighting for different behaviours. *Wingard, Berkman and Brand* use both methods in their longitudinal investigation of health practices and health outcomes.

The method of assessing health behaviour is another important issue in this area. The reliability and validity of the measurements of health behaviour are critical to the success of such investigations, and a range of methods have been used to estimate the level of behaviour. In some international comparsion studies *per capita* indices have been used, as in Keys's (1970) study of dietary fat and heart disease. In other cases, the behaviour can be assessed from public records (e.g. the use of records of breast screening attendance by *Calnan*). Self-reports of behaviours such as smoking, diet or exercise provide the most realistic method of assessment in much health behaviour research. As the public becomes more aware of the negative reactions of health professionals to people with 'unhealthy' lifestyles, increasing care will be needed to obtain accurate information. In some cases it is possible to supplement self-reports by information from other family members and thereby increase the reliability of the behavioural data. In other cases, biochemical confirmation or validation can be used, for example in the use of serum cholesterol to support reported changes in diet or the assessment of plasma thiocyanate to confirm reports of cigarette consumption (*Farquhar et al.*).

Interventions to promote health behaviours now represent a major activity in the area of public health. Few adults can be unaware of at least some of the prevailing advice across the spectrum of behaviours including quitting smoking, avoiding fatty foods, using condoms, wearing seatbelts and attending cancer screening. However, only a minority follow all such recommendations and many follow none. Publicity about the links between behaviour and health or public advice about health behaviour can appear to be comparatively ineffective in achieving behaviour change. For example, the benefits of exercise have been publicised for decades, but the evidence suggests little public response in the UK and even a decline in both exercise participation and fitness in children (Sports Council, 1992). Likewise, fruit has been promoted as health-enhancing for a very long time, yet consumption has risen marginally, if at all, and a substantial proportion of the adult population rarely, if ever, eat fruit (Gregory *et al.*, 1990). Nevertheless, the evidence from a range of social trends suggests that the public *do* respond to advice about health promotion. In response to advice on the adverse health effects of tobacco, smoking prevalence declined from 45% to 30% in the UK between 1974 and 1990, and to even lower levels in the highest social status groups. Dietary changes have also been pronounced with brown bread consumption increasing and butter consumption decreasing strikingly in response to public health advice (Ministry of Agriculture, Fisheries and Food, 1991).

Controlled intervention studies have also provided compelling evidence that health behaviours are susceptible to influence through health promotion. Mass media campaigns, combined where possible with environmental and legislative support, may offer a cost-effective approach, since coverage is wide and no identification of individual targets is necessary. The North Karelia Project, started after Finland was shown to have exceptionally high levels of heart disease, was directed towards reducing smoking, reducing fat intake and increasing detection of hypertension. The five-year results suggested a modest but significant change in behaviour and a decline in cardiovascular disease relative to the control population (Puska *et al.*, 1985). Likewise, in the Stanford Heart Disease Prevention Project (*Farquhar et al.*) the communities exposed to media campaigns showed significant changes in health habits. The alternative approach is to target high-risk groups, which has the advantage that the study population may perceive the intervention to be personally relevant, but has the disadvantage of needing an expensive screening procedure to select the subjects (Rose, 1985). The Multiple Risk Factor Intervention Trial (MRFIT Research Group, 1982) involved one of the largest controlled interventions with high-risk subjects for coronary heart disease. A sample of 12 000 men who smoked or had raised cholesterol or hypertension were assigned randomly either to a special intervention condition or to a control group (usual care). Unexpectedly, the control group showed considerable improvement in health habits and cardiovascular risk, and over the intervention period there were no mortality differences between the intervention and control groups. However, there were differences in morbidity, which, while not as spectacular as mortality changes, reinforce the position that rigorous health promotion is effective in changing behaviour.

Health-related behaviour and mortality

The paper by *Wingard, Berkman and Brand* evaluates the relationship between seven behaviours and mortality, as well as a health practices index based on the sum of five of the behaviours. The data for this analysis came from the Alameda County study that was described in Section 1 (*Berkman and Syme*). Demographic data were collected at interview and the health behaviour data were based on questionnaire responses. In the first report, Belloc and Breslow (1972) showed strong relationships between health practices and health status. Since then, information on mortality has strengthened the conclusions. In the analysis described in this reading, mortality data were obtained for the nine-year- follow-up period from the California Death Registry. Age-adjusted mortality rates were found to be related to each of the health practices except meal patterns, with relative risks ranging from 1.2 to 1.9. The use of the health practices index showed higher death rates among those with poor health practices for all-cause mortality as well as individually for cancer, coronary heart disease and other circulatory diseases. As noted earlier, the use of an index which combines a number of behaviours has been criticised (Slater and Linder, 1988), but it does nevertheless capture and quantify the idea of a healthy lifestyle. The specific behavioural factors which are included might have been different if the study had been conceived in the 1990s. Diet is the most obvious omission, with avoidance of fat and other healthy dietary practices being included in more recent health behaviour profiles (Wardle and Steptoe, 1991).

Data from the Alameda County Human Population Laboratory have been very influential in establishing links between behaviour and health status, initially in terms of cross-sectional relationships and subsequently from longitudinal data. The basic cross-sectional phase of the study has been replicated in a similar study of adults in Michigan (Brock *et al.*, 1988), and endorses epidemiological associations between lifestyle factors and mortality from major causes such as cancer, cardiovascular disease and accidents (Amler and Dull, 1987). The same patterns of heightened risk associated with less 'healthy' behaviour were found in an older subgroup of the Alameda County subjects (Kaplan *et al.*, 1987).

The challenge with this, as with other data sets in which behaviour and health are compared, lies in identifying the direction of the causal effects. While there is good reason to expect that physical activity, for example, might promote good health and longevity, it is also true that ill-health could curtail physical activity. An effect of this kind would exaggerate the apparent health-benefits of exercise. Similarly, low body weight predicts poorer longevity, but perhaps because as-yet-undetected disease is compromising appetite. Two steps are often taken to minimise this effect. In some cases, subjects with any evidence of ill-health are excluded from the study. The other strategy is to exclude deaths which occur close to the original assessment time. The demonstration in *Wingard et al.*'s paper that mortality is still raised in people with poor health practices, even after excluding deaths in the first five years, increases the confidence with which causal conclusions can be drawn.

Among the most interesting observations on the Alameda study is that health behaviours were related to a wide range of illnesses and causes of death. This suggests a pervasive influence rather than disease-specific effect. This has important implications for the possible mechanisms – some of which are explored in other sections.

Health beliefs and health behaviour

The issue of why some people, but not others, have healthy lifestyles or healthy practices has attracted considerable attention from social psychologists who have put forward a number of social cognition models. The models have in common an emphasis on a rational decision process leading to health behaviour, in which perceived costs are weighed against perceived advantages. At the simplest level, beliefs in the value of the particular behaviour are related to the probability of practice of that behaviour, and consistent relationships emerge across a wide range of belief–behaviour associations (Steptoe and Wardle, 1992). The Health Belief Model (Becker, 1974) was among the first to propose that health behaviour can be predicted from the individual's appraisal of the risks and benefits of compliance. Across a range of behaviours from attendance at immunization to weight loss, there has been a wealth of evidence that people's evaluation of their susceptibility to the relevant condition, the severity of the condition, the efficacy of the recommended behaviour and the barriers to compliance determine whether or not they will comply. The Theory of Reasoned Action (Ajzen and Fishbein, 1980) has similar components but also incorporates the individual's perception of the social pressures to perform the behaviour.

These and other social cognition models have provided a valuable theoretical background within which the cognitive influences on health behaviour have been evaluated, and from which interventions have been derived. However, *Calnan* points out in the next reading that many of these studies have collected data on attitudes and behaviour at the same time – thus reducing the prospects for drawing causal inferences from the data. *Calnan* himself examined the relationship between a range of variables deriving from the Health Belief Model and later attendance either at mammography or breast self-examination classes. The initial interviews were carried out at least one month before the arrival of the invitation to attend the breast screening service. The results produced strong support for the predictive value of cognitive variables. Health motivation, perceived vulnerability to breast cancer and belief that the benefits of screening outweigh the costs, were among the best discriminators between attenders and non-attenders. A recent study which used a very similar prospective design to evaluate attendance at breast screening broadly replicated these findings (Sutton *et al.*, 1994). Again, beliefs about the benefits of breast screening and perceived risk of breast cancer were the best predictors of attendance.

Calnan's study has the advantage of employing objective criteria of health behaviour (attendance at clinics or classes) rather than relying on self-report. However, in common with other studies, the health belief variables do not explain a large proportion of the variance. This is perhaps to be expected in a situation where many unpredictable environmental factors must almost certainly play an influential role. More generally, the commonly voiced criticism that cognitive models are of limited value because they only explain a small proportion of the variance is perhaps not justified. Health behaviours are clearly affected by a host of factors ranging from macroeconomic conditions and cultural background to social and family habits and practices (Cohen and Henderson, 1988). It is improbable that analysis at any single level will provide a complete explanation. Health beliefs are important because they may be more amenable to change than many of the structural social determinants of health-related behaviour (Weinstein, 1987).

Morbidity and mortality as endpoints

Decisions about the appropriate endpoints in health behaviour research have been controversial. They include overall mortality, disease-specific mortality, morbidity, quality of life, and risk factor changes. Mortality statistics (such as those collected in the Alameda County study) attract least criticism, since death registrations are likely to be complete and incontrovertible, but overall mortality may obscure changes in the pattern of causes of death. Disease-specific mortality figures depend on the registered cause of death being accurate, and where there is no standardised method of establishing the cause of death, there can be variability in diagnostic practices. Morbidity data represent 'softer' endpoints, depending as they do on the processes whereby people seek and receive diagnoses, but may provide a more sensitive index of behavioural interventions. Some scientists have preferred the 'harder' endpoint of mortality, and in the absence of any effect on mortality have discounted morbidity effects and denied the importance of behaviour to health (McCormick and Skrabanek, 1988). A number of important studies have failed to show evidence that behavioural interventions affect all-cause mortality and, in some cases, even mortality benefits for the target condition have been minimal (e.g. MRFIT Research Group, 1982). However, in their reading, *Fries, Green and Levine* put forward the idea that life expectancy in the developed world has reached, or is close to reaching, its limit. When this upper boundary is approached, treatment or prevention of one condition only permits mortality from another, so length of life is not extended, and reduction in mortality rate is a remote and possibly unrealistic target. Improvement in health and quality of life in the later years may provide a more appropriate target for health promotion (see also Olshansky *et al.*, 1990).

Fries et al. identify considerable scope for what they call the 'compression of morbidity'. Good health practices and good medical care can prolong the proportion of life associated with excellent health, and may abbreviate the proportion associated with disabling morbidity. This view has important implications for outcome assessments in health promotion. Measures of morbidity such as functional disability and quality of life may provide more effective demonstrations of the potency of new treatments or preventive programmes than will mortality data. In MRFIT, morbid events were reduced by 16% in the intervention compared with the control group, and comparable effects have been found in other intervention trials which have failed to find effects on mortality. This approach has yet to find favour in behavioural epidemiology, where one of the claims to status has been the apparent ability of psychosocial factors to prolong life. It also increases the difficulty and subjectivity of investigations, since the assessment of factors such as health status, functional ability and quality of life all require more intensive effort than searching death certificates. Nevertheless, there may be considerable gains to be made. A shift of perspective from quantity to quality could prove to be an important emerging theme in years to come.

Community education and risk reduction

The paper from *Farquhar and his colleagues* describes results from the Stanford Heart Disease Prevention Project, one of the most influential community programmes designed to improve cardiovascular health. Three comparable communities in California were identified. Tracy was the control community, in which no new initiatives were implemented, while the intervention communities (Gilroy and Watsonville) had intensive mass-media campaigns designed to increase knowledge and motivation in relation to dietary change and smoking cessation. In Watsonville, high-risk groups were given additional face-to-face instruction. In each city there were annual interviews concerning knowledge and behaviour, measures of lipids and blood pressure, and plasma thiocyanate validations for cigarette consumption. An overall coronary risk index was computed from age, sex, cholesterol, weight, smoking and the electrocardiogram. The results showed that the intervention communities became more knowledgeable, ate less fat, smoked less and achieved lower cholesterol and blood pressure, although they did not change weight. In terms of the high risk subjects, there was clear evidence for the most change in the intensive interaction group (Watsonville).

The Stanford study has shown that behaviours can be changed and that mass-media campaigns are an appropriate vehicle for change. Out of this study grew the larger Stanford Five City Project (Farquhar *et al.*, 1985) which also used community education methods applied to a range of community groups. In this study, mortality and morbidity are being monitored as well as behaviour change, and reductions of around 15% in estimated mortality risk have been observed (Farquhar *et al.*, 1990). Other comprehensive, community-based cardiovascular prevention projects have produced similar beneficial effects on behaviour change and are now reaching the point of adoption as routine in public health. The growing implementation of cardiovascular prevention may have costs as well as benefits. Economic costs for mass-media campaigns are not inconsiderable. The cost/benefit ratio for new information may increase further as the sheer mass of health information available to the public reaches saturation. Most adults today receive a wealth of health advice, in magazines and newspapers, on the radio and TV, on billboards, in doctors' and dentists' surgeries, on cigarette packets, on foods, in supermarkets, and even in leaflets direct to the home. Health psychology may need to consider the impact of health-related information on self-perception of health and well-being. Barsky (1988) has referred to the 'Paradox of Health' whereby subjective evaluation of illness has increased despite improvements in the population's health. One explanation for this may be that the emphasis on the steps which individuals can take to improve their health, and the sometimes exaggerated claims for the efficacy of any particular step, lead to an impression that perfect health should be accessible to all. By comparison, the *status quo* can appear to be unsatisfactory. The challenge posed by these findings is to develop ways of increasing the levels of health behaviour without increasing the extent of worry about health. One possible route is to increase the environmental support for healthy behaviours as an alternative to targeting individuals' effort.

School-based primary prevention

The logic of primary prevention suggests that the earlier the intervention the more effective it would be. An ideal situation would be one in which children would never adopt unhealthy lifestyles. An added incentive for interventions with children derives from the expectation that habits acquired in childhood will persist into later life. Early prevention of adverse health habits has been investigated most extensively in the smoking field, where there have been many school-based interventions designed to forestall smoking uptake in children. The Houston project (Evans et al., 1981) reported lower levels of smoking among the group who had received a multi-media intervention designed to heighten awareness of the harm of smoking and to teach skills in resisting it. In the context of the Five City Project, school-based nutrition and smoking programmes have been initiated (Altman et al., 1987). The reading from *Walter, Vaughan and Wynder* describes a school-based intervention directed towards cigarette smoking and diet. The teacher-based 'know your body' programme was incorporated into the school curriculum. The results showed favourable effects for both saturated fat consumption and smoking uptake in the intervention schools. An earlier analysis indicated that these effects were coupled with higher levels of physical activity and greater health knowledge in the intervention schools (Walter et al., 1988).

School-based interventions are now being evaluated widely, and target not only diet, physical activity and smoking, but behaviours such as the use of seat belts (Morrow, 1989). A potential drawback stems from the fact that school-based interventions are not universally successful and, in some cases, considerable effort is spent for few returns (Murray *et al.*, 1992). Negative results may undermine the willingness of school systems to expend efforts in health education and disease prevention. One explanation could be that the proposed benefits of health behaviour (e.g. prevention of premature death, freedom from chronic cardiovascular disease in the later decades) may not be sufficiently attractive to young people. Health is typically valued less by younger than older people, while factors such as fashion, appearance and socialising are more significant influences in the young. It could be argued that if even the best intervention outcome is only a limited period of healthy behaviour over the lifespan, then this might be more profitable it it is carried out close to the years of morbidity in late middle-age. However, on the positive side, school-based interventions offer an unparalleled opportunity for health education. Health education can be incorporated into the school curriculum with comparative ease, and imparted in a fashion suited to the abilities of the recipients. A generation of young people possessing the basic knowledge about behaviour and health should enhance the prospects of promoting healthier lifestyles both in youth and later in life.

References

Ajzen, I. and Fishbein, M. (1980). *Understanding Attitudes and Predicting Social Behaviour*. Englewood Cliffs, NJ: Prentice-Hall.

Altman, D. G., Fortmann, S. P. and Farquhar, J. W. (1987). Cost-effectiveness of three smoking cessation programs. *American Journal of Public Health*, **77**, 162–5.

Amler, R. W. and Dull, H. B. (eds.) (1987). *Closing the Gap*. New York: Oxford University Press.

Barsky, A. J. (1988). The paradox of health. *New England Journal of Medicine*, **318**, 414–18.

Becker, M. H. (ed.) (1974). *The Health Belief Model and Personal Health Behaviour*. New Jersey: Slack.

Belloc, M. and Breslow, L. (1972). Relationship of physical health status health practices. *Preventive Medicine*, **1**, 409–21.

Brock, B. M., Haefner, D. P. and Noble, D. S. (1988). Alameda County Redux: replication in Michigan. *Preventive Medicine*, **17**. 483–95.

Cohen, D. R. and Henderson, J. B. (1988). *Health, Prevention and Economics*. Oxford: Oxford University Press.

Department of Health (1992). *The Health Of The Nation*. London: HMSO.

Doll, R. and Bradford-Hill, A. (1954). The mortality of doctors in relation to their smoking habits. *British Medical Journal*, **1**, 1451–5.

Evans, R. I., Rozelle, R. M., Maxwell, S. E., Raines, B. E., Dill, C. A. and Guthrie, T. J. (1981). Social modeling films to deter smoking in adolescents. Results of a three-year field investigation. *Journal of Applied Psychology*, 66, 399–414.

Farquhar, J. W., Fortmann, S. P., Maccoby, N., Haskell, W. B., Williams, P. T., Flora, J. A., Taylor, C. B., Brown, B. W., Solomon, D. S. and Hulley, S. B. (1985). The Stanford Five City Project: design and methods. *American Journal of Epidemiology*, 122, 323–43.

Farquhar, J. W., Fortmann, S. P., Flora, J. A., Taylor, C. B., Haskell, W. L., Williams, P. T., Maccoby, N. and Wood, P. D. (1990). Effects of communitywide education on cardiovascular disease risk factors. *Journal of the American Medical Association*, 264, 359–65.

Fontham, E. T. H. (1990). Protective dietary factors and lung cancer. *International Journal of Epidemiology*, 19 (supl. 1), S32–S42.

Gregory, J., Foster, K., Tyler, H. and Wiseman, M. (1990). *The Dietary and Nutritional Survey of Adults*. London: HMSO.

Kaplan, G. A., Seeman, T. E., Cohen, R. D., Knudsen, L. P. and Guralnik, J. (1987). Mortality among the elderly in the Alameda County Study: behavioral and demographic risk factors. *American Journal of Public Health*, 77, 307–12.

Keys, A. (1970). *Coronary Heart Disease in Seven Countries*. New York: American Heart Association Monograph No. 29.

McCormick, J. and Skrabanek, P. (1988). Coronary heart disease is not preventable by population interventions. *Lancet*, ii, 839–41.

Ministry of Agriculture, Fisheries and Food (1991). *Fifty Years of the National Food Survey*. London: HMSO.

Morrow, R. (1989). A school-based program to increase seatbelt use. *Journal of Family Practice*, 29, 517–20.

MRFIT Research Group (1982). MRFIT: risk factor changes and mortality results. *Journal of the American Medical Association*, 248, 1465–77.

Murray, D. M., Perry, C. L., Griffin, G., Harty, K. C., Jacobs, D. R., Schmid, L., Daly, K. and Pallonen, U. (1992). Results from a statewide approach to adolescent tobacco use prevention. *Preventive Medicine*, 21, 449–72.

Olshansky, S. J., Carnes, B. A. and Cassel, C. (1990). In search of Methuselah: estimating the upper limits of human longevity. *Science*, 250, 634–40.

Puska, P., Nissinen, A., Tuomilehto, J., Salonen, J. T., Koskela, K., McAlister, A., Kottke, T. E., Maccoby, N. and Farquhar, J. W. (1985). The community-based strategy to prevent coronary heart disease: conclusions from the ten years of the North Karelia Project. *American Review of Public Health*, 6, 147–93.

Rose, G. (1985). Sick individuals and sick populations. *International Journal of Epidemiology*, 14, 32–8.

Slater, C. H. and Linder, S. H. A. (1988). A reassessment of the additive scoring of health practices. *Medical Care*, 26, 1216–27.

Sports Council (1992). *National Fitness Survey*. London: Sports Council and the Health Education Authority.

Steptoe, A. and Wardle, J. (1992). Cognitive predictors of health behaviour in contrasting regions of Europe. *British Journal of Clinical Psychology*, 31, 485–502.

Sutton, S., Bickler, G., Aldridge, J. and Saidi, G. (1994). Prospective study of predictors of attendance for breast screening in inner London. *Journal of Epidemiology and Community Health*, **48**, 65–73.

US Department of Health and Human Services (1990). *Healthy people 2000*. Washington DC: USDHHS.

van Griensven, G. J. P., de Vroome, E. M. M., Goudsmit, J. and Coutinho, R. A. (1989). Changes in sexual behaviour and the fall in incidence of HIV infection among homosexual men. *British Medical Journal*, **298**, 218–21.

Walter, H. J., Hofman, A., Vaughan, R. D. and Wynder, E. L. (1988). Modification of risk factors for coronary heart disease: five-year results of a school-based intervention trial. *New England Journal of Medicine*, **318**, 1093–100.

Wardle, J. and Steptoe, A. (1991). The European Health and Behaviour Survey: rationale, methods and results from the United Kingdom. *Social Science and Medicine*, **33**, 925–36.

Weinstein, N. D. (ed.) (1987). *Taking Care: Understanding and Encouraging Self-Protective Behavior*. New York: Cambridge University Press.

A multivariate analysis of health-related practices: a nine-year mortality follow-up of the Alameda County Study

Deborah L. Wingard, Lisa F. Berkman and Richard J. Brand

Department of Community and Family Medicine, M-007, University of California, San Diego, La Jolla, CA 92093, USA; Department of Epidemiology and Public Health, Institute for Social and Policy Studies, Yale University, New Haven, CT, USA; Department of Biomedical and Environmental Health Sciences, Program in Biostatics, School of Public Health, University of California, Berkeley, CA, USA

Abstract

Wingard, D. L. (Dept. of Community and Family Medicine, School of Medicine, U. of California, San Diego, CA 92093), L. F. Berkman and R. J. Brand. A multivariate analysis of health-related practices: a nine-year mortality follow-up of the Alameda County Study. *Am J Epidemiol* 1982;116:765–75.

Associations between several common health-related practices and a variety of health outcomes have been reported. However, the independent associations between each of these practices and mortality from all causes have not been assessed. In the present report, a multiple logistic analysis of seven potentially health-related practices (individually and in a summary index) and mortality from all causes is conducted, using data from the Human Population Laboratory Study of a random sample of 6928 adults living in Alameda County, California in 1965 and a subsequent nine-year mortality follow-up. Many covariables such as physical health status and socioeconomic status are simultaneously analyzed. The health-related practices examined are: 1) never smoking; 2) regular physical activity; 3) low alcohol consumption; 4) average weight status; 5) sleeping seven to eight hours/night; 6) not skipping breakfast; and 7) not snacking between meals. The analysis reveals that five of the practices are associated with lower mortality from all causes. Neither eating breakfast nor not snacking have significant independent associations with lower mortality. After covariable adjustment, respondents who reported few low-risk practices have a relative risk of 2.3 ($p < 0.001$) when compared with those who had many low-risk practices. Mortality risks for possible combinations of health-related practices are discussed.

Reprinted from Wingard, D. L., Berkman, L. F. and Brand, R. J. A multivariate analysis of health-related practices: a nine-year mortality follow-up of the Alameda County Study. *American Journal of Epidemiology*, **116**, 765–75, 1982.

alcohol drinking; exertion; longevity; longitudinal studies; mortality; sleep; smoking

In the last 20 years, a considerable body of evidence has accumulated which indicates that certain common behaviors, notably cigarette smoking, alcohol consumption, and physical inactivity, play an important role in the development of disease. Since its beginning, the Human Population Laboratory has had a strong commitment to conducting research in this area. Based on cross-sectional data, Belloc and Breslow (1) reported an association between good physical health status and seven potentially health-related practices: never smoking, physical activity, moderate or no alcohol consumption, average weight, sleeping seven or eight hours/night, eating breakfast, and not snacking between meals. In subsequent work, these same health-related practices have been found to be associated with low six- and nine-year mortality risk (2, 3).

Data from other sources also suggest that these practices are associated with a wide variety of health outcomes (4). Religious groups that avoid the use of tobacco, alcohol, coffee, and tea have low rates of cancer (5), coronary artery disease (6), and respiratory system disease (7). Prospective studies in Framingham (8) and by the American Cancer Society (9) indicate that physical inactivity, obesity, and smoking are associated with high morbidity and mortality. Studies of longshoremen also reveal a substantial association between cigarette smoking, abnormal weight status, and physical inactivity and subsequent fatal heart attacks (10–12).

The majority of research in this area, however, focuses on the morbidity or mortality risk of single practices. For example, numerous studies since the work by Doll and Hill (13) demonstrate a relationship between cigarette smoking and poor health status (14–16). Other studies of the effects of alcohol on health (17, 18) indicate that alcoholics have higher mortality rates than the general population (19, 20) and that heavy alcohol consumption is associated with higher mortality rates (21). More recent research indicates that alcohol consumption may be negatively associated with coronary heart disease mortality (22, 23), but positively associated with cancer mortality (23), especially when linked with smoking (24). Research also demonstrates that physical inactivity (25) and obesity (26, 27) are associated with an increase in morbidity and mortality, especially from cardiovascular difficulties. Very little research, however, has been done on the mortality risk associated with different sleeping patterns, skipping breakfast, and snacking between meals.

Since the work cited above predominately considers each habit individually or in a summary index, the independent contribution of each potentially health-related practice to mortality risk, after adjustment for other practices, is difficult to assess. Further, many studies fail to control for original health status or demographic and social variables that are related to subsequent health-related practices. The following multivariate analyses consider simultaneously the nine-year mortality risk of each of seven potentially health-related practices, original health status, and several demographic and social variables, in an effort to determine the independent relationship of each habit to health. In keeping with previous reports from the Human Population Laboratory (1–3), mortality prediction based on a summary index of health practices is also presented.

Materials and methods

Study population

The data presented in this report are based on information gathered by the Human Population Laboratory of the California State Department of Health Services. In 1965, the department surveyed a stratified systematic sample of Alameda County housing units. Institutionalized populations were not included. The sampling procedure, explained in greater detail elsewhere (28), resulted in the selection of 4452 occupied housing units. An enumerator visited each of these units, gathered demographic data on household members of all ages, and left a questionnaire for all persons aged 20 years or over, or younger people who were married. Identified as eligible for the study were 8023 adults. Of these, 6928 (86 per cent) returned questionnaires. When compared to respondents, the nonrespondents include slightly more older people, males, whites, retired, single, and widowed persons. However, the differences between respondents and nonrespondents are small, and respondents have been judged to be a fairly representative sample of adults in the county (29). The present analysis is restricted to the 2229 men and 2496 women who were between 30 and 69 years of age in 1965.

Mortality follow-up

Mortality data were collected for the nine-year period from 1965 to 1974. To obtain death certificates of those who had died within the state, a computer-matching file was created with the California Death Registry (30). Out-of-state death clearance information was obtained for those respondents who moved out of state during this period. Through these methods, death certificates were obtained for 211 men and 160 women respondents aged 30 to 69 years in 1965. Death rates for nonrespondents were higher than for respondents in the first two years of follow-up, and then equalized (30). An extensive follow-up survey in 1974 located all but 149 respondents or 3 per cent of the present sample. Since those lost to follow-up did not differ markedly on health measures as determined in the 1965 survey, their death rate is probably similar to the whole sample. The collection of mortality data, therefore, seems fairly complete and unbiased.

Variables studied

The seven health-related practices identified in earlier reports by the Human Population Laboratory (1–3) are analyzed in the present report. They include information about cigarette smoking, physical inactivity, alcohol consumption, weight status, sleeping patterns, skipping breakfast, and snacking between meals. Each of the first five are dichotomized for ease of analysis and to replicate the approach of earlier reports from the Human Population Laboratory. The last two variables concerning eating habits are not dichotomized, since preliminary analyses revealed no consistent trend. Categorization of each variable is presented in table 1.

A health practices index, similar to that reported in earlier Human Population Laboratory studies, is constructed from five practices which exhibit an association with mortality risk (see Results). It includes information about cigarette smoking, physical inactivity, alcohol consumption, weight status, and sleeping patterns. For each practice, the category associated with the lowest mortality risk is assigned one point, while the category associated with the highest mortality risk received none. Points from the five practices are totalled for the index, which ranges from 0 to 5. The index is then divided into three categories: low, 0–2; medium, 3; and high, 4–5. This replicates earlier work and allows for an easier analysis. The index is based on the *a priori* hypothesis that it is the number of healthy behaviors that counts rather than an attempt to construct an index based on mortality rates. Therefore, the relative risk associated with the extreme categories of the health practices index, i.e., low to high, will not be the same as the relative risk determined from the combined risk of the individual health-related practices. An index based on those risks, to be tested in another data set, would use the logistic coefficients determined in this study to weight each health-related practice.

Seven demographic and social variables implicated as mortality risk factors and associated with health practices are controlled for in the following analyses. Included are age, sex, race, socioeconomic status, use of health services, life satisfaction, and a social network index. Since health may influence which health-related practices a person adopts, health status in 1965 is also included in the following analyses. Classification of each of the above variables is presented in table 1.

Table 1. *Classification of variables influencing mortality, Alameda County, CA, 1965–1974*

Variable (codes)	Categories	Remarks
Health-related practices		
Cigarette smoking (0.1)	Never; ever	
Physical inactivity (0, 1)	Active; inactive	Based on the frequency (often, sometimes, never) and presumed strenuousness of leisure time participation in active sports, swimming or long walks, physical exercise, gardening, and/or hunting or fishing
Alcohol consumption (0, 1)	Low; high ($\geq$45 drinks/month)	Based on frequency of drinking (no. of times/week) and amount consumed (usual no. of drinks/sitting) for beer, wine, and liquor combined; dichotomization based on studies of drinking practices by Calalan and Cisin (31)
Weight status (0, 1)	Average weight (9.9% underweight to 29.9% overweight); extreme underweight or overweight	Measured by the Quetelet index, weight in pounds/(height in inches)^2, categories based on Metropolitan Life Insurance reports (32) of desirable weights
Sleeping patterns (0, 1)	7 or 8 hours/night; $\leq$6 or $\geq$9 hours/night	Based on usual no. of hours slept/night
Skipping breakfast (1–3)	Never; sometimes; often	
Snacking (1–3)	Never; sometimes; often	
Demographic and social variables		
Age (30–69)	Years	
Sex (1, 2)	Female; male	
Race (0, 1)	White; other	

Table 1 (cont.)

Variable (codes)	Categories	Remarks
Socioeconomic status (1–5)	Five groups, high to low class	Based on education and household income; Berkman (33)
Use of health services (1–3)	Often; sometimes; rarely	Based on visits to a doctor or dentist when not ill; Berkman (33)
Life satisfaction (1–3)	High; moderate; low	Based on 9 questions about satisfaction with aspects of one's life, such as marriage or job; Berkman (33)
Physical health status (1–4)	Healthy; symptoms; chronic condition; disabled	Derived from extensive checklist of health problems, coded by most serious condition; Belloc et al. (34)
Social network index (1–4)	Four groups, many to few social connections	Based on marital status, contacts with friends and relatives, church and group membership; Berkman and Syme (35)

Statistical analyses

Two stages of analysis are included in this report. The first stage consists of a series of univariate computations of sex-specific nine-year mortality rates for categories of each potentially health-related practice. These rates are used for within-practice and within-sex comparisons. The mortality rates are age-adjusted by the indirect method. The second stage of analysis presents relative mortality risks for each variable controlled for all other variables by a multiple logistic risk model (36). In this model, the mortality risk (R) for k risk factors ($x_1, x_2 \ldots x_k$) is represented by the equation:

$$R = \frac{1}{1 + e^{-(B_0 + B_1 x_1 \ldots + B_k x_k)}}$$

The logistic coefficients $(B_0, B_1 \ldots B_k)$ are estimated by the method of maximum likelihood. Discriminant analysis (37) is used to provide initial values, followed by Gauss-Newton iteration (38). The quantity $\ln(R/(1-R))$ is called the logit of R and is the transformation from which this model derives its name.

An approximate relative risk (odds ratio) per unit change in level of risk factor, x_i, is e^{B_i}. More generally, $e^{(D x_i B_i)}$ approximates the relative risk per D units of change in the level of risk factors, x_i, and can be used to determine the relative risk of the highest vs. the lowest category of a variable.

The multiple logistic risk model assumes that any multicategorical factor as scaled in the analysis is associated with the dependent variable in a logistic manner. Therefore, a preliminary, univariate analysis of the mortality risk of each multicategorical variable was conducted. If the pattern of the mortality risk associated with each successive category of the variable did not follow a logistic curve, that variable was not included in its multicategorical form. If a likelihood ratio test of the logistic pattern was rejected at $p \le 0.20$, the scaled variable was replaced by a collection of dichotomous variables—one for each subcategory, except for one set aside as a reference subcategory. In the present analysis, two multi-categorical variables, use of health services and physical health status, were replaced by appropriate dichotomous variables.

While the multiple logistic model determines the independent relative risk of each potentially health-related practice, it should be noted that this analysis allows only a general comparison of practices. Each relative risk is dependent on the categorization of that variable. A different cutoff point for alcohol consumption, for example, might yield a different relative risk.

The multiple logistic risk model also imposes definite constraints on risk patterns that can emerge from data analysis. To assess the goodness-of-fit of the model to the data, observed and expected numbers of deaths were compared after grouping subjects by decile of estimated risk. This provides some indication of the adequacy of the model for multivariate prediction.

Results

Mortality risk of individual health-related practices

Age-adjusted mortality rates for each of the seven potentially health-related practices examined are presented in table 2. Note that for both men and women, mortality rates are higher in the expected category for each of the first five practices, and in every case the difference is statistically significant for at least one sex. However, skipping breakfast

Table 2. *Age-adjusted mortality rates from all causes by individual health-related practices: adults aged 30–69 years, Alameda County, CA, 1965–1974*

Health-related practice	Mortality rates (per 100)			
	Men		Women	
	%	n	%	n
Cigarette smoking				
Never	5.5	564*	4.9	1140*
Ever	10.9	1665	7.9	1356
Physical inactivity				
Active	8.0	1568*	3.9	1399*
Inactive	12.0	661	8.6	1097
Alcohol consumption				
Low	8.6	1748*	6.3	2277*
High	13.2	481	8.5	219
Weight status				
Average weight	9.2	1928	5.7	1875*
Under or overweight	11.6	301	8.3	621
Sleeping patterns				
7 or 8 hours/night	8.2	1745*	5.5	1910*
≤6 or ≥9 hours/night	13.6	484	8.8	586
Skipping breakfast				
Never	8.7	1548	6.0	1634
Sometimes	12.8	361	8.3	497
Often	9.8	320	6.5	365
Snacking				
Never	8.9	660	6.6	579
Sometimes	9.3	1020	6.6	1196
Often	10.6	549	5.9	721
Total	9.5	2229	6.4	2496

*Difference between categories statistically significant at $p \leq 0.01$.

and snacking are not consistently or significantly associated with mortality.

Mortality risk of individual health-related practices by the logistic model

Approximate relative risks as determined by a multiple logistic analysis are presented in table 3 for all seven potentially health-related practices and the various adjustment variables. Note that the effect of skipping breakfast and snacking are again clearly small and insignificant, with 95

Table 3. *Independent mortality risks for individual health-related practices by multiple logistic analysis: adults aged 30–69 years. Alameda County, CA, 1965–1974*

Variables (high/low risk category)	Logistic coefficient	Approximate relative mortality risk			
		Per unit increase	High vs. low	95% CI* for high vs. low	p-value
Cigarette smoking (ever/never)	0.6246	1.9	1.9	1.4–2.4	<0.001
Physical inactivity (inactive/active)	0.3060	1.4	1.4	1.1–1.7	0.015
Alcohol consumption (high/low)	0.4187	1.5	1.5	1.1–2.1	0.008
Weight status (under or over/average)	0.1628	1.2	1.2	0.9–1.6	0.253
Sleeping (≤6 or ≥9 hours/7 or 8 hours)	0.2545	1.3	1.3	1.1–1.7	0.043
Skipping breakfast (often/never)	−0.0095	1.0	1.0	0.7–1.4	0.915
Snacking (often/never)	0.0694	1.1	1.1	0.8–1.6	0.396
Age (69/30 years)	0.0846	1.1	27.1	16.1–45.5	0.000
Sex (male/female)	0.5499	1.7	1.7	1.3–2.2	<0.001
Race (other/white)	0.2780	1.3	1.3	1.0–1.8	0.088
Socioeconomic status (low/high)	0.0479	1.0	1.2	0.8–1.9	0.413
Health services (sometimes/often)	0.0665	1.1	1.1	0.8–1.4	0.525
Health services (rarely/often)	0.1562	1.2	1.2	0.9–1.6	0.317
Life satisfaction (low/high)	0.1527	1.2	1.4	1.0–1.9	0.071
Health (disabled/healthy)	1.1144	3.0	3.0	2.1–4.5	0.001
Health (chronic condition/healthy)	0.1583	1.2	1.2	0.8–1.6	0.342
Health (symptoms/healthy)	−0.0419	1.0	1.0	0.6–1.4	0.832
Social networks (few/many)	0.2487	1.3	2.1	1.5–3.0	<0.001
Intercept	−9.9836				

*CI, confidence interval.

per cent confidence intervals that include 1.0. Abnormal weight status has an approximate relative risk of 1.2 and is not statistically significant. Of the other four practices, smoking has the highest relative risk, 1.9, and all four are significant.

Relative mortality risks for various combinations of health-related practices can be computed from information in table 3. For example, to determine the relative risk of smoking and physical inactivity, one may calculate the natural antilogarithm of the sum of their logistic coefficients: $e^{(0.6246+0.3060)} = 2.6$. Similarly, the absolute mortality risk for an individual person can be determined by inserting the appropriate logistic coefficients (B) and categorical values (x) into the risk equation. For example, the

Table 4. *Changes in the relative mortality risk for the health practices index, with adjustment by 11 multiple logistic analyses: adults aged 30–69 years, Alameda County, CA, 1965–1974*

Adjustment variables	Approximate relative mortality risk	
	Per unit increase	Highest vs. lowest risk category
Unadjusted	1.88	3.52
Sex	1.87	3.50
Age	1.85	3.42
Age, sex	1.85	3.41
Age, sex, race	1.82	3.32
Age, sex, socioeconomic status	1.83	3.35
Age, sex, health services	1.82	3.31
Age, sex, life satisfaction	1.76	3.08
Age, sex, physical health status	1.65	2.73
Age, sex, social network index	1.73	3.00
All eight variables	1.52	2.31

nine-year mortality risk of a white male, 55 years old, of lower-middle class, with moderate use of health services, moderately satisfied with life, with symptoms of poor health, several social connections, and who smokes, is 9.3 per cent.

Mortality risk of the health practices index

As expected, the health practices index is also associated with mortality risk. Those with few low-risk practices have over three times the death rate of those with many low-risk practices (see first entry in table 4).

To determine if the health practices index predicts mortality independently of other known mortality risk factors, a series of 11 separate multivariate analyses of the relative mortality risk for the health practices index were conducted. As presented in table 4, each analysis includes a different combination of adjustment factors, although most include the standard adjustment variables, age and sex. In every case, the relative risk of mortality associated with the health practices index is reduced, whether comparing the two extreme categories (high or low) or the per unit increase from any category to the next. Adjustment for health status in 1965 reduces the relative risk more than any other factor. Adjustment for all eight factors, seen more fully in table 5, reduces the overall relative risk from 3.5 to 2.3.

Table 5. *Independent mortality risks for the health practices index by multiple logistic analysis: adults aged 30–69 years, Alameda County, CA, 1965–1974*

Variables (high/low risk category)	Approximate relative mortality risk				
	Logistic coefficient	Per unit increase	High vs. low	95% CI* for high vs. low	*p*-value
Health practices index (low/high)	0.4196	1.5	2.3	1.7–3.1	<0.001
Age (69/30 years)	0.0808	1.1	23.4	14.5–37.8	0.000
Sex (male/female)	0.6651	1.9	1.9	1.5–2.5	<0.001
Race (other/white)	0.2505	1.3	1.3	0.9–1.8	0.119
Socioeconomic status (low/high)	0.0552	1.1	1.3	0.8–2.0	0.340
Health services (sometimes/often)	0.0659	1.1	1.1	0.8–1.4	0.505
Health services (rarely/often)	0.1597	1.2	1.2	0.9–1.6	0.304
Life satisfaction (low/high)	0.1484	1.2	1.3	1.0–1.9	0.077
Health (disabled/healthy)	1.1090	3.0	3.0	2.1–4.4	<0.001
Health (chronic condition/healthy)	0.1683	1.2	1.2	0.8–1.6	0.310
Health (symptoms/healthy)	−0.0142	1.0	1.0	0.7–1.4	0.942
Social networks (few/many)	0.2543	1.3	2.1	1.5–3.1	<0.001
Intercept	−9.9012				

*CI, confidence interval.

Adequacy of the multiple logistic risk model

An assessment of the goodness-of-fit of the model to the data is presented in figure 1, demonstrating a generally good agreement between observed and expected deaths in each decile of risk.

Cause of death

To determine whether health practices predict mortality for different causes of death, cause-specific mortality rates for the health practices index were examined (see table 6). For both men and women, the index predicts age-adjusted mortality rates for each cause listed: ischemic heart disease, other circulatory disease, cancer, and all other causes combined.

Discussion

The foregoing analyses demonstrate that four of the seven potentially health-related practices examined are associated with a low mortality risk after adjustment for the other practices, several demographic and social variables, as well as original health status. These four are: never smoking, physical activity, low alcohol consumption, and sleeping seven or eight

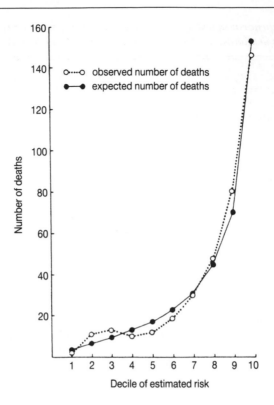

Figure 1. Observed and expected numbers of deaths by decile of estimated risk, as predicted by the multiple logistic model, Alameda County, CA, 1965–1974.

hours/night. A fifth practice, maintaining average weight status, has a slight, nonsignificant association with mortality. Two variables, skipping breakfast and snacking between meals, demonstrate no substantial or significant association with mortality after multivariate adjustment.

When an association is found in a univariate analysis, it may be a direct association or indirect through another variable. In the latter case, multivariate analysis that includes this other variable will eliminate or reduce the association. Whatever association remains after adjustment may be direct (independent) association, or it may be due to incomplete control because of misclassification or crude scaling of the confounding variable. The association may also result from some bias. One can only conclude that an association that remains after adjustment is consistent with a causal interpretation.

Even when an association is eliminated or reduced, that variable could still be important to health. What matters is whether the indirect association reflects a coincidental or causal relationship involving the

Table 6. *Age-adjusted cause-specific mortality rates by health practices index: adults aged 30–69 years, Alameda County, CA, 1965–1974*

Health practices index	Cause-specific mortality rates (per 100)					n
	Ischemic heart disease	Other circulatory disease	Cancer	All other	Total	
Men						
Low	5.2	2.2	2.6	5.7	16.0	404
Medium	4.4	1.5	1.9	3.1	10.9	748
High	2.2	0.5	1.5	1.6	5.8	1077
Total	3.6	1.1	1.8	2.9	9.5	2229
Women						
Low	4.2	1.4	2.6	3.8	11.9	426
Medium	1.4	1.1	2.0	2.6	7.1	809
High	0.7	0.6	1.4	1.1	3.9	1261
Total	1.6	1.0	1.8	2.1	6.4	2496

other variable. For example, the univariate association of alcohol consumption and mortality may be coincidental, reflecting smoking habits. Research has demonstrated that persons who consume moderate to large amounts of alcohol also tend to be smokers (39). The high mortality rates among alcohol consumers may be entirely due to smoking habits. However, the present multivariate analysis suggests that the association between alcohol consumption and mortality involves some pathways that do not involve smoking, since adjustment does not eliminate the alcohol-mortality association.

Indirect relationships are not all coincidental, but may reflect causal associations with a third variable. For example, the mortality risk associated with physical inactivity is reduced after adjustment for other factors such as weight status. While these variables could represent coincidental relationships, they may also reflect indirect causal relationships. Physical activity may induce weight loss, which in turn lowers mortality risk. In this interpretation, physical activity would be indirectly associated with lower mortality risk by causing changes in other risk factors.

In the present analysis, skipping breakfast and snacking between meals have no substantial association with mortality after multivariate adjustment. This indicates that the weak age-adjusted association seen with mortality may be indirect involving pathways of the other variables. These results may also indicate that these variables do not measure significant aspects of eating habits. Perhaps total quantity and types of food eaten are more important than the frequency or times of consumption.

The health practices index used in the present report is constructed from information concerning five practices: cigarette smoking, physical inactivity, alcohol consumption, sleeping patterns, and weight status. This differs from previous reports of the Human Population Laboratory in that the variables about skipping breakfast and snacking are omitted, because, as just noted, they are not associated with mortality after accounting for other factors.

In this analysis, the health practices index is associated with mortality risk after accounting for original health status and other demographic and social factors. These variables do not entirely explain why persons scoring high on the health practices index have the lowest mortality rates. While including health status in 1965 in the logistic model may not completely control for the influence of health status on behaviors, the finding of an association after such adjustment reinforces a causal interpretation of the association between the health-related practices and mortality. In addition, in another report of these data (3), the relationship between a health practices index and mortality was evident throughout the period of follow-up. While the relationship diminished some over time, a substantial gradient remained during the last four years, 1971–1974. If the relationship was entirely due to self-selection of behaviors according to original health status, one would expect the association with mortality to diminish more dramatically.

The foregoing analyses demonstrate that several behaviors are independently associated with mortality rates from all causes. The fast analysis also demonstrates that they are associated with several cause-specific mortality rates. If these practices influence resistance to illness, the entire spectrum of health would be affected, including morbidity as well as mortality. Analysis of health status in those surviving nine years in this same population indicates that health practices are associated with later morbidity as well as mortality (40). Similar findings in other univariate and multivariate studies of morbidity (15–18, 25, 40) and mortality (1–27) and the adequacy of fit of the multiple logistic model to these data, are consistent with the hypothesis that certain behaviors play an important role in promoting longevity and delaying illness and death.

Acknowledgements

This work was supported by the National Center for Health Services Research Grant No. 00368, and by Biomedical Research Grant 5-S07-RR05441, from the National Institutes of Health to the School of Public Health, University of California, Berkeley.

The authors gratefully acknowledge the staff of the Human Population Laboratory, California State Department of Health Services, for their assistance and support in the preparation of the manuscript.

References

1. Belloc NB, Breslow L. Relationship of physical health status and health practices. Prev Med 1972;1:409–21.
2. Belloc NB. Relationship of health practices and mortality. Prev Med 1973;2:67–81.
3. Breslow L, Enstrom JE. Persistence of health habits and their relationship to mortality. Prev Med 1980;9:469–83.
4. Berkman LF, Wingard DL. The impact of health practices on mortality. In: Berkman L, Breslow L, eds. Health and ways of living: some social and behavioral predictors of mortality. New York: Oxford Press (in press).
5. Enstrom JE. Cancer mortality among Mormons. Cancer 1975;36:825–41.
6. Wynder EL, Lemon FR, Bross IJ. Cancer and coronary artery disease among Seventh-Day Adventists. Cancer 1959;12:1016–28.
7. Lemon FR, Walden RT. Death from respiratory system disease among Seventh-Day Adventist men. JAMA 1966;198:136–46.
8. Kannel WB. Habits and heart disease. In: Palmore E, Jeffers FC, eds. Prediction of life span. Lexington, MA: D. C. Heath and Company, 1971.
9. Hammon EC, Garfinkel L. Coronary heart disease, stroke and aortic aneurysm: factors in the etiology. Arch Environ Health 1969;19:167–82.
10. Paffenbarger RS, Hale WE. Work activity of longshoremen as related to death from coronary heart disease and stroke. N Engl J Med 1970;282:1109–14.
11. Paffenbarger RS Jr, Hale WE, Brand RJ, et al. Work-energy level, personal characteristics, and fatal heart attack: a birth-cohort effect. Am J Epidemiol 1977;105:200–13.
12. Paffenbarger RS Jr, Brand RJ, Sholtz RI, et al. Energy expenditure, cigarette smoking, and blood pressure level as related to death from specific diseases. Am J Epidemiol 1978;108:12–18.
13. Doll R, Hill AB. Mortality in relation to smoking: ten years' observations of British doctors. Br Med J 1964;1:1399–1410, 1460–7.
14. Kahn HA. The Dorn Study of smoking and mortality among U.S. veterans: report on eight and one-half years of observation. Natl Cancer Inst Monogr 1966;19:1–26.
15. World Health Organization. Smoking and disease: the evidence reviewed. WHO Chron 1975;29:402–8.
16. US Department of Health, Education and Welfare, Public Health Service, Center for Disease Control. The health consequences of smoking—1975. Washington, DC: US GPO, 1976. (DHEW publication no. (CDC) 76-8704.)
17. US Department of Health, Education and Welfare, Public Health Service, National Institute of Alcohol Abuse and Alcoholism. Alcohol and health, new knowledge. Washington, DC: US GPO, 1975. (DHEW publication no. (HSM) 72-9099.)

18. Aarens, M, Cameron T, Roizen R, et al. Alcohol, casualties and crime. Special Report to the National Institute on Alcohol Abuse and Alcoholism, November 1977.

19. Pell S, D'Alonzo CA. A five-year mortality study of alcoholics. J Occup Med 1973;15:120–5.

20. Schmidt W, DeLint J. Causes of death of alcoholics. Q J Studies Alcohol 1972;33:171–85.

21. Room R, Day N. Alcohol and mortality. Special Report to the National Institute on Alcohol Abuse and Alcoholism, March 1974.

22. Yano K, Rhoads LG, Kagan A, et al. Dietary intake and risk of coronary heart disease in Japanese men living in Hawaii. Am J Clin Nutr 1978;31:1270–9.

23. Marmot M, Rose G, Shipley J, et al. Alcohol mortality: a u-shaped curve. Lancet 1981;1:580–2.

24. Rothman K. Alcohol. In: Fraumeni J, ed. Persons at high risk of cancer: an approach to cancer etiology and control. New York: Academic Press, 1975:139–50.

25. Froelicher VF. The effects of chronic exercise on the heart and on coronary atherosclerotic heart disease: a literature survey. Report SAM-TR 76-6 to the USAF School of Aerospace Medicine, February 1976.

26. Society of Actuaries. Build and blood pressure study, 1959. Vol. I and II. Chicago: Society of Actuaries, 1959.

27. Levinson ML. Obesity and health. Prev Med 1977;6:172–80.

28. California State Department of Public Health. Alameda County population 1965. Berkeley: California State Department of Public Health, 1966.

29. Hochstim JR. Health and ways of living—the Alameda County Population Laboratory. In: Kessler I, Levin ML, eds. The community as an epidemiological laboratory. Baltimore: Johns Hopkins University Press, 1970;149–76.

30. Belloc N, Arellano M. Computer record linkage on a survey population. Health Serv Rep 1973;88:344–50.

31. Cahalan D, Cisin JH. American drinking practices: summary of findings from a national probability sample. II. Measurement of massed versus spaced drinking. Q J Studies Alcohol 1968;29:642–56.

32. Metropolitan Life Insurance Company. New weight standards for men and women. Stat Bull Metropol Life Ins Co 1959;40:1–4.

33. Berkman LF. Social networks, host resistance and mortality: a follow-up study of Alameda County residents. Ph.D. dissertation. Berkeley: University of California Press, 1977.

34. Belloc NB, Breslow L, Hochstim JR. Measurement of physical health in a general population survey. Am J Epidemiol 1971;93:328–36.

35. Berkman LF, Syme SL. Social networks, host resistance, and mortality: a nine-year follow-up study of Alameda County residents. Am J Epidemiol 1979;109:186–204.

36. Rosenman MH, Brand RJ, Sholtz RI, et al. Multivariate prediction of coronary heart disease during 8.5 year follow-up in Western Collaborative Group Study. Am J Cardiol 1976;37:903–10.

37. Truett J, Cornfield J, Kannel W. A multivariate analysis of the risk of coronary heart disease in Framingham. J Chronic Dis 1967;20:511–24.

38. Walker SH, Duncan DB. Estimation of the probability of an event as a function of several independent variables. Biometrika 1967;54:167–79.
39. Cahalan D, Cisin IH, Crossley HM. American drinking practices: national study of drinking behavior and attitudes. New Brunswick: Rutgers Center of Alcohol Studies, 1969.
40. Wiley JA, Camacho TC. Life-style and future health: evidence from the Alameda County Study. Prev Med 1980;9:1–21.

The Health Belief Model and participation in programmes for the early detection of breast cancer: a comparative analysis

Michael Calnan

Health Services Research Unit, George Allen Wing, University of Kent, Canterbury, Kent, England

Abstract

Extravagant claims have been made about the power of the Health Belief Model (HBM) to explain both decisions to adopt patterns of health behaviour and to use preventive health services. However, studies where information on beliefs are collected before information on behaviour are not common. The analyses presented here are based on prospective studies examining how far the variables which make up the HBM predict attendance at (i) a class teaching breast self-examination and (ii) a clinic providing mammography. The results show that different dimensions of the HBM are amongst the best predictors of attendance at each of the different services although the overall variance explained by the HBM in both sets of analysis was small.

Introduction

Extravagant claims have been made about the power of the Health Belief Model (HBM) to explain decisions to use preventive health services [1] and decisions to adopt patterns of health behaviour [2, 3]. However, much of its support has come from studies where data on beliefs and behaviour are collected at the same time. These studies have shown strong correlations between beliefs and behaviour although it is difficult to judge if beliefs produce behaviour or vice versa as there is evidence to show that individuals sometimes rationalise their beliefs and feelings to fit with their behaviour [4].

The best way of testing if beliefs produce behaviour is to ensure that information about beliefs are collected before the behaviour occurs. The few prospective studies which do this have been less supportive to the HBM [5]. However, these prospective studies have also suffered from a fundamental weakness in that they have studied behaviour which is relatively common such as the use of dental services and where the prospective participants could have used the service previously. Thus, their beliefs may have been modified by their previous contact with the service. Studies examining the explanatory power of the Health Belief Model should ideally focus on use of a service which is relatively novel to the participants. However, if this is impractical, then some attempt should be made to allow for previous contact with the service when the relationship between beliefs and behaviour is examined.

One area where there has been strong evidence of an association between health beliefs and participation in preventive programmes is in the early detection of cancer. For example, a recent study [6] showed that while attenders and non-attenders at a breast screening clinic were equally well informed about breast cancer, non-attenders were more likely to be afraid of breast cancer being found and to be anxious that their lives would be disrupted if cancer was identified compared with the attenders. Another study [7] showed that women who participated in a breast screening programme felt more vulnerable to breast cancer and were more concerned about its severity than the non-participants.

Studies of factors associated with the practice of breast self-examination also identify the importance of health beliefs. For example, Haran *et al.* [8] found that those who practice breast self-examination are more likely to view breast cancer as the most worrying illness to which women are prone. One study [9] showed that women's belief in the efficacy of the early detection of breast cancer to reduce the danger from the disease was found to be the strongest correlate of the ability to perform breast self-examination. However, none of these studies nor those examining use of breast screening clinics were prospective and none of them attempted to take into account previous health behaviour.

Theoretical model

The aim of the study presented here is to examine the social, psychological and demographic factors, using a prospective design, which are associated with women's decisions to participate or not to participate in two different types of programme for the early detection of breast cancer. The two different types of method of early detection of breast cancer which will be examined in this study are those which are currently being evaluated in a comparative multi-centre trial which is being carried out in the U.K. [10]. The two methods being evaluated are mammography with physical examination and breast self-examination. The former is being provided in a clinic which women in two centres are being invited to attend, and women in two other centres are being invited to attend a class where they are taught how to carry out BSE effectively and on a regular basis.

The specific objective is to examine the power of the HBM for explaining attendance at the clinic providing mammography and attendance at the BSE class. This analysis is not only important for assessing the value of the HBM for explaining use of screening services, but also will show whether the HBM is more useful for explaining use of a certain type of service. Attendance at a breast screening clinic providing mammography has considerably different implications for the participant than attendance at a class teaching BSE. In the case of breast screening the participant is passive and dependent on the medical detection of abnormalities whereas, in the case of attendance at the class, the participant is taught how to play a more active role in the identification of abnormalities. Also, while both types of service are not common in the UK, women appear to be more familiar with the principle of medical screening than being taught by a professional how to do BSE, even though they are not unfamiliar with the idea of BSE itself [11].

The framework of the Health Belief Model as proposed by Becker and Maiman [2] was used to define the relevant variables to be studied. However, certain recent modifications have been made. Two factors have been added to the Health Belief Model. First, locus of control [12] is believed to be an important factor in explaining health behaviour, in that the more the person feels powerless to control his or her life, or the more fatalistic the person is, the less likely he or she is to comply with officially recommended health actions. However, more recently this general concept has been questioned and it has been suggested that an individual's specific feelings of control over getting the disease in question is a more sensitive measure of personal control over health [13]. The second factor is the availability of social support and social networks. Studies of general health behaviour [14] and of use of breast screening facilities [15] have shown that those women who are socially well integrated are more likely to participate in preventive health programmes than those who are less well integrated.

As well as these factors identified in the most recent version of the Health Belief Model, other factors have also been shown to explain decisions to use preventive health services. First, there is the health status of the individual in that it has been hypothesised that those people who have poor health or some kind of disability may be more or less likely to participate in preventive programmes [16]. Secondly, it has been suggested that an individual's self-esteem may influence decisions to adopt patterns of health behaviour. For example, those people with low self-esteem might be less likely to feel that protection of health is worthwhile and thus be less likely to participate [17]. The third factor which is said to be influential in people adopting patterns of health behaviour is social pressure. This can be direct pressure by friends, relatives or neighbours to make certain decisions [18] or can occur through what is called 'normative' pressure, which is inherent in the cultural values available to the individual [19].

The study design adopted in this study lends itself to be a particular stringent test of the HBM as the information on health beliefs was collected at least one month before the women received an invitation to attend the class or attend the clinic. The invitation itself could be seen as one of the enabling factors or cues for actions which are said to be necessary to trigger off decisions to participate. The only data collected retrospectively were that on the impact of others on the decision to attend the class (for full details see [20]).

Methods

Research design

The study was carried out in two health districts which were included in the main trial [10]. The health district (BSE district) where women were being invited to attend a BSE class was situated in a large provincial city in the Midlands in England, whereas the health district where women were invited to attend the breast screening clinic was situated in a city in Southern England. A comparison of the socio-demographic characteristics of the samples from the two districts shows some differences [21]. Women in the sample from the district in the Southern city were more likely than their counterparts who lived in the district in the Midlands to come from a background where the head of the household was in a professional or semi-profesional occupation and to have left school after 16 years. All women aged between 45 and 64 who are registered with general practitioners serving the districts were included in the trial. No estimate is available for the proportion of women in this age group who live in these two districts and who are not registered with general practitioners. However, other studies have shown [22] that in provincial areas the proportion of the population who are not registered with a GP is seldom above 4%. Each woman in the BSE district was invited to attend a BSE class, held in a hospital clinic in the centre of town. The class itself consisted of a short instructional film and a talk by a nurse, followed by a discussion. Each woman in the breast screening district was invited to attend a clinic providing mammography and physical examination carried out by medically trained personnel.

Random samples of women were selected from the age/sex registers serving the districts. One thousand, one hundred and fifty women were randomly selected in the BSE district but due mainly to inaccuracies in the GP registers the sample that was originally selected (89 women's addresses could not be traced and another 170 were found to have moved or were not known at the address) was reduced to 825. Similar inaccuracies were found in the breast screening district and the original sample of 1222 was reduced to 854. In this sample 68 of the women's addresses could not be traced and another 225 had either moved out of the area or were not known at the address.

The two samples of women were interviewed with the same questionnaire in their own homes at least one month before they received their invitations to attend one or other of the two services. The interview schedules were administered by trained interviewers unconnected with the breast screening team or the BSE education team. Respondents had no prior knowledge that they were to be interviewed and the interview was introduced to them as a study about women's beliefs and feelings in relation to breast cancer and its early detection. Data on whether the women attended the class or the clinic or neither were subsequently derived from information collected in the main trial.

Six-hundred and seventy-eight (82%) of the 825 women in the BSE district were successfully interviewed. Of these 678, 45% subsequently attended the class which is a slightly lower rate of attendance than that found for the whole cohort (51%). The sample interviewed was representative of attenders and non-attenders in that there was only a small difference in the participation rate in the interview study between class attenders (83%) and the non-attenders (81%).

Six-hundred and fifty-four (77%) of the 854 women were successfully interviewed. Of the 654, 471 women (72%) subsequently attended the clinic, which was higher than the attendance rate for the whole cohort (69%) and 139 (21%) did not. There was no information on attendance for 44 women (7%) who had been interviewed. The analysis was carried out on the 610 where there was information on attendance. There was a difference in participation rates in the survey between attenders (84%) and non-attenders (64%).

Scales and indices

Data on [all] variables were available for both samples of women. These variables included measures of socio-demographic characteristics (see Table 1), health beliefs (see Table 2), health status, social networks,

Table 1. *Socio-demographic characteristics and attendance/non-attendance at the (i) breast screening clinic and (ii) the class teaching BSE (χ^2 value)*

Socio-demographic characteristics	Attendance at breast screening	Attendance at BSE class
1. Social class	2.5 (4 d.f.)	23.0 (3 d.f.)‡
2. School leaving age	3.7 (4 d.f.)	10.1 (4 d.f.)*
3. Age	7.3 (4 d.f.)	1.5 (3 d.f.)
4. Marital status	13.2 (3 d.f.)†	8.3 (3 d.f.)*
6. Employment status	6.5 (4 d.f.)	4.3 (4 d.f.)

*$P < 0.05$; †$P < 0.01$; ‡$P < 0.001$.

Table 2. *Dimensions of Health Beliefs and attendance/non-attendance at the (i) breast screening clinic (ii) class teaching breast self examination (χ^2 values)*

Health belief dimensions	Attendance breast screening	Attendance at class
Health motivation		
7. Concern about health	5.4 (2 d.f.)	0.6 (2 d.f.)
8. Willingness to seek medical care	1.7 (3 d.f.)	4.2 (3 d.f.)
9. Ever had a cervical smear	22.5 (3 d.f.)‡	25.7 (3 d.f.)‡
10. Use of dentist	19.5 (2 d.f.)‡	34.0 (2 d.f.)‡
11. Previous use of breast screening	1.1 (2 d.f.)	0.8 (2 d.f.)
12. Pattern of personal health behaviour (index of behaviour and knowledge— smoking, diet, exercise, seat belt use)	24.7 (8 d.f.)†	32.8 (8 d.f.)‡
Value of Illness Threat Reduction		
13. Perceived vulnerability to breast cancer	12.9 (2 d.f.)†	33.1 (2 d.f.)‡
14. Type of person who tends to get ill	10.6 (3 d.f.)*	2.2 (2 d.f.)
15. Concern about breast cancer	12.0 (4 d.f.)*	13.2 (4 d.f.)†
16. Past experience with breast symptoms	2.3 (1 d.f.)	5.8 (1 d.f.)*
17. Knowledge of someone with breast cancer	0.2 (1 d.f.)	8.1 (1 d.f.)†
Probability that Compliant Behaviour will Reduce the Threat		
18. Perceived costs and Benefits	8.0 (3 d.f.)*	6.9 (3 d.f.)
19. Faith in medicine	0.8 (2 d.f.)	1.8 (2 d.f.)
20. Control over health (general)	3.4 (4 d.f.)	8.0 (4 d.f.)
21. Control over health (specific)	0.6 (1 d.f.)	1.0 (1 d.f.)

*$P < 0.05$; †$P < 0.01$; ‡$P < 0.001$.

Table 3. *Additional variables and attendance/non-attendance at* (i) *a breast screening clinic and* (ii) *a class teaching BSE* (χ^2 *values*)

Independent variables	Attendance at breast screening	Attendance at a BSE class
State of Health		
22. Self assessment of health	14.3 (4 d.f.)†	3.3 (3 d.f.)
23. Presence of impairment	9.4 (2 d.f.)†	3.7 (2 d.f.)
24. Intention to attend	42.6 (1 d.f.)‡	11.0 (1 d.f.)
25. Social pressure to attend	0.7 (1 d.f.)	5.4 (1. d.f.)*
Social Support		
26. (i) Presence of confiding relationship	9.4 (3 d.f.)*	0.2 (3 d.f.)
27. (ii) Network of close friends	11.3 (3 d.f.)*	13.4 (3 d.f.)†
28. Self-esteem	6.1 (2 d.f.)*	5.7 (2 d.f.)
Practice of BSE		
29. (i) Frequency	15.4 (3 d.f.)†	38.0 (1 d.f.)‡
30. (ii) Technique	5.9 (1 d.f.)*	0.8 (1 d.f.)
31. Feelings that should participate in breast screening	24.6 (2 d.f.)‡	—
32. Time since last breast screen	6.3 (2 d.f.)*	—
33. Knowledge of BSE	—	9.9 (1 d.f.)†
34. Confident doing it right	—	5.6 (1 d.f.)*
35. Confident can identify abnormality	—	11.6 (1 d.f.)‡
36. Previous contact with BSE education	—	6.8 (1 d.f.)†
37. Image of BS examiner	—	0.3 (2 d.f.)

*$P < 0.05$; †$P < 0.01$; ‡$P < 0.001$.

self-esteem and previous practice of breast self-examination (see Table 3). Many of the variables were indices constructed from a number of different questions. However, the measure of perceived vulnerability to breast cancer was a scale which had been validated previously [23]. All but two of these variables were defined in exactly the same way. The two variables which were defined differently were perceived costs and benefits of BSE/breast screening (18) and social pressure (25). The index measuring perceived costs and benefits of BSE was made up from an eight statement scale which was a modified version of a scale previously validated by Stillman (for full details see [23]). The index measuring perceived costs and benefits of breast screening was as follows: women who said that they had heard of breast screening or routine checkups of the breasts were allocated one point; those who felt it was a good idea were allocated 1 point; and those who said that they were not worried about any aspects of it were allocated 1 point. Thus, the index ran from 0 to 3 points, with the highest scorers being those who felt breast screening was beneficial and had no 'costs'.

The pressure to attend the class was taken from a question in a follow-up survey which asked both non-attenders and attenders if they had received any encouragement or discouragement to attend. However, social pressure to attend the breast screening clinic was taken from a question given in the first survey, which asked if they had ever discussed breast screening with their friends.

In addition to these 30 variables a further 5 variables were included *only* in the analysis of the attendance at the BSE class, and a further two were included *only* in the analysis of attendance at the screening clinic (see Table 3).* These latter two were a question which asked the women if they thought they 'should' have their breasts regularly examined more often than they did at the time of the interview (31). This variable was used as a crude indicator of 'normative pressure', although an element may be contained in the variable measuring intention to take part. The other variable exclusively used in the analysis of attendance at screening was the time since the women had had their last breast screening (if any) (32).

Variables exclusively used in the analysis of attendance at the BSE class were the extent to which women felt that they carried out BSE in the right way (34), and the confidence that they had about their ability to detect a breast abnormality if it was there (35). Questions on the respondent's knowledge of BSE (33) and their previous experience with BSE education, such as leaflets, was also included (36). A further variable measured the stereotypes that women hold (if any) about the person who carries out BSE in that it was hypothesised that those who see the breast self-examiner in a positive or attractive manner were more likely to attend than those who did not (37).

A behavioural item (24) was also included in *both* sets of analysis which was intention to take part in the classes or attend for breast screening.

Statistical analysis

The relationships between each of the 35 variables and attendance/non-attendance at the class were examined independently using a χ^2 test. Then, the variables were analysed in combination, using linear discriminant analysis to identify the strongest predictors of attendance at the class. Similar but separate analyses were carried out examining the relationship

*Full tabulations for each of these variables against attendance can be obtained on application direct to the author.

between attendance/non-attendance at the breast screening clinic and the 32 independent variables.

In the linear discriminant analyses of attendance at the BSE class, social pressure to attend (25) was excluded from the analysis because it was based on retrospective data. Marital status is a nominal variable and was represented in the discriminant analyses by the introduction of three dummy variables taking the value of 1, if married, widowed or divorced/separated respectively. The variable Ethnic Group (5) was excluded from all the analyses as the numbers of non-whites in both samples was small ($N = 7$).

Results

Tables 1, 2 and 3 show the statistical relationships* between the independent variables and the two outcome variables.

Socio-demographic characteristics

Table 1 shows the statistical relationships between attendance/non-attendance at the two services and socio-demographic characteristics. The socio-demographic profile of the non-attender at the breast screening clinic was one who was more likely to be single or widowed and be aged over 60, whereas the profile of the non-attender at the BSE class was more likely to be divorced or separated, have left school before 16 years of age and come from a background where the head of household was in a semi-skilled or unskilled occupation (IV + V).

Health beliefs

Health motivation

Attenders at the class teaching BSE and attenders at the breast screening clinic shared the same characteristics in relation to the health motivation dimension (see Table 2). Both groups were more likely than non-attenders to have been for a cervical smear (whether it was deliberately sought or not), both were more likely to go regularly to the dentist for checkups and both were more likely to have a pattern of personal health behaviour which complied with officially recommended health actions. However, non-attenders at breast screening were more likely to have had mammography previously than attenders, although this difference was not statistically significant. The reverse trend was found for the class teaching BSE although this difference was not statistically significant either.

Value of illness threat reduction

Both groups of attenders were more likely than non-attenders to feel vulnerable to breast cancer and be concerned about breast cancer (see Table 2). In the case of concern about breast cancer, there was a similar trend for both groups in that those who felt moderately or highly concerned (1 pt+) were more likely to attend than those with little or no concern about getting breast cancer.

However, in the case of perceived vulnerability, the pattern was different in that attenders at the breast screening clinic were more likely than non-attenders to have shown moderate and high levels of vulnerability to breast cancer. But attenders at the class teaching BSE were more likely to feel highly vulnerable to breast cancer than non-attenders.

The three remaining variables measuring different elements of this dimension differed markedly in their relationship to attendance/non-attendance at the two services (see Table 2). Those women who said that they were the type of person who was more likely to get ill were more likely to attend the breast screening clinic than those who felt the same or less vulnerability to illness as anyone else. No similar difference was found for attendance at the class. However, women who either had past experience with an abnormality in their breast which they thought was serious, or had known personally someone who had had breast cancer, were more likely to attend the BSE class than those who had neither direct nor indirect experience. No similar statistically significant relationship was found between these variables and attendance at the breast screening clinic.

Probability that compliant behaviour will reduce the threat

Both groups of attenders were more likely than non-attenders to feel that the benefits of breast screening or BSE outweighed the costs in that attenders were more likely to score moderate-to-high or high on the respective scales measuring the perceived value of the service compared with non-attenders, even though the relationship between this variable and attendance at the class was not statistically significant (see Table 2).

State of health

Women who said that they had very good or good health were more likely to attend for breast screening than those whose health was rated as fair to poor. Women who said that they had an impairment that restricts them in a lot of things that they would like to do were less likely to attend for breast screening than those who had a lesser impairment or no impairment. No variations in attendance at the class teaching BSE were found to be associated with the state of the respondents' health (see Table 3).

Intention to attend

Not surprisingly, those women who said that they intended to attend for breast screening or they intended to attend the class teaching BSE were much more likely to attend both services than those who said that they had no specific intention to attend (see Table 3).

Social pressure to attend

Women who said that they were encouraged to attend the class teaching BSE were more likely to attend than those who reported no encouragement or discouragement. However, this information was collected some time after possible attendance and thus there may be inaccuracies in recall, and respondents' reports may have been coloured by their subsequent attendance or non-attendance at the class.

No significant relationship was found between this variable and attendance at the breast screening clinic (see Table 3).

Social support

Both groups of attenders were more likely to have at least one close friend compared with non-attenders (see Table 3). Those with no confiding relationship or a confiding relationship with a female only were less likely to attend for breast screening than those who reported having a confiding relationship with a husband or boyfriend. A similar trend was found for attendance at the BSE class, although the relationship was less marked.

Self-esteem

Those women who said they were not a confident sort of person (low self-esteem) were more likely to attend for breast screening than those who said that they were a confident person and those who could not say. Once again a similar trend was found amongst attenders/non-attenders at the class, although the difference was not statistically significant (see Table 3).

Practice of BSE

These women who said that they carried out BSE at least once a month were more likely to attend both the services than those who carried out BSE less often than once a month or never carried it out at all (see Table 3). While those whose BSE technique was defined as adequate (for full details see [20]) were more likely to attend the breast screening clinic than those whose technique was not adequate, there was no significant relationship between level of BSE technique and attendance at the BSE class.

Additional factors and relationships with attendance at breast screening clinic (*see Table 3*)

Women who said that they should have their breasts examined more often than they did at the time of the interview were more likely to attend the breast screening clinic than those who said their breasts were examined often enough. This appears to be compatible with the finding that women who reported having breast screening within the last 2 years were less likely to have attended the breast screening clinic than those who had never experienced breast screening or had been screened at least 2 years before.

Additional factors and relationships with attendance/non-attendance at the class teaching BSE (*see Table 3*)

Women who had heard of BSE and who said they had previously seen BSE education such as leaflets, were more likely to have attended the class than those who had not heard of BSE or seen any education about it.

Women who were either not sure about their ability to detect an abnormality or about whether they were carrying out BSE in the right way were also more likely to be attenders than those who were more certain about their BSE technique.

There was no significant relationship between 'the image' of the breast self-examiner (if any) and attendance at the class.

Discriminant analyses

In order to identify the group of variable which distinguished between attenders and non-attenders at the breast screening clinc, 31 variables were included (excluding ethnic group) as independent variables in a linear discriminant analysis. Similarly, 33 variables (excluding ethnic group and social pressure to attend), were included in another discriminant analysis to find out which group of variables best discriminated between attendance/non-attendance at the BSE class. The results for both analyses are given in Table 4, which shows the combination of the variables which increased the discrimination between the groups significantly. A positive sign for the discriminant score shows a positive association between the variable and attendance.

The best discriminators for attendance at the breast screening clinic were different to those for attendance at the BSE class (see Table 4). The best discriminators for attendance at the breast screening clinic was intention to attend for breast screening followed by three variables measuring use of preventive health services, which were use of dentist for checkups, previous use of breast screening (women who had previously had mammography were less likely to attend) and previous use of cervical smear.

In contrast, ten significant discriminators were identified in the analysis of attendance at the class teaching BSE and intention to attend the class was not amongst them (see Table 4). The best discriminator (according to the order in which they entered the analysis and levels of statistical significance) was personal health behaviour followed by perceived vulnerability to breast cancer, number of close friends, control over health in general (those who felt more control were less likely to attend), Marital Status (divorced/separated less likely to attend), regular dental checkups, previous use of cervical smear, age (younger age groups more likely to attend), Marital Status (widowed less likely to attend than the rest) and self-esteem (confident person less likely to attend).

There was a large value of Wilk's Lambda (see Table 4), an inverse measure of the remaining variance, in both analyses suggesting that much of the difference between the groups of attenders and non-attenders at both types of service remains unexplained.

As the variable intention to take part in the breast screening is believed to provide a bridge between beliefs and behaviour it may be concealing the effects of other health belief variables. Therefore, a subsidiary analysis was carried out only on the sample of women invited for breast screening, excluding the intention variable. This analysis identified five significant discriminators and they were in the order in which they were entered into the analysis: previous use of cervical smear, use of dentist for checkups, previous use of breast screening (those who had been screened in the last two years were less likely to attend), perceived vulnerability to breast cancer and perceived costs and benefits of breast screening. The figure for Wilk's Lambda was 0.87.

As 'intention to attend the breast screening clinic' was the best discriminator and is a behavioural item, an analysis was carried out with

Table 4. *Comparison of discriminant analyses for attendance at breast screening with attendance at BSE class*

	Attendance at breast screening				Attendance at BSE class		
Step	Variable	Significance of change in discriminant function	Standardised discriminant score	Step	Variable	Significance of change in discriminant function	Standardised discriminant score
1.	Intention to attend for breast screening (24)	$P < 0.001$	0.54	1.	Personal health behaviour (12)	$P < 0.001$	0.35
2.	Use of dentist for regular checkups (10)	$P < 0.01$	0.36	2.	Perceived vulnerability to BC (13)	$P < 0.01$	0.29
3.	Previous use of breast screening (11)	$P < 0.05$	−0.29	3.	Social support: close friends (27)	$P < 0.01$	0.24
4.	Previous use of cervical smear (9)	$P < 0.05$	0.23	4.	Control over health in general (20)	$P < 0.01$	−0.28
				5.	Marital status (div/sep vs rest) (4)	$P < 0.05$	−0.41
				6.	Regular dental checkups (10)	$P < 0.05$	0.20
				7.	Previous use of cervical smear (9)	$P < 0.05$	0.20
				8.	Age (3)	$P < 0.05$	0.28
				9.	Marital status (widow vs rest) (4)	$P < 0.05$	−0.42
				10.	Self-esteem (28)	$P < 0.05$	−0.21

Wilks Lambda = 0.85; $N = 524$

Wilks Lambda = 0.82; $N = 503$

this as the dependent variable. The results of the analysis showed that 'perceived vulnerability to breast cancer' was the best discriminator, followed by previous use of cervical smear, whether the respondent felt that they should have their breasts examined more often than they did, Marital Status (married women were more likely to say that they intended to attend compared with other groups), BSE frequency, personal health behaviour, faith in medicine, perceived costs and benefits of breast screening and previous experience of breast screening (those who had been for breast screening in the last 2 years were less likely to say they intended to attend). The analysis gave a value for Wilk's Lambda of 0.73.

Discussion

It has been argued that the amount of variance in behaviour explained by the health belief variables in the HBM is quite small [24] and the predictive power of the HBM is generally low [14]. The results from this analysis of the value of the HBM for explaining participation in two different services for the early detection of breast cancer supports these statements. However, even though the overall variance explained in both sets of analyses was low, it must be remembered that variables other than those from the HBM were also included in the analyses and these too were of limited explanatory value. Also, the health belief variables were amongst the best discriminators, particularly in the analysis of take up of screening. However, this might be expected given the eclectic nature of the HBM which in its extended form embraces a wide range of factors with no coherent theoretical framework [24].

While the predictive power of the HBM for explaining attendance at the screening clinic and the BSE class was in both cases low, different health belief variables were associated with the different services. In the case of preventive health services the best discriminators (excluding intention to attend) were those associated with previous positive health activities and previous use of more general preventive services (regular dental checkups) were as important as use of specific cancer screening services (use of cervical smear). Specific beliefs about breast cancer and about breast screening were of importance, but to a lesser extent, and only when intention to attend was excluded from the analysis.

It must be remembered that the strongest discriminator between attendance and non-attendance at the breast screening clinic was intention to attend. This suggests that intention to attend is identifying other aspects which influence decisions to use the screening clinic than those being measured in the HBM. One of these may be normative pressure although this was only measured very crudely in this study. Thus, the findings support Fishbein and Ajzen's [19] proposition that a specific behaviour is determined by that person's intention to perform that behaviour. Fishbein and Ajzen [19] also state that intention to take part is made up of two dimensions: (i) attitude towards the behaviour in question (i.e. attendance at the screening clinic) and (ii) subjective 'norm' concerning that behaviour which is defined as the individual's perception of the social pressure put on her by salient individuals to perform, or not to perform, that behaviour. The analyses also provided some support for this second proposition in that two of the best discriminators were variables measuring beliefs about the consequences of the behaviour (perceived vulnerability to breast cancer) and normative pressure. However, these findings must be interpreted cautiously as the measure of normative pressure (ought to have breasts examined more often) was crude and there was no direct measure of *attitudes* towards attendance.

Evidence reported previously [21] showed that women preferred the prospect of attending breast screening to that of attending classes teaching breast self-examination, mainly because they had much more faith in the ability of professional medical staff to detect abnormalities than themselves. However, they also showed a preference for breast screening because they preferred the private and personal setting of the screening clinic. The relative unattractiveness of a class teaching breast self-examination, at least relative to attendance at a breast screening clinic, suggests there was little normative pressure to attend the class. This may account for intention to attend the class not being amongst the best discriminators.

The novelty of the concept of a class teaching breast self-examination might explain why there was a wide range of different factors which best discriminated between attendance and non-attendance. However, the strongest discriminators were elements from the Health Belief Model. In contrast to breast screening, attendance at a class teaching breast self-examination was more closely associated with personal health behaviour than previous use of preventive services, which might be expected given the emphasis in the class on self-examination. However, perceived vulnerability to breast cancer was also a strong discriminator. This might be explained by the need for additional influences to motivate people (who are already health 'conscious') to attend a service which is relatively unattractive. Perceptions of being 'at risk' may be one of the major motivating forces in these circumstances.

The results from these analyses cast doubt on the value of the HBM for predicting use of different types of services for the early detection of breast cancer. The results also suggest a need for a change in focus in the study of health behaviour, and to explore the importance of other factors such as the role of normative pressure. In addition, the analysis of attendance at the BSE class highlighted the importance of marital status and age and suggests a need to explore the relationship between the status associated with being married or being elderly, and the way people think about health and its protection. Alternatively, the results may indicate the need to critically examine some of the assumptions about health and health beliefs which are inherent in the HBM. Evidence from recent ethnographic studies shows that lay models of health and its control do not match up with those of the HBM. For example, the approach adopted in the HBM assumes that the general public as a whole shares the same definitions of health, and this definition is congruent with official medical definitions. However, recent evidence [25, 26] has suggested that not only are there a range of definitions of health held by the general public which might vary according to the social and economic status of the person, but that lay definitions differ sometimes markedly from medical definitions. Evidence from another ethnographic study [27] which examined the way different groups conceptualise threats to their health suggests that the notion of perceived vulnerability to a disease is problematic. The study showed that definite feelings of vulnerability were rare, although they tended to be found when the respondent felt there were good reasons for it, such as the presence of signs and symptoms.

Acknowledgements

I would like to thank Dr Price, Professor Blamey and their staff at the two centres for their help in the organisation of this study. Thanks also go to Dr J. Chamberlain and Susan Moss for their help with various aspects of the analysis and to Chandra Nagarajah for carrying out the computing. I am grateful to Social and Community Planning Research for providing their team of interviewers and to the Department of Health and Social Security for sponsorship for the study.

References

1. Rosenstock I. Why people use health services. *Milbank Meml Fund Q*. **44**, 94, 1966.
2. Becker M. H. and Maiman L. A. Socio-behavioural determinants of compliance with health and medical care recommendation. *Med. Care*, **13**, 10, 1975.
3. Rosenstock K. The Health Belief Model and preventive health behaviour. *Hlth Educ*. Monogr., **2**, 354, 1974.
4. McKinlay J. B. Some approaches and problems in the study of the use of services—an overview. *J. Hlth soc. Behav*. **13**, 115, 1972.
5. Weisenberg M., Kegeles S. S. and Lund A. K. Children's health beliefs and acceptance of a dental preventive activity. *J. Hlth soc. Behav*. **21**, 59, 1980.
6. French K., Porter A., Robinson S., McCallum F., Howie J. and Roberts M. Attendance at a breast screening clinic: a problem of administration or attitudes? *Br. med. J*. **285**, 617, 1982.

7. Fink R, Shapiro S. and Lewis R. The reluctant participant in a breast screening programme. *Publ. Hlth Rep.* **83**, 479, 1968.
8. Haran D., Hobbs P. and Pendleton L. L. An evaluation of a programme teaching breast self-examination for the early detection of breast cancer. In *Research in Psychology and Medicine* (Edited by Osborne *et al.*), Vol. II, pp. 101–109. Academic Press, London, 1979.
9. Manfredi C., Warnecke R. B., Graham S. and Rosenthal S. Social psychological correlates of health behaviour: knowledge of breast self-examination techniques among black women. *Soc. Sci. Med.* **11**, 433, 1977.
10. U.K. Trial of Early Detection of Breast Cancer Group. Trial of early detection of breast cancer: description of method. *Br. J. Cancer* **44**, 618, 1981.
11. George W. D., Gleave E. W., England P. C. *et al.* Screening for breast cancer. *Br. med. J.* **2**, 858, 1976.
12. Wallston K. and Wallston B. Locus of control and health: a review of the literature. *Hlth Educ. Monogr.* **6**, 107, 1978.
13. King J. The impact of patients' perceptions of high blood pressure on attendance at screening. *Soc. Sci. Med.* **16**, 1074, 1982.
14. Langlie J. K. Social networks, health beliefs and preventive health behaviour. *J. Hlth soc. Behav.* **18**, 244, 1977.
15. Van Den Heuvel W. J. A. Participants and non-participants in a mammography mass screening: who is who? In *Breast Cancer* (Edited by Brand P. C. and van Keep P. A.), pp. 91–96. M.T.P. Press, London, 1978.
16. Schwoon D. R. and Schmoll J. H. Motivation to participate in cancer screening programmes. *Soc. Sci. Med.* **13A**, 283, 1979.
17. Vermost L. Factors affecting participation in screening programmes. In *Breast Cancer* (Edited by Brand P. D. and van Keep P. A.), pp. 91–96. M.T.P. Press, London, 1978.
18. Hobbs P., Eardley A. and Wakefield J. Motivation and education in breast cancer screening. *Publ. Hlth* **91**, 221, 1977.
19. Fishbein M. and Ajzen I. *Belief, Attitude, Intention and Behaviour. An Introduction to Theory and Research.* Addison-Western, Boston, 1975.
20. Calnan M., Chamberlain J. and Moss S. Compliance with a class teaching breast self-examination: the impact of the class on the practice of BSE and on women's beliefs about breast cancer. *J. Epid. Communit. Hlth* **37**, 264, 1983.
21. Calnan M. Women and medicalisation. *Soc. Sci. Med.* **18**, 561, 1984.
22. Calnan M. The hospital accident and emergency department: what is the role? *J. soc. Pol.* **11**, 483, 1982.
23. Stillman M. Women's health beliefs about breast cancer and breast self-examination. *Nurs. Res.* **26**, 121, 1977.
24. Kegeles S. S. Review of the Health Belief Model and personal health behaviour. *Soc. Sci. Med.* **14C**, 227, 1981.
25. Blaxter M. and Peterson L. *Mothers and Daughters: A Three-Generational Study of Health Attitudes and Behaviour.* Heinemann, London, 1982.
26. Williams R. Concepts of health: an analysis of lay logic. *Sociology* **17**, 185, 1983.
27. Calnan M. and Johnson B. Health, health risks and inequalities: a study of women's perceptions (unpublished paper). Health Services Research Unit, University of Kent, 1984.

Health promotion and the compression of morbidity

James F. Fries, Lawrence W. Green and Sol Levine

Department of Medicine, Stanford University School of Medicine, Stanford, CA 94305, USA; and Henry J. Kaiser Family Foundation, Menlo Park, CA 94025, USA

Health promotion activities have come under attack because of experimental evidence that reduction of cardiovascular risk does not appreciably affect total mortality.[1] Reviewing the results, McCormick and Skrabanek[2] are sceptical about health promotion in general. Their arguments embody the assumption, often shared by proponents, that the purpose of health promotion is life extension. In our opinion, the primary purpose of most health promotion activities in developed societies is to improve quality of life, to "compress" morbidity,[3-6] and to extend *active* life expectancy.[7] The compression of morbidity is illustrated in the figure. Extension of life itself can be a realistic goal as long as the aim is to prevent deaths that occur reasonably early—for example, by seat-belt laws and preventive measures in infancy.[8] There also remain opportunities to lessen mortality in developing societies and in disadvantaged populations where improvements of social conditions and personal risk factors have lagged behind those in more favoured groups. But, for health promotion in general, we must face some new facts.

The disturbing new facts

Life expectancy

Looking at the most recent and best performed trials of primary prevention of cardiovascular disease—the MRFIT Study,[9] the Lipid Research Clinics Study,[10] the Physician's Aspirin Study,[11] and the Helsinki Heart Study[12]—we agree with McCormick and Skrabanek that there is no effect whatsoever upon total mortality (table I). This lack of effect is unlikely to be due to a counterbalancing mortality from side-effects of drugs since it is seen also in trials of diet or exercise.[1]

Reprinted from Fries, J. F., Green, L. W. and Levine, S. Health promotion and the compression of morbidity. *Lancet*, i, 481–3, 1989.

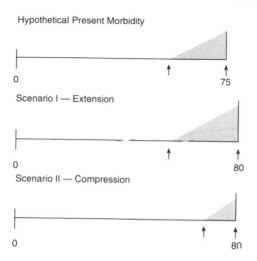

Hypothetical Present Morbidity

0   75

Scenario I — Extension

0   80

Scenario II — Compression

0   80

Compression of morbidity. The future of population health is dependent upon relative movement of the two arrows, the first representing the average age of initial onset of disease or infirmity and the second representing average age at death. If the first moves more rapidly than the second, there is compression of morbidity.

Epidemiological data support these observations. It is commonly stated that if atherosclerosis, the cause of 49% of all deaths in the United States, were eliminated, the average life expectancy would rise 8–10 years. However, in Japan there is essentially no atherosclerosis, and the Japanese national average serum cholesterol is very low. The average Japanese does live a little longer than the average American, but the difference in life expectancy at advanced ages is only a few months, not 8 or 10 years. (Higher incidence of other diseases in Japan, such as gastric carcinoma and stroke, does not begin to account for this observation.) Similarly, natural experiments on good health practices have been underway in the United States over many years. In Utah, because of the pervasive presence of the Mormon Church, smoking and drinking rates are very far below national averages. Economically and educationally favoured groups, such as physicians, have modified risk factors well in advance of the general population and in directions reflecting the most recent knowledge (physician cigarette smoking in the United States is now down to 6%). Yet, the mortality statistics from Utah, after adjustment for race mix, are not particularly impressive. Doctors live barely longer than their high-school classmates of the same race. These observations should give us pause. In our society, overall total mortality rates are becoming stubbornly resistant to either preventive or curative interventions.

Table I. *Major randomised trials of primary prevention*

Trial	No of men	Duration (yr)	Deaths			Coronary deaths			Morbid events			Morbidity/ mortality
			Intervention	Control	Diff (%)	Intervention	Control	Diff (%)	Intervention	Control	Diff (%)	
1. MRFIT	12 866	7	265	260	−5 (−2)	115	124	9 (7)	1366	1628	262 (16.1)‡	262/−5
2. LRC	3806	7	68	71	3 (4)	44	32	12 (27)	906	1112	206 (18.5)‡	206/3
3. Physicians	22 071	5	110	115	5 (4)	5	18	13 (72)†	173	239	66 (28)†	66/5
4. Helsinki	4081	5	45	42	−3 (−7)	14	19	5 (26)	45	71	26 (37)*	36/−3

* = p < 0.05; † = p < 0.01; ‡ = < 0.001. Morbid events: trial 1, angina pectoris, intermittent claudication, congestive heart failure, peripheral vascular disease, stroke, accelerated hypertension, left ventricular hypertrophy, impaired renal function, total non-fatal coronary events; trial 2, definite or suspect non-fatal coronary, positive exercise test, angina, coronary bypass surgery, congestive heart failure, intraoperative myocardial infarction, resuscitated coronary collapse, transient ischaemic attack, brain infarct, intermittent claudication; trial 3, non-fatal coronary, non-fatal stroke; trial 4, non-fatal coronary.

Risk-factor modification

If a man has several risk factors for early death, it is thus an error to assume that modification of the risk factors will substantially extend his life. The health professions fell into this trap for several reasons. Risk factor models were developed from data that are now old, and derived from high-risk populations at a time when there was more scope for improvements in life expectancy. With ageing of our population, the models have failed to include a term for "senescence"—the increasing frailty which inherently increases the imminence of all types of fatal event. And, the "independence assumption" embedded in competing risk models is obviously inappropriate; the modellers generally assume that escape from one hazard leaves an individual at average risk for the next hazard, whereas in reality the spared individual is typically at higher risk.

Trends in life expectancy

Life expectancy in the United States has risen in this century from 47 to 75 years. During the 1970s, the rate of increase continued strong as major chronic illnesses declined by as much as 40%. In the 1980s, these rates of increase have declined sharply (table II). The most favoured populations, such as women who have already reached age 65, have a life expectancy today which is exactly the same (18·6 years) as it was in 1979. The reasons are complex, but the largest factor is likely to be the increasing role of senescent changes. Another factor may be the inclusion of weaker individuals into the group who survive to age 65. At any rate, this firming of the upper life expectancy boundary provides a natural opportunity for the "compression of morbidity".

Duration of benefit from risk factor improvement

Here is another new and uncomfortable fact for risk factor theorists. The standard multiple risk logistic functions do not allow for the need to weight recent events. Thus, risk for lung cancer is said to increase with the number of pack-years of cigarette smoking that have been acumulated. If you stop smoking, the risk factor model holds you at your highest accumulation. Epidemiological data show otherwise. Risk of heart attack after stopping cigarette smoking returns to normal in 2 years.[13] Risk of lung cancer after stopping cigarette smoking returns to normal in 10 years.[14] Atherosclerotic lesions on the inside of blood vessels can be reversed by diet and exercise. It is not too far from the facts to conclude that only recent bad habits hurt you. Similarly, and unhappily, only recent good works helps. You lose cardiovascular fitness and

Table II. Changes in life expectancy, US, 1976–86

	1976	1977	1978	1979	1980	1981	1982	1983	1984	1985	1986
From birth											
All	72.9	73.3	73.5	73.9	73.7	74.2	74.5	74.6	74.7	74.7	74.8
Change	0.3	0.4	0.2	0.4	–0.2	0.5	0.3	0.1	0	0	0.1
Males	69.1	69.5	69.6	70.0	70.0	70.4	70.9	71.0	71.2	71.2	71.3
Females	76.8	77.2	77.3	77.8	77.4	77.8	78.1	78.1	78.2	78.2	78.3
Male/female gap	7.7	7.7	7.7	7.8	7.4	7.4	7.2	7.1	7.0	7.0	7.0
From age 65											
All	16.1	16.4	16.4	16.7	16.4	16.7	16.8	16.7	16.8	16.8	16.9
Change	0.5	0.3	0	0.3	–0.3	0.3	0.1	–0.1	0.1	0	0.1
Males	13.7	13.9	14.0	14.2	14.1	14.3	14.5	14.5	14.6	14.6	14.8
Females	18.1	18.3	18.3	18.6	18.4	18.6	18.7	18.6	18.6	18.6	18.6
Male/female gap	4.4	4.4	4.3	4.4	4.3	4.3	4.2	4.1	4.0	4.0	3.8

Sources: *Health, United States, 1986* DHHS Pub No (PHS) 87–1232; *Statistical Bulletin, Metropolitan Life* vol **68**, pp. 8–14, 1987; *Statistical Bulletin, Metropolitan Life* vol. **67**, pp. 18–23, 1988; *Monthly Vital Statistics Report* vol **35**, no 13, 1987.

muscular strength very rapidly after you stop exercising—perhaps within a month or so. Your calcium, oestrogen, and exercise programme to maintain bone calcium and prevent osteoporosis works only as long as you continue it.[15] These observations greatly complicate calculation of the effects of risk factors. Because the only data available on this ebb and flow of underlying health status are rough estimates and the estimates are drawn from various sources, it is difficult to know how to combine them. One can be certain, however, that if risk factor models do not capture the effects of recent trends in individual risk factors, they give wrong answers.

The pleasant new realities

Prevention can reduce morbidity

In every randomised clinical trial of primary prevention, effects on morbidity have far exceeded effects on mortality (table I). In the MRFIT study, for example, morbid events such as angina pectoris and congestive heart failure were reduced by 16% in the intervention group despite a small (non-significant) excess of deaths in the intervention group. Studies of this kind have *not* been negative; rather they have focused too strongly on mortality. Even when some forms of morbidity have been considered, investigators have overlooked the effects on the quality of life. Contrary to what McCormick and Skrabanek allege, population interventions can be very successful in improving health.

Prevention can reduce medical expenditure

Bad health habits cost everyone money. For a long time, data were not available to link health habits with medical utilisation and costs. Now material from Control Data Corporation strongly ties health habits to medical utilisation. In univariate analyses, a bad habit such as cigarette smoking is likely to increase yearly medical costs by 20–50% and lifetime medical costs by nearly as large a factor.[16] In controlled trials,[17,18] simple but well-conceived health promotion interventions have reduced medical utilisation from 7–37%.

Prevention can act even late in life

Part of the bad news was that the benefits of health promotion cannot be "banked"—ie, the gains evaporate. The reverse side of this observation is more important. In 2 years you can have stronger bones[15] and cleaner arteries. After 8–10 years, you can reduce your cancer risks to essentially normal.[14] From these facts some might conclude that programmes of heart health or cancer prevention should be switched from the young to the old. After all, if the school child is half a century away from his first infirmity, prevention of atherosclerosis and lung cancer may seem relatively unimportant (seat-belt use and avoidance of drugs or alcohol are more urgent). Some will counter that school health promotion is valuable for establishing lifelong habits.

However, it is in the pre-senior and senior populations that the greatest leverage from health promotion practices directed at chronic and degenerative diseases is to be obtained. The events to be prevented are now only a few years away. Costs and chance of illness are very much higher. Even small changes in these populations yield big and rapid differences in health and economic endpoints. Unfortunately, little health promotion effort has been directed at such people.[19]

New directions for preventive medicine

It may be hard to accept that immortality will not be achieved by a Pritikin diet or that, no matter how far you jog, you will not live to be 140. But the opportunities afforded by the new perspectives are exciting. They require a change of focus from quantity to quality of life—"Add life to your years, not years to your life".

As life-style practices continue to improve and as mortality rates at advanced ages decline more slowly, there may be disillusionment about the link between risk factors and health. It is critically important to recognise that the dividends of prevention are mainly in reduction of the population illness burden and enhancement of the quality of life, and that these are very large dividends indeed. We must dampen our enthusiasm for technical precision in individual health prophecy. Not only are the available data too weak and too oddly drawn; the models that employ these data are themselves inadequate to the task. Changes in some standard risk factors in an individual over time can provide a useful indication of trends in the future health of that individual, as long as the emphasis is on reduction of morbid events—such as sick days, hospital days, or symptomatic markers—upon the quality and not upon the duration of life. The primary purpose of population interventions, risk assessment, and risk reduction in developed societies is to compress morbidity and to improve the quality and vigour of life.

Acknowledgements

This work was supported in part by a grant to ARAMIS from the National Institutes of Health (AM21393).

References

1. Oliver MF. Reducing cholesterol does not reduce mortality. *J Am Col Cardiol* 1988; **12**: 814–17.
2. McCormisk J, Skrabanek P. Coronary heart disease is not preventable by population interventions. *Lancet* 1988; ii: 839–41.
3. Fries JF. Aging, natural death, and the compression of morbidity. *N Engl J Med* 1980; **303**: 130–36.
4. Fries JF. Vitality and aging. New York: Freeman, 1981.
5. Fries JF. The compression of morbidity. *Milbank Mem Fund Q* 1983; **61**: 397–419.
6. Fries JF. Aging, illness, and health policy: implications of the compression of morbidity. *Perspect Biol Med* 1988; **31**: 407–28.
7. Katz S, Branch L, Branson MH, et al. Active life expectancy. *N Engl J Med* 1983; **309**: 1218–24.
8. Williams AF, Lund AK. Seat belt use laws and occupant crash protection in the United States. *Am J Publ Health* 1986; **76**: 1438–42.
9. Multiple Risk Factor Intervention Trial Research Group. Coronary heart disease death, non-fatal acute myocardial infarction and other clinical outcomes in the multiple risk factor intervention trial. *Am J Cardiol* 1986; **58**: 1–13.
10. Lipid Research Clinics coronary primary prevention trial results. I. Reduction of incidence of cornary heart disease. *JAMA* 1984; **251**: 351–64.
11. The Steering Committee of Physicians' Health Study Research Group Preliminary report: findings from the aspirin component of the ongoing Physician's Health Study. *N Engl J Med* 1988; **381**: 262–64.
12. Frick MH, Elo O, Haapa K, et al. Helsinki Heart Study: Primary-prevention trial with gemfibrozil in middle-aged men with dyslipidiemia. *N Engl J Med* 1987; **316**: 1237–45.
13. Hermanson B, Omenn GS, Kronmal RA, Gersh BJ. Beneficial six-year outcome of smoking cessation in older men and women with coronary artery disease. *N Engl J Med* 1988; **319**: 1365–69.
14. Fielding JE. Smoking health effects and control. *N Engl J Med* 1985; **313**: 491–498.
15. Lane NE, Bloch DA, Hubert HB, Jones H, Simpson U, Fries JF. Running, osteoarthritis, and bone density: initial two-year longitudinal study. *JAMA* (in press).
16. Milliman and Robertson Inc. Health risks and behavior: the impact on medical costs. Control Data Corporation, 1987.
17. Lorig K, Kranes RC, Richardson N. A workplace health education program which reduces outpatient visits. *Med Care* 1985; **9**: 1044–54.
18. Vickery DM, Kalmer H, Lowry D, Constantine M, Loren W. Effect of self-care education program on medical visits. *JAMA* 1983; **250**: 2952–56.
19. Green LW, Gottlieb NH. Health promotion for the aging population: approaches to extending active life expectancy. In: Hogress JR, ed. Health care for an aging society. New York: Churchill Livingstone, 1989: 139–54.

Community education for cardiovascular health

John W. Farquhar, Nathan Maccoby, Peter D. Wood,
Janet K. Alexander, Henry Breitrose, Byron W. Brown, Jr,
William L. Haskell, Alfred L. McAlister, Anthony J. Meyer,
Joyce D. Nash and Michael P. Stern

*Stanford Heart Disease Prevention Program, Stanford University,
Stanford, California 94305, USA*

Summary

To determine whether community health education can reduce the risk of
cardiovascular disease, a field experiment was conducted in three northern
California towns. In two of these communities there were extensive mass-media
campaigns over a 2-year period, and in one of these, face-to-face counselling was
also provided for a small subset of high-risk people. The third community served
as a control. People from each community were interviewed and examined before
the campaigns began and one and two years afterwards to assess knowledge and
behaviour related to cardiovascular disease (e.g., diet and smoking) and also to
measure physiological indicators of risk (e.g., blood-pressure, relative weight, and
plasma-cholesterol). In the control community the risk of cardiovascular disease
increased over the two years but in the treatment communities there was a
substantial and sustained decrease in risk. In the community in which there was
some face-to-face counselling the initial improvement was greater and health
education was more successful in reducing cigarette smoking, but at the end of the
second year the decrease in risk was similar in both treatment communities. These
results strongly suggest that mass-media educational campaigns directed at entire
communities may be very effective in reducing the risk of cardiovascular disease.

Introduction

Cigarette smoking, high plasma-cholesterol concentrations, and high
blood-pressure are important risk factors for premature cardiovascular
disease.[1][2] In 1972 we began a field experiment in three northern

Reprinted from Farquhar, J. W., Maccoby, N., Wood, P. D., Alexander, J. K.,
Breitrose, H., Brown, B. W., Haskell, W. L., McAlister, A. L., Meyer, A. J.,
Nash, J. D. and Stern, M. P. Community education for cardiovascular health.
Lancet, i, 1192–5, 1977.

California communities to attempt to modify these risk factors by community education.

The mass media, face-to-face instruction, or combinations of the two may be used in community education campaigns. The habits influencing cardiovascular risk factors are complex and longstanding ones, are often reinforced by culture, custom, and continual commercial advertising, and are unlikely to be strongly influenced by mass media alone.[3-6] Face-to-face instruction and exhortation also have a long history of failure, particularly when aimed at producing permanent changes in diet[7] and smoking habits.[8] The disappointing results of a very limited attempt to reduce cardiovascular risk with a direct mail and lecture campaign reinforced pessimism about the possibility of changing health behaviour through public education.[9]

After considering the powerful cultural forces which reinforce and maintain the health habits that we wished to change, and in view of the failure of past health education campaigns, we decided to use an untested combination of an extensive mass-media campaign plus a considerable amount of face-to-face instruction. We also included three elements often ignored in health campaigns: (1) the mass-media materials were devised to teach specific behavioural skills, as well as offering information and affecting attitude and motivation; (2) both the mass-media approaches and, in particular, the face-to-face instruction used established methods of achieving changes in behaviour and self-control training principles; and (3) the campaign was designed after analysis of the knowledge deficits and the media-consumption patterns of the intended audience. Our goal was to develop and evaluate methods for achieving changes in smoking, exercise, and diet that would be both cost-effective and applicable to large population groups.

Research procedure

Three roughly comparable communities in northern California were selected for study. Tracy was selected as a control because it was relatively distant and isolated from media in the other communities. Gilroy and Watsonville, the other two communities, share some media channels (television and radio), but each town has its own newspaper. Watsonville and Gilroy received fundamentally similar health education over two years through a mass-media campaign. Additionally, in Watsonville high-risk people received intensive face-to-face instruction. Two-thirds of this group was randomly assigned to the intensive-instruction treatment group (w-i.i.) and one-third which received health education through the media only, was used as a control group (w-r.c.).

Data were gathered from a random (multi-stage probability) sample of

Table I. *Demographic characteristics and survey-response rates in each of three communities*

Characteristics of community groups	Tracy	Gilroy	Watsonville
Entire town (1970 census):			
Population (total)	14 724	12 665	14 569
Population (35–59 yr)	4 283	3 224	4 115
Mean age of 35–59 yr olds	47.0	46.2	47.6
Random sample (ages 35–59):			
Original sample	659	659	833
Natural attrition (migration or death)	74	79	107
Potential participants for all 3 surveys	585	580	726
Participants completing 1st and 3rd survey	418	427	449
Percent of potential participants	72	74	62
Mean age at Oct., 1972 (yr)	46.9	45.8	48.4
Spanish speaking or bilingual (%)	9.0	26.2	17.3

35–59-year-old men and women through interviews conducted in a survey centre set up in each of the three communities. These annual interviews were designed to measure both knowledge about heart-disease and individual behaviour related to cardiovascular risk. Knowledge was measured by a 25-item test of factors associated with coronary heart-disease. Daily intake of cholesterol, saturated and polyunsaturated fats, sugar, and alcohol were estimated,[10] and the daily rate of cigarette, pipe, and cigar smoking was recorded. Plasma-thiocyanate assay[11] indicated that only about 4% of those reporting abstinence may have given inaccurate reports.

Coincident with each annual interview, we also measured plasma total cholesterol and triglyceride concentrations, systolic and diastolic blood-pressure, and relative weight. Blood was collected into disodium E.D.T.A. 'Vacutainers' after a fast of 12–16 h. Plasma-total-cholesterol concentrations were determined by the procedures of the Lipid Research Clinics Program[12] and were adjusted for systematic variation in blood-sampling method.[13] Blood-pressure was determined by means of a standard mercury manometer with the cuff on the right arm and the patient sitting with the arm at heart level. Two measurements were recorded after the subject had been seated for several minutes and the second, taken approximately one minute after the first, was used for analysis. A different person measured blood-pressure in each community and all staff were trained in a standard manner. Other measurements made included plasma-renin and urinary sodium.[14][15] Results were sent to participants and their physicians.

The overall risk of coronary heart-disease developing within 12 years was estimated by a multiple logistic function incorporating the person's age, sex; plasma-cholesterol concentration, systolic blood-pressure, relative weight, smoking-rate, and electrocardiographic findings.[16]

The mass media and counselling campaigns were designed to produce awareness of the probable causes of coronary disease and of the specific measures which may reduce risk and to provide the knowledge and skills necessary to accomplish and maintain recommended behaviour changes. Dietary habits recommended for all participants were those which, if followed, would lead to substantial reduction of saturated fat, cholesterol, salt, sugar, and alcohol intake. We also urged reduction in body-weight through caloric reduction and increased physical activity. Cigarette smokers were educated on the need and methods for ceasing or at least reducing their daily rate of cigarette consumption.

The mass-media campaign in Gilroy and Watsonville consisted of about 50 television spots, three hours of television programming, over 100 radio spots, several hours of radio programming, weekly newspaper columns, newspaper advertisments and stories, billboards, posters, and printed material posted to participants. A campaign was also created for the sizeable population of Spanish speakers. The media campaign began two months after the initial survey and continued for nine months in 1973, was withheld for three months during the second survey, and then continued for nine more months in 1974.

Two-thirds (113) of the Watsonville participants whom we identified as being in the top quartile of risk of coronary heart-disease[16] were randomly selected for counselling. 107 attended counselling sessions and 77 high-risk individuals and 34 spouses completed all three interviews and examinations. These individuals, and their physicians, were informed by letter of their relatively high risk of coronary heart-disease (the letter was regarded as part of the "treatment"). They and their spouses were invited to participate in the instruction programme that was launched six months after the first baseline survey and was conducted intensively over a 10-week period through group classes and home counselling sessions. In the summer months of the second year, at a less intensive level, individuals were counselled about special problems (e.g., smoking and weight-loss) and were encouraged to maintain previous changes. The counsellors were graduate students in communication, physicians, and specialist helth educators trained in behaviour modification techniques. Pre-tested protocols were used.[17]

The intensive instruction programme was designed[18–21] to achieve the same changes that were advocated in the media campaign. The strategy was to present information about the behaviour which influences risk of coronary heart-disease, to stimulate personal analysis of existing behaviour, to demonstrate desired skills (e.g., food selection and preparation), and to guide the individual through practice of those skills and gradually withdraw instructor participation.

Results

Baseline values were remarkably uniform. Both the media and media plus face-to-face instruction had significant positive effects on all variables except relative weight after the two years of campaigning (fig. 1). (However, relative weight was significantly lower among the Watsonville intensive-instruction group after one year.) Thus, for risk-factor knowledge, saturated-fat intake, cigarette use, plasma-cholesterol, and systolic blood-pressure there were slight-to-moderate changes in the expected direction. When the last three variables (and relative weight) were incorporated into the risk equation the net difference in estimated total risk between control and treatment samples was 23–28%. This difference is in part attributable to the fact that the greatest change occurred in individuals with the highest plasma-cholesterol and blood-pressure. Face-to-face intensive instruction (Watsonville i.i.) in high-risk subjects increased knowledge gain and the extent of reduction of smoking but not other variables. Reasons for the changes in blood-pressure are not yet clear but include a probable interaction between weight-loss and enhanced adherence to antihypertensive medications, the latter being an unintended consequence of exposure to health education.[22]

Changes in knowledge and risk factors produced in the first year in Watsonville and Gilroy were not only maintained, but improved further during the second year (fig. 2). Groups which received counselling show a greater decrease at the end of the first year than that in the media-only groups. But in the second year the groups exposed only to the media show further substantial gains and the apparent difference between the effects of media and media plus face-to-face instruction is reduced. The parallel relation of the two media-only groups (Gilroy and Watsonville reconstituted) indicates that the media campaigns had similar effects on risk in the two treatment communities.

Discussion

Unlike the subjects of previous studies of giving up smoking[8] and weight reduction,[7] our participants were randomly selected from open populations, thus providing a better basis for generalisations about future public-health education efforts. But since we were able to recruit only

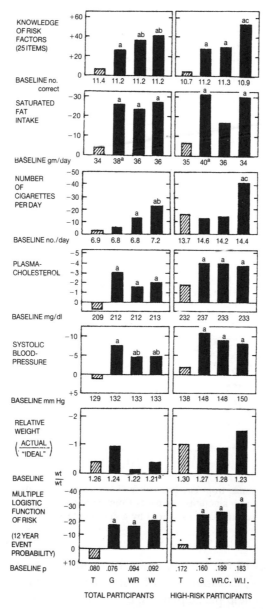

Fig. 1. Absolute baseline values and percentage change in selected variables after two years in control (shaded) or treatment (dark) groups. See table II for definition of groups. a=P<0·05 for baseline or differences in percentage change of control versus treatment. b=P<0·05 for differences in percentage change within treatment G versus W (total) or WR, c=P<0·05 for differences in percentage change within treatment W-R.C. versus W-I.I.

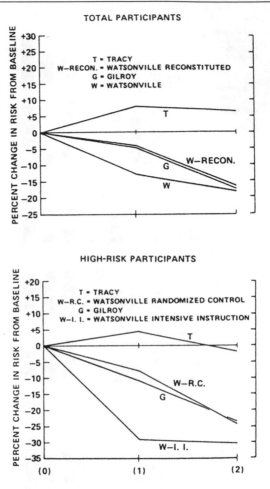

Fig. 2. Percentage change from baseline (0) in risk of coronary heart-disease after 1 and 2 years of health education among participants from three communities. Groups are defined in table II. Cardiovascular risk is measured by a multiple logistic function of risk factors.

about two-thirds of the total samples of eligible participants selected in the three surveys, extrapolation of our results may be limited. Also we were not able to help participants learn to achieve sustained weight-loss.

In general the changes in knowledge, behaviour, and physiological endpoints that were observed in the first year of treatment were maintained, and even improved in the second year of study. Intensive face-to-face instruction and counselling seem important for changing refractory behaviour such as cigarette smoking and for inducing rapid change of dietary behaviour. But we must also learn how to use these methods to correct obesity, and to employ them effectively with limited

Table II. *Composition and treatment of 9 participant groups in communities*

Group	Treatment*	
Tracy total participants (n = 384)	s	
Tracy high risk† (n = 95)	s	
Gilroy total participants (n = 397)	s + m.m.	
Gilroy high risk† (n = 94)	s + m.m.	
Watsonville total participants (n = 423)	s + m.m.	(for n = 312 participants)
	s + m.m.	(for 2/3 of high-risk
	+ i.i	participants and spouses n = 111)
Watsonville intensive instruction (w-i.i)† (n = 77)	s + m.m. + i.i	(2/3 of high-risk group randomly assigned to receive i.i.)
Watsonville randomised control (w-r.c.)† (n = 40)	s + m.m.	(1/3 of high-risk group randomly assigned not to receive i.i.)
Watsonville reconstituted (wr)‡ (n = 423)	s + m.m.	(weighted probability sample with i.i. group excluded)

*s = Surveying and feedback of results (annual), m.m. = mass media, i.i. = Intensive instruction programme.
†Participants in the initial survey at Watsonville, Gilroy, and Tracy whose examination results placed them in the top quartile of risk of coronary heart-disease according to a multiple logistic function of risk factors.
‡To correct for bias resulting from exclusion of intensively instructed subjects— i.e., high-risk persons and their spouses—means for remaining subjects in high-risk and lower-risk groups were weighted to compensate for the differential numbers of excluded subjects in the two risk strata. Resulting weighted means were called means of the reconstituted sample—i.e., sample reconstituted after exclusion of intensively instructed subjects.

resources (e.g., by training volunteer instructors). Mass media are potentially much more cost-effective than face-to-face education methods. Our results show that mass media can increase knowledge and change various health habits, but we believe that the power of this instrument could be considerably enhanced if we can find ways to use mass media to stimulate and coordinate programmes of interpersonal instruction in natural communities (such as towns and factories) and to deliver forms of specialised training and counselling about weight-loss and smoking avoidance.

Prevention of the premature cardiovascular disease epidemic of industrialised countries will require national purpose, planning, and action. It seems that part of this effort—i.e., persuading people to alter their life styles—can be achieved at reasonable cost.

Acknowledgements

This investigation was supported by grant HL 14174 (Stanford Specialised Center for Research in Arteriosclerosis) and contract NIH 71-2161-L (Stanford Lipid Research Clinic) from the National Heart, Lung and Blood Institute.

References

1. American Heart Association: Intersociety Commission for Heart Disease Resources, *Circulation*, 1970, **42**.
2. Blackburn, H. *in* Progress in Cardiology, (edited by P. Yu and J. Goodwin); vol. III, p. 1. Philadelphia, 1974.
3. Griffiths, W., Knutson, A. *Am. J. publ. Hlth*, 1960, **50**, 515.
4. Bauer, R. A. *Am. Psychol.* 1964, **19**, 319.
5. Cartwright, D. *Hum. Relat.* 1951, **4**, 381.
6. Robertson, L. S., Kelley, A. B., O'Neill, B., Wixom, C. W., Eisworth, R. S., Haddon, W. *Am. J. Publ. Hlth*, 1974, **64**, 1071.
7. Stunkard, A. J. *Psychosom. Med.* 1975, **37**, 195.
8. Bernstein, D., McAlister, A. L. *Addict. Behav.* 1976, **1**, 89.
9. Aronow, W. S., Allen, W. H., De Cristofaro, D., Ungermann, S. *Circulation*, 1975, **51**, 1038.
10. Fetcher, E. S., Foster, N., Anderson, J. T., Grande, F., Keys, A. *Am. J. clin. Nutr.* 1967, **20**, 475.
11. Butts, W. C., Kuehneman, M., Widdowson, G. M. *Clin. Chem.* 1974, **20**, 1344.
12. Department of Health, Education and Welfare (N.I.H.) 75-628. Manual of Laboratory Operations, Lipid Research Clinics Program, Lipid and Lipoprotein Analysis, Bethesda, 1974.
13. Stern, M. P., Farquhar, J. W., Maccoby, N., Russell, S. H. *Circulation*, 1976, **54**, 826.
14. Lucas, C. P., Holzwarth, G. J., Ocobock, R. W., Sozen, T., Stern, M. P., Wood, P. D. S., Haskell, W. L., Farquhar, J. W. *Lancet*, 1974, **ii**, 1337.
15. Lucas, C. P., Holzwarth, G. J., Ocobock, R. W., Sozen, T., Stern, M. P., Wood, P. D. S., Haskell, W. L., Farquhar, J. W. *Angiology*, 1975, **26**, 31.
16. Truett, J., Cornfield, J., Kannel, W. *J. chron. Dis.* 1967, **20**, 511.
17. Meyer, A. J., Henderson, J. B. *Prev. Med.* 1974, **13**, 225.
18. McGuire, W. J. *in* Handbook of Social Psychology (edited by G. Lindzey and E. Aronson); p. 136, Menlo Park, California, 1969.
19. Bandura, A. Principles of Behaviour Modification; New York, 1969.
20. Thoreson, C., Mahoney, M. Behavioural Self-Control. New York, 1974.
21. McAlister, A. L., Farquhar, J. W., Thoreson, C. E., Maccoby, N. *Hlth Educ. Monogr.* 1976, **4**, 45.
22. Curry, P. J., Haskell, W., Stern, M. P., Farquhar, J. W. CVD Epidemiology Newsletter no. 20, p. 48. Council in Epidemiology, American Heart Association, January, 1976.

Primary prevention of cancer among children: changes in cigarette smoking and diet after six years of intervention

Heather J. Walter, Roger D. Vaughan and Ernst L. Wynder

H. J. Walter and R. D. Vaughan (Division of Child Health) and E. L. Wynder, American Health Foundation, New York, USA

Abstract

A study of the effectiveness of an intervention program designed to favorably modify behaviors hypthesized to be related to the future development of cancer was initiated among 1,105 eligible children in 15 schools in the vicinity of New York City. Schools were assigned to either an intervention or a nonintervention group. Subjects in schools in the intervention group received each year, from fourth through ninth grade, a teacher-delivered curriculum focusing on diet and prevention of cigarette smoking. After 6 years of intervention, the rate of initiation of cigarette smoking was significantly lower among subjects in intervention schools than among those in nonintervention schools. There was a significant net decrease in reported intake of saturated fat and a significant net increase in reported intake of total carbohydrate among subjects in intervention schools compared to those in nonintervention schools. These findings, if replicated, suggest that such programs are feasible and acceptable and may have a favorable effect on diet and prevention of cigarette smoking in children. [J Natl Cancer Inst 81:995–999, 1989]

Cancer is the second leading cause of mortality in the United States today, accounting for ≈20% of all adult deaths (*1*). The age-adjusted cancer mortality rates for sites other than the respiratory tract (cancers of which are primarily attributed to cigarette smoking) have remained generally stable over the past 30–40 years (*2*).

Considerable effort has been expended over this period to elucidate the environmental and genetic factors initiating and promoting the development of cancer. In the course of this research, evidence has accumulated implicating behavioral causative or promoting factors, particularly

Reprinted from Walter, H. J., Vaughan, R. D. and Wynder, E. L. Primary prevention of cancer among children: changes in cigarette smoking and diet after six years of intervention. *Journal of the National Cancer Institute*, **81**, 995–9, 1989, cigarette smoking and diet. Some researchers suggest that these two factors contribute to the development of up to 70% of all cancers (*3*). Specifically, tobacco smoking is associated with increased risk for cancers of the lung, larynx, mouth, esophagus, bladder, kidney, and pancreas (*4*), and excessive intake of dietary fat has been linked to the development of cancers of the breast, colon, and prostate (*5*). A low intake of certain components of dietary fiber may be related to increased risk for colorectal cancer (*6*).

Exposure to these environmental factors begins in childhood or adolescence. The diets of American children mimic those of adults; currently, children consume ≈40%, 15%, and 45% of their calories as total fat, saturated fat, and total carbohydrate, respectively (*7*), in contrast to the recommended intakes of 25%, 10%, and 60% (*8*). Adolescence is the modal period for the initiation of cigarette smoking (*9*), and once the smoking habit is established, it has been estimated that fewer than one-third of smokers quit successfully (*10*). Accordingly, experts in preventive medicine increasingly are considering pediatric populations to be appropriate targets for the primary prevention of cancer through the modification of patterns of behavior believed to increase cancer risk (*11*).

The study described herein was intiated to evaluate, over a 6-year period, the effectivenesss of a school-based, teacher-delivered program targeted at the favorable modification of cigarette smoking and dietary behaviors among a cohort of 1,105 children in the New York City area. The earlier findings of this program have been published elsewhere (*12–14*). The results of the program at the end of the intervention period are presented in this paper.

Methods

Subjects and settings

The eligible study population consisted of students who were in the fourth grade in 1979 in all 15 elementary schools in four school districts in Westchester County, a suburban area adjacent to New York City. The mean age of these subjects at baseline was 8.9 years; 51.5% were male. Racial/ethnic distribution was 79.3% white, 13.8% black, 2.2% Hispanic, and 4.7% other (primarily Asian or Pacific origin). The median family income in 1983 was $55,904.

Study design

The investigation was a 6-year intervention study with two treatment groups. At baseline, 485 subjects in eight schools randomly were assigned to the intervention group; 620 subjects in seven schools were assigned to the nonintervention group. The intervention group received, beginning in the fourth grade and continuing consecutively through the ninth grade, a special curriculum (entitled "Know Your Body") aimed at reducing the risk of developing chronic disease. The comparison group did not receive the special curriculum.

Intervention methods

The special curriculum (*13*) targeted voluntary risk-reducing behavioral changes in the areas of diet, physical activity, and cigarette smoking. Curriculum development was guided by principles derived from social learning theory (*15*) and the health belief model (*16*). Cognitive development theory (*17*) provided a framework for the adaptation of these constructs to the maturational stage of the child.

The nutrition component of the curriculum promoted the adoption of a diet reduced in total and saturated fat intake and increased complex carbohydrate and fiber intake (*5*). Specific dietary recommendations included eating fewer fatty meats, whole-fat dairy products, fat-rich bakery goods, fried foods, and fat-rich sauces and dressings; and eating more whole-grain breads and cereals, legumes, fresh fruits and vegetables, and lower-fat meats and dairy products. Foods high in fat and low in complex carbohydrate and fiber content were designated as "Stop" foods in the lower grades and as "Hold Back" foods in the upper grades, whereas foods low in fat and high in complex carbohydrate and fiber content were categorized as "Go" or "Best Choice" foods.

The cigarette smoking prevention component promoted abstinence from the use of tobacco. The content of this component was based on previous research identifying three major factors believed to influence adolescents' decisions regarding smoking; namely, health beliefs, psychological influences, and social influences (*18*).

The health beliefs section featured biofeedback experiments demonstrating the immediate effects of smoking a cigarette on heart rate, blood pressure, hand tremor, peripheral skin temperature, and expired carbon monoxide level. Students also learned about the potential long-term health consequences of cigarette smoke inhalation, such as impaired respiratory function, cancer, and heart disease. In the psychological influences section, students explored the effects of self-image, values, stress, and anxiety on smoking-related decisions. Skills training in this section included alternative stress management techniques, such as progressive muscle relaxation and mental imagery. The social influences section focused on parental modeling, peer pressure, and media influences in relation to initiation of cigarette smoking. Training in decision making, communication, and assertiveness skills was emphasized.

The special curriculum was taught in intervention school classrooms for approximately 2 hours per week throughout each school year by the regular teacher, who had been trained by the research staff. Teacher training emphasized the behavioral orientation of the program and demonstrated teaching strategies derived from social learning theory, such as modeling, rehearsal, practice, reinforcement, and cuing (*19*). Adherence to the special teaching protocols was ascertained through a system of teacher monitoring conducted by the research staff.

Measurements

The prevalence of cigarette smoking was measured among consenting intervention and nonintervention subjects at study baseline by determining individual levels of serum thiocyanate (a metabolite of hydrogen cyanide) according to the method of Butt et al. (*20*), and at termination by levels of saliva continine (a metabolite of nicotine) according to the method of Haley et al. (*21*). The biochemical indicator was changed because of the greater sensitivity and specificity of the cotinine test (*21*) and because the cotinine test eliminated the need for venipuncture. The blood or saliva specimens were collected by trained professional personnel in the schools. Subjects with serum thiocyanate levels $\geqslant 100$ μmol/L or with detectable saliva cotinine levels were classified as current cigarette smokers.

Independent subsample populations of consenting intervention and nonintervention subjects were randomly selected for the 24-hour dietary recall interview, which was conducted at study baseline and at termination to estimate current diet. The proportions of gender and ethnicity groups in the subsample populations were similar to those in the entire population. Subjects interviewed at termination were drawn from the cohort of subjects who were eligible for participation at baseline. The 30–40-minute interviews were conducted by trained dieticians in the schools and followed a modified protocol of Frank et al. (*22*). Subjects were asked to recount all foods and beverages consumed in the previous 24 hours. Telephone calls were made to parents or housekeepers who prepare the child's food to obtain supplemental information on food preparation techniques and types of food consumed, if deemed necessary by the interviewer. School lunch portions were weighed by the interviewers to obtain accurate quantities. Prepackaged snack items were recorded with nutrient amounts obtained from package labels. Food amounts estimated with the use of portion models were converted to either fluid ounces or other common volume measurements, gram weights, or proportion of standard units recognized by a computer program. Calculations were standardized by supplemental guides developed specifically for use with the food models. The nutrient composition of subjects' self-reported dietary intake was analyzed using the Highland View Hospital-Case Western Reserve University Nutrient Data Base (Revision 7, May 1983).

Data analysis

Of the 1,105 eligible subjects, 911 (82.4% overall, 92.1% of intervention subjects, and 74.9% of nonintervention subjects) participated in the baseline examination. Of the 911 participants, 593 (65.1% overall, 69.3% of intervention subjects, and 61.0% of nonintervention subjects) had measurement data recorded at both study baseline and at termination 6 years later. The unit of intervention in this study was the school; thus, the school (rather than the student) was used as the unit of analysis. To determine the effectiveness of the intervention, the average changes in cigarette smoking and dietary intake over the 6-year course of the investigation were compared between schools in the intervention and nonintervention groups. The percentages of biochemically verified current cigarette smokers in each school were averaged across schools within treatment groups. At study termination, the differences in the mean rate of initiation of cigarette smoking among subjects in intervention and nonintervention schools were compared using the t-test. One hundred fifty-three and 188 subjects at baseline and termination, respectively, participated in the 24-hour dietary recall interview, for a 95% participation rate. The mean dietary values for individual subjects in each school were averaged across schools within treatment groups. The mean changes in the dietary values between baseline and termination among subjects in intervention and nonintervention schools were computed. The differences in change between these two groups were compared using a linear regression model.

Results

Table 1 presents the demographic characteristics of subjects in the intervention and nonintervention groups. Previously published data have demonstrated that study participants did not differ significantly from nonparticipants with respect to health knowledge and behaviors measured at baseline (*13*). The mean serum thiocyanate concentrations at baseline did not differ significantly ($P = .824$) between subjects for whom data were collected at both baseline and termination (35.6 μmol/L) and subjects lost to follow-up (35.2 μmol/L). Previously published data have demonstrated that subjects lost to follow-up also did not differ significantly from subjects remaining in the cohort with respect to height, blood

Table 1. *Demographic characteristics at baseline of participating subjects in intervention and nonintervention schools*

	Baseline	
Characteristic	Intervention (n = 8)	Nonintervention (n = 7)
No. of subjects	447	464
Age (mean, in yr)	8.9	8.9
Gender %		
Male	54.1	46.9
Female	45.9	53.1
Ethnic origin (%)		
White	89.8	78.9
Black	2.8	15.1
Other (primarily Hispanic)	7.4	6.0

Table 2. *Baseline and termination school mean percentages of cohort subjects classified biochemically as current cigarette smokers*

	Baseline (mean ± SD)		Termination (mean ± SD)	
Subjects	Intervention (n = 8)	Nonintervention (n = 8)	Intervention (n = 8)	Nonintervention (n = 7)
All	0.0 ± 0.0	0.0 ± 0.0	3.5 ± 4.3	13.1 ± 5.2*
Males	0.0 ± 0.0	0.0 ± 0.0	0.0 ± 0.0	12.4 ± 12.9†
Females	0.0 ± 0.0	0.0 ± 0.0	8.3 ± 9.7	16.3 ± 13.4

*$P < .005$.
†$P < .05$.

pressure, plasma total and high-density lipoprotein cholesterol, postexercise pulse recovery index, ponderosity index, and knowledge levels (*14*).

Table 2 presents the baseline and termination school mean percentages of subjects classified according to the biochemical indicators as current cigerette smokers. In the fourth grade, the percentage of subjects in both treatment groups classified as smokers was zero. By the ninth grade, the rate of initiation of cigarette smoking was significantly less (73.3%) among subjects in intervention schools than among those in nonintervention schools. The intervention effect appeared to be stronger among males. An additional analysis, in which adjustment for percentage of white subjects by school was made, yielded essentially identical results.

Table 3 presents the baseline school means in grams per 1,000 kilocalories of reported 24-hour nutrient intake and the changes in these means between baseline and termination. By the ninth grade, there was a significant net decrease (19.4%) in reported intake of saturated fat and a significant net increase (9.5%) in reported intake of total carbohydrate among subjects in intervention schools compared to those in nonintervention schools. There also was a favorable net reduction (9.8%) in reported intake of total fat. Among males, there was a significant $(P < .05)$ net increase in reported intake of total carbohydrate. Among females, there were significant $(P < .05)$ net decreases in reported intake of total and saturated fat and significant $(P < .05)$ net increases in total carbohydrate and crude fiber. An additional analysis, in which adjustment for percentage of white subjects by school was made, yielded essentially identical results.

Discussion

The main finding from this school-based intervention study aimed at the primary prevention of chronic disease is that the program appears to be effective in favorably modifying the two major behavioral factors—cigarette smoking and diet—implicated in the development of cancer. However, prior to a discussion of these findings, some methodological issues must be considered.

The external validity of the study may be threatened by the nonparticipation of a proportion of subjects at study baseline and by loss of a proportion of subjects to follow-up. However, the participation and cohort retention rates were relatively high. Moreover, participants were shown not to differ significantly from nonparticipants with respect to baseline prevention-related knowledge and behaviors, and subjects lost to follow-up were shown not to differ significantly from subjects remaining in the cohort with respect to baseline levels of risk factors for chronic disease. Thus, the findings from this study may be largely generalizable to similar populations of largely white, middle- to upper-middle-class schoolchildren.

The internal validity of the study may be compromised by differential rates of attrition between subjects in the two treatment groups. However, the proportions of subjects lost to follow-up did not differ significantly between the intervention and nonintervention groups, thus rendering it unlikely that differential loss to follow-up affected the estimates of the intervention effect.

Since a relatively small number of schools were involved in this study, the analysis by school has limited statistical power. Moreover, the small number of units available for randomization may also account in part for

Table 3. Baseline school means (in grams per 1,000 kilocalories) and school mean changes between baseline and termination in reported nutrient intake of subsamples of cohort subjects

Nutrient	Baseline (mean ± SD)		Changes between baseline and termination (mean ± SD)		Difference between groups (mean ± SD)
	Intervention (n = 8)	Nonintervention (n = 7)	Intervention (n = 8)	Nonintervention (n = 7)	
Total fat	35.7 ± 2.4	36.8 ± 5.3	−1.0 ± 2.7	+2.6 ± 5.4	−3.6 ± 2.2
Saturated fat	13.2 ± 1.8	13.9 ± 3.3	−1.9 ± 2.0	+0.8 ± 3.2	−2.7 ± 1.0*
Polyunsaturated fat	5.2 ± 1.2	5.0 ± 1.1	+0.3 ± 1.4	+1.5 ± 3.2	−1.2 ± 1.2
Total protein	39.5 ± 5.2	38.5 ± 5.0	−2.6 ± 7.2	+0.9 ± 4.4	−3.5 ± 3.4
Animal protein	26.6 ± 4.6	25.2 ± 6.7	−2.5 ± 6.8	+2.3 ± 6.7	−4.8 ± 3.7
Plant protein	8.4 ± 1.2	8.5 ± 2.4	+0.5 ± 1.6	+0.3 ± 2.8	+0.8 ± 1.2
Total carbohydrate	133.5 ± 7.8	131.2 ± 12.6	+5.4 ± 11.1	−7.1 ± 9.9	+12.5 ± 4.9*
Refined carbohydrate	18.0 ± 9.5	17.2 ± 6.7	+9.6 ± 15.0	+7.2 ± 9.3	+2.4 ± 7.0
Crude fiber	1.3 ± 0.2	1.3 ± 0.6	+0.2 ± 0.4	−0.1 ± 0.5	+0.3 ± 0.2

*P < .05.

the ethnicity differences between the two treatment groups. However, analyses in which adjustments for percentage of white subjects by school were made yielded results similar to the observed estimates.

Cigarette smoking is the single most important modifiable factor contributing to morbidity and mortality in the United States today (*23*). Despite widespread knowledge of the harmful effects of tobacco use, adolescents continue to adopt the smoking habit. Cigarette smoking among teenagers is reported to increase fivefold between the seventh and ninth grades, and by age 18, ≈25% of youths are said to smoke regularly (*9*).

Early smoking prevention research conducted among adolescents tended to focus on the adverse long-term health consequences of tobacco use (*24*). While some of these studies reported favorable effects on knowledge and attitudes, few demonstrated change in the target behavior. Recent studies suggest that more promising smoking prevention programs are those that focus primary attention on the psychosocial factors that influence the initiation of the smoking habit and provide training in assertiveness and other social skills that are hypothesized to deter initiation (*25*). These studies have demonstrated reductions in the rate of initiation of cigarette smoking ranging from 30% to 75% (*25*), although not all studies verified smoking status biochemically.

Several previous programs attempting to alter dietary patterns among children and adolescents also have reported encouraging results, demonstrating favorable changes in target food preferences and consumption (*26–28*). In contrast to these other studies, this study assessed dietary change through the analysis of nutrient intake. The 24-hour dietary recall interview, although subject to overreporting and underreporting, has not been shown to suffer from systematic bias, and it is believed to be one of the more feasible methods for estimating the current diet of large groups of subjects (*29*).

The "Know Your Body" intervention program, which originally was designed for middle and junior high school students, was terminated at the experimental stage of adolescent smoking behavior (ninth grade). Thus, a major question remaining is whether the favorable effect on smoking initiation observed to date can be maintained through the high school years, when adoption and maintenance of smoking behaviors occur. A currently funded follow-up study will track these subjects through the 12th grade in an attempt to address this question.

In summary, a longitudinal intervention study aimed at the primary prevention of chronic disease was initiated among fourth-grade students in Westchester County, New York. After 6 years of intervention, the program was shown to be feasible, acceptable to students, parents, and the school system, and effective in favorably modifying behaviors hypothesized to influence the future development of cancer. If these findings can be replicated among sociodemographically diverse populations of schoolchildren, it would suggest that programs such as this may have the potential to reduce the population risk for the second leading cause of death in the United States.

Acknowledgements

Supported by Public Health Service grant HL-21891 from the National Heart, Lung, and Blood Institute, National Institutes of Health, Department of Health and Human Services.

We acknowledge Drs. Christine Williams, Charles Arnold, and Nancy Haley; Patricia Connelly, Stephanie Converse, Kathryn Kost, Rebecca Patterson, and other "Know Your Body" staff; and the Byram Hills, Rye, Scarsdale, and White Plains school districts for their contributions.

References

(1) AMERICAN CANCER SOCIETY: Cancer Facts and Figures. New York: Am Cancer Soc., 1984

(2) NATIONAL CENTER FOR HEALTH STATISTICS: Vital Statistics in the United States. Mortality, vol II (Parts A and B, published annually), 1950–1980. Washington, DC: US Govt Print Off

(3) DOLL R, PETO R: The causes of cancer: Quantitative estimates of avoidable risks of cancer in the United States today. JNCI 66:1191–1308, 1981

(4) U.S. DEPARTMENT OF HEALTH AND HUMAN SERVICES: The health consequences of smoking. Cancer. A report of the Surgeon General. DHHS Publ No. (PHS)82-50179. Washington, DC: US Govt Print Off, 1982

(5) COMMITTEE ON DIET, NUTRITION, AND CANCER, NATIONAL ACADEMY OF SCIENCES: Diet, Nutrition, and Cancer. Washington, DC: Natl Acad Press, 1982

(6) REDDY BS: Colon cancer: Future directions. *In* Dietary Fiber. Basic and Clinical Aspects (Vahouny GV, Kritchevsky D, eds). New York: Plenum Press, 1986, pp 543–552

(7) BERENSON GS, MCMAHAN CA, VOORS AW, ET AL: Cardiovascular risk factors in children. The Early Natural History of Atherosclerosis and Essential Hypertension. New York: Oxford Univ Press, 1980

(8) IACONO JM, MCKEOWN-EYSSEN GE: Recommendations of the fat and fiber groups from the workshop on new developments on dietary fat and fiber in carcinogenesis (optimal types and amounts of fat or fiber). Prev Med 16:592–595, 1987

(9) JOHNSTON LD, O'MALLEY PM, BACHMAN JG: Use of licit and illicit drugs by America's high school students: 1975–1984. DHHS Publ No. (ADM) 85-1394. Washington, DC: US Govt Print Off, 1985

(10) KABAT GC, WYNDER EL: Determinants of quitting smoking. Am J Public Health 77:1301–1305, 1987

(11) IAMMARINO NK, WEINBERG AD: Cancer prevention in the schools. J Sch Health 55:86–95, 1985

(*12*) WALTER HJ, HOFMAN A, BARRETT LT, ET AL: Coronary heart disease prevention in childhood: One-year results of a randomized intervention study. Am J Prev Med 2:239–245, 1986

(*13*) WALTER HJ, HOFMAN A, BARRETT LT, ET AL: Primary prevention of cardiovascular disease among children: Three year results of a randomized intervention trial. *In* Cardiovascular Risk Factors in Childhood: Epidemiology and Prevention (Hetzel BS, Berenson GS, eds). Amsterdam: Elsevier North Holland Biomed 1987, pp 161–181

(*14*) WALTER HJ, HOFMAN A, VAUGHAN RD, ET AL: Modification of risk factors for coronary heart disease: Five-year results of a school-based intervention trial. N Engl J Med 318:1093–1100, 1988

(*15*) BANDURA A: Social Learning Theory. Englewood Cliffs, NJ: Prentice Hall, 1977

(*16*) ROSENSTOCK I: The health belief model and preventive health behavior. Health Educ Monogr 2:354–386, 1974

(*17*) PIAGET J, INHELDER B: The Psychology of the Child. New York: Basic Books, 1969

(*18*) McALISTER AL, PERRY C, MACCOBY N: Adolescent smoking: Onset and prevention. Pediatrics 63:650–658, 1979

(*19*) PARCEL GS, BARANOWSKI T: Social learning theory and health education. Health Educ May/June 14–18, 1981

(*20*) BUTT WC, KUEHNEMAN M, WIDDOWSON GM: Automated method for determining serum thiocyanate to distinguish smokers from non-smokers. Clin Chem 20:1344–1348, 1974

(*21*) HALEY NJ, AXELRAD CM, TILTON KA: Validation of self-reported smoking behavior: Biochemical analyses of cotinine and thiocyanate. Am J Public Health 73:1204–1207, 1983

(*22*) FRANK GC, BERENSON GS, SCHILLING PE, ET AL: Adapting the 24-hour recall for epidemiologic studies of schoolchildren. J Am Diet Assoc 71:26–31, 1977

(*23*) RAVENHOLT RT: Tobacco's impact on twentieth-century U.S. mortality patterns. Am J Prev Med 1:4–17, 1985

(*24*) GOODSTADT MS. Alcohol and drug education. Health Educ Monogr 6:263–279, 1978

(*25*) BOTVIN GJ: Substance abuse prevention research: Recent developments and future directions. J Sch Health 56:369–374, 1986

(*26*) COATES TJ, JEFFERY RW, SLINKARD LA: Heart healthy eating and exercise: Introducing and maintaining changes in health behaviors. Am J Public Health 7:15–23, 1981

(*27*) COATES TJ, BAROFSKY I, SAYLOR KE: Modifying the snack food consumption patterns of inner city high school students: The Great Sensations study. Prev Med 14:234–247, 1985

(*28*) PERRY CL, MULLIS RM, MAILE MC: Modifying the eating behavior of young children. J Sch Health 55:399–402, 1985

(*29*) CARTER RL, SHARBAUGH CO, STAPELL CA: Reliability and validity of the 24-hour recall. J Am Diet Assoc 79:542–546, 1981

Section 5

Coping with illness and disability

Readings

Active coping processes, coping dispositions, and recovery from surgery.
   F. Cohen and R. S. Lazarus. *Psychosomatic Medicine*, **35**, 375–89, 1973.

The impact of denial and repressive style on information gain and rehabilitation outcomes in myocardial infarction patients.
   R. E. Shaw, F. Cohen, B. Doyle and J. Palesky. *Psychosomatic Medicine*, **47**, 262–73, 1985.

Reduction of postoperative pain by encouragement and instruction of patients: a study of doctor–patient rapport.
   L. D. Egbert, G. E. Battit, C. E. Welch and M. K. Bartlett. *New England Journal of Medicine*, **270**, 825–7, 1964.

Psychological response to breast cancer: effect on outcome.
   S. Greer, T. Morris and K. W. Pettingale. *Lancet*, **ii**, 785–7, 1979.

The effects of choice and enhanced personal responsibility for the aged: a field experiment in an institutional setting.
   E. J. Langer and J. Rodin. *Journal of Personality and Social Psychology*, **34**, 191–8, 1976.

Introduction

Illness, disability, and in some cases treatment itself, can represent major threats to psychological adjustment. The growing prevalence of chronic disease in the ageing western population is increasing the numbers of people who need to adapt to living with conditions which are never likely to be cured, but only controlled, by medical treatment. The physical problems related to illness or treatment have the potential ιο curtail work, leisure activities or social life. Painful or life-threatening conditions can also take a severe emotional toll; research on cancer patients has suggested that as many as 50% may have sufficiently severe symptoms to warrant a diagnosis of psychiatric disorder (Derogatis *et al.*, 1983). Patients with heart disease have also been shown to have raised depression and anxiety and impaired quality of life (Wiklund *et al.*, 1984). Medical research has been directed principally towards management of symptoms or pathological processes, while the cognitive-emotional processes involved in coping with illness have attracted comparatively little attention. However, with the development of health psychology there has been a growing interest in how people cope with illness and disability, both in terms of the best strategies to ameliorate the stress of illness, and the mechanisms whereby coping behaviour might influence the development of illness. Some of the research on the psychophysiological mechanisms which link coping behaviour to physiology and pathology is discussed in Section 2, while the papers in this section illustrate the clinical utility of the coping concept.

Coping research in health psychology draws on a number of different psychological traditions. There is a strong body of animal research which has investigated the influences of coping strategies in relation to their effects on neuroendocrine markers of stress (Levine, 1983). In this field, coping is defined in terms of responses which can be shown to minimise neuroendocrine stress responses, so the emphasis is on *successful* coping. Research in the psychodynamic tradition also analyses coping in terms of success, with coping being defined in terms of activation of defence mechanisms, and thereby the prevention of distress. Defence mechanisms such as repression or denial have been explored extensively in relation to their contribution to the amelioration of stress responses (*Shaw et al.*). In both of these models, coping need not be either effortful or conscious. The alternative approach views coping as the repertoire of responses brought into play by the organism in order to manage stressful situations. In this model, coping is defined as the spectrum of cognitive and behavioural efforts which are directed towards a successful adaptation to stressful situations (Lazarus and Folkman, 1984). This approach to coping is not predicted on the notion of success – indeed some strategies may fail.

The readings in this section describe a range of applications of coping and related concepts in the field of health and illness and a number of important themes are illustrated. The distinction between coping as a *process*, i.e. the particular strategies adopted in that situation, and coping style as a *disposition* or *trait*, is one issue which has attracted a good deal of research attention. Repression–sensitisation (Byrne, 1964) is an important dispositional measure of coping style which developed from the psychoanalytic tradition. Assessment is by questionnaire and individuals are allocated a position along the dimension of repression–sensitisation (R-S) in relation to their responses to questions about their usual emotional reactions. One problem with the R-S scale is that the concept of sensitisation is closely related to anxiety itself and may therefore confound interpretation of studies on the moderating effect of coping style. A more recent development is the monitoring–blunting dimension, assessed by means of a questionnaire that specifies particular stressful situations (e.g. a visit to the dentist) and then offers a set of response options such as 'try to go to sleep' (a *blunting* option) or 'watch the dentist's movements' (a *monitoring* option, see Miller and Mangan (1983)). The balance of monitoring versus blunting choices across the eight situations is one index of coping style. Again this is a trait concept, because the assessment is not specific to the situation under investigation, but unlike the R-S scale it addresses the actual behaviours elicited in stressful situations rather than general responses to stress. A higher monitoring score has been associated with a more adverse emotional response to stressful medical procedures in the short term (Miller and Mangan, 1983; Wardle *et al.*, 1993) and with less satisfaction with communication in medical settings (Steptoe *et al.*, 1991).

The process approach to coping depends upon establishing the coping activities used in the particular situation in question. It has the advantage that it recognises that the adoption of one or another strategy may depend on its perceived applicability to the particular situation. The Ways of Coping checklist was developed by Folkman and Lazarus (1980) to evaluate coping responses to daily life stresses, and has been revised by Vitaliano *et al.* (1985). The checklist includes items such as 'talked to others', 'tried to forget the whole thing' or 'prayed for guidance', each of which is rated in terms of how much it has been used in relation to a particular stressor. In other studies, coping processes are operationalised in terms of the individual's specific behaviour in the situation, e.g. seeking or not seeking knowledge about a medical condition (*Cohen and Lazarus*), or expressing fatalistic versus optimistic attitudes (*Greer et al.*).

In coping research a distinction is drawn between actions or thoughts that are intended to ameliorate the emotional reaction, such as confiding in a friend or taking tranquillisers (*emotion-focused coping*), and those which are directed towards modification of the source of stress (*problem-focused coping*), such as planning a new way of approaching the problem (Steptoe, 1991). In the context of illness, problem-focused coping might relate to seeking information about alternative treatments, while emotion-focused coping might concern the use of distraction as a way of diminishing emotional distress. Strategies may change over the course of a stressful encounter, tending more towards *emotion-focused* coping at times where the emotional reaction is strong and towards *problem-focused* coping at a later stage. These coping responses should not be seen as immutable, since one of the important developments of recent years has been the demonstration that health benefits may accrue from modifying coping patterns. The readings in this section illustrate the impact of extending coping options both in acute medical settings (*Egbert et al.*) and in response to chronic conditions of institutional care (*Langer and Rodin*).

Coping style, coping processes and responses to treatment

In the early scientific literature on coping, overt emotional distress in response to illness or medical procedures was thought to index a mature recognition of the seriousness of an event compared with denial-based responses. Janis (1958) reported that patients who showed little apprehension prior to surgery (i.e. denied their fear) had a worse post-surgical adjustment. This was attributed to the absence of the 'work of worrying'. However, the status of denial as an immature, ineffective, or even pathological means of coping with medical stress has not been consistently supported. Indeed, the weight of evidence favours avoidant strategies in minimising short-term distress (Suls and Fletcher, 1985), at least in situations where actions are unlikely to change the outcome.

Cohen and Lazarus's paper focuses on a comparatively short-term stressor (surgery and post-operative recovery). The study evaluates the relationship between coping and recovery from major surgery using measures both of coping style and coping activities in the specific situation. Coping style was assessed pre-operatively using the R-S scale and an interview including items developed by Janis. Coping strategies were judged on the basis of interviewer ratings. The interviewer judged vigilance and avoidance in terms of patients' knowledge about their condition and its treatment and their willingness to discuss their thoughts about the operation. Recovery from surgery was assessed in terms of hospital stay length, medication usage and psychological reactions. Clear relationships between avoidant behaviour and recovery emerged, with avoiders (those who had less knowledge and were less willing to discuss their thoughts) having the best, and vigilant patients the worst, outcome. Interestingly, coping style was unrelated to any aspect of outcome. These results suggested that avoidant behaviour (a process measure) was a better predictor of outcome than avoidance as a disposition. Such a finding might be expected if dispositions are understood as a set of response tendencies which may or may not be expressed depending on the circumstances. Disposition is likely to be maximally predictive of outcomes assessed with a similarly broad brush. The issue of mapping levels of measurement of dependent and independent variables (i.e. general to general and specific to specific) is one which arises across the spectrum of individual difference research.

Cohen and Lazarus's finding that vigilant coping practices are associated with a poorer clinical outcome is one which has been replicated in a number of other studies (Miller *et al.*, 1988; Levenson *et al.*, 1989). A body of research is now investigating the mechanisms whereby vigilant coping strategies might adversely influence underlying physiological processes (see Section 2). However, the 'work of worrying' has not been entirely relegated to the status of an outmoded coping strategy. A number of studies have suggested that the benefits of a vigilant coping style emerge more clearly when the threat is prolonged (Suls and Fletcher, 1985; Holmes and Stevenson, 1990). One explanation for this may be that over the longer term, accurate appraisal of threat and its impact can promote acquisition of information and the use of new and better ways of coping. Avoidant or denying strategies by contrast may limit exposure to novel approaches to managing the illness.

Coping style and rehabilitation after myocardial infarction

Patients who have survived one heart attack remain at considerable risk of a second one, with more than ten times the risk of death over the next year compared with age-matched controls. Even among survivors there can be persistent morbidity and a severely impaired quality of life. Rehabilitation programmes offer the best hope of secondary prevention and are used widely. They usually incorporate advice on smoking cessation, exercise and diet and in some cases extending to stress management or modification of Type A behaviour (see Section 6), but the efficacy of many programmes is modest. *Shaw, Cohen, Doyle and Palesky* have evaluated the argument that a denying coping style could be a factor which adversely affects responses to rehabilitation (by reducing the learning of new material related to heart attack). The subjects were 30 men and women who had been admitted to coronary care units and were recommended for rehabilitation. As in the reading from *Cohen and Lazarus*, both process and trait measures of coping were included. Denial was assessed by structured interview, the R-S scale and by the related Weinberger *et al.* (1979) measure in which repressive coping is operationalised as a high social desirability score combined with a low anxiety score. Cardiac knowledge was assessed in relation to heart anatomy and physiology, heart disease symptoms, risk factors and treatment. Denial was assessed shortly after moving from the acute coronary care unit, and cardiac knowledge before and after the rehabilitation programme. Six months after discharge, behaviour was assessed in terms of both psychosocial functioning and compliance with treatment. In the hospital, there was evidence that a denying coping style was associated with lower information gain over the rehabilitation period, although the effects were more clearcut for denial as assessed by interview (the process measure) than the R-S or Weinberger (dispositional) measures. At follow-up, repressive coping as a style was associated with a poorer behavioural outcome, but only among patients with high levels of cardiac risk knowledge.

Other studies have also shown that while denial may be associated with more rapid recovery in the early phase, the long-term prognosis is impaired by poor treatment adherence and limited lifestyle change in patients who fail to acknowledge the severity of their condition (Levine *et al.*, 1987; Havik and Maeland, 1988). The 'mismatch' between coping style and information found in *Shaw et al.*'s study has been reported in studies where information level is manipulated experimentally. In an early study, Andrew (1970) found that repressors in a 'high-information' condition had a slower post-surgical recovery than in the 'low-information' condition. In a more recent study of responses to cardiac catheterisation, Ludwick-Rosenthal and Neufeld (1993) randomised subjects to high- or low-information conditions. Subjects who were classified as 'monitors' showed best adjustment to catheterisation in the high-information condition, while 'blunters' did best in the low-information condition.

Pre-operative intervention and post-operative pain

Following Janis's (1958) work on pre-surgical anxiety and post-surgical pain, there has been considerable interest in strategies which enable surgical patients to cope more successfully with the inevitable post-operative pain. Janis had shown that patients who had known what to expect after surgery remembered the operative procedures more favourably. This suggested that provision of information could have a positive effect on post-operative stress. The notion was first tested systematically by *Egbert and his colleagues* who conducted an evaluation of the benefits of information about post-operative pain in 97 abdominal surgery patients randomised to information or control groups. The controls had the normal pre-operative visit from the anaesthetist to describe the anaesthetic procedures. The information group was given the same basic information, but was also told about the anticipated post-operative pain and was given instructions on how to cope with it, including a recommendation to ask for medication if needed. Nursing staff and surgeons were blind to the group allocation. The results showed that post-operative narcotic use was significantly lower in the information group than in the controls, and that information subjects were also discharged from hospital sooner than the controls. This clear and careful demonstration of the clinical efficacy of information was a remarkable stimulus to research in this area, and to developments in clinical practice that have progressively increased the availability of information to patients. Other work has consistently confirmed the value of information in reducing pain and distress during stressful medical procedures (Johnson and Leventhal, 1974; Melamed and Siegel, 1975).

In subsequent research on preparation for surgery, one important issue has concerned whether information alone is adequate or whether the combination of information and coping advice, as used in *Egbert et al.*'s study, is necessary for the best outcome. The balance of the evidence supports the view that the combined preparation produces the optimum effect (Mathews and Ridgeway, 1984). The other issue is that of matching the amount of information to the patient's coping style. As discussed above, information appears to be most effective for patients who have a monitoring coping style (Auerbach, 1989). One explanation for this may be that information facilitates the natural coping processes for these individuals. This idea is supported by Ludwick-Rosenthal and Neufeld's (1993) finding that the levels of problem-focused coping are higher when coping style and information level are matched. Matching might thereby be more important for stressors which are susceptible to problem-focused coping and less salient for others.

Coping style and cancer survival

The idea that mental activity can influence bodily function has been accepted widely in relation to functional psychophysiological changes such as blood pressure or heart rate, and many neuroendocrine pathways have been delineated (see Section 2). However, the relationship between psychological factors and cancer has proved much more difficult to establish. *Greer, Morris and Pettingale*'s paper was a landmark in the area. They evaluated the psychological adjustment of women with breast cancer three months after mastectomy. Women were categorised as showing denial (17% of the total group), fighting spirit or vigilant optimism (17%), stoic acceptance (56%) or hopelessness (9%). There was no relationship between the psychological measures and tumour mass at the time of assessment. After five years, only 10% of the women in the denial or fighting spirit groups had died compared with 31% of those showing stoicism and 80% of the hopeless subjects. These findings persisted in a 10-year follow-up (Pettingale *et al.*, 1985).

A finding as striking and unexpected as this demands replication (Watson and Ramirez, 1991). A study of women with advanced disease failed to replicate any relationship with survival (Cassileth *et al.*, 1985), but in a careful replication of *Greer et al.*'s study, Dean and Surtees (1989) found that denial, as identified three months post-operatively, appeared to be protective. However, the fighting spirit group was no different from the other two groups with a poor prognosis, nor was denial as assessed pre-operatively related to survival. The authors interpreted this finding as casting doubt on the results and, by implication, the whole idea that psychological responses could be related to cancer survival. There is no doubt that the role of psychological factors in cancer is elusive. Studies such as *Spiegel et al.*'s (see Section 6), which have shown a positive impact on survival of psychological treatment, clearly suggest that this is a very important area to explore but findings have not been entirely consistent (Linn *et al.*, 1982). The increased understanding of the ways in which stress can influence immune function (outlined in Section 2) provides an important biological background; however, it would be premature to suggest that the role of psychosocial factors in the progression of cancer is yet established on the basis of this work.

Personal control and health outcome

One mechanism whereby active coping might influence health is through control (or at least perceived control) over the stressor. There is an extensive animal literature documenting the toxicity of uncontrollable stress (see Section 2). The human literature is more complex, although there is broad agreement that control, also sometimes described as self-efficacy, can be associated with better health outcomes (Steptoe and Appels, 1989). *Johnson and Hall*'s reading in Section 1 illustrates the protective effect of control over decisions in the workplace. *Langer and Rodin*'s paper is a fine example of the empirical evaluation of the utility of control in a real-life situation where issues of control may be central to survival. Their intervention was directed towards nursing home residents, a group in whom there has been concern that the loss of control associated with being 'put in a home' could be responsible for a deterioration in well-being. Control was operationalised in terms of the environmental demands for participation in decisions and activities. In the intervention group, participation in decision making was emphasised in relation to a number of aspects of life in the home. The comparison group was reminded about the range of help the staff could give to them. These subjects therefore had the same privileges, but they were awarded passively. Unfortunately (for the study) perceived control did not increase in the intervention group. Nevertheless the intervention subjects were improved on a wide range of measures including self-rated mood and activity, nurse-rated activity, and general improvement, after three weeks of the intervention. By contrast the majority of the control subjects had deteriorated. In an 18-month follow-up (Rodin and Langer, 1977), the differences between the two groups persisted on the nurses ratings. Health was also better in the intervention group, and mortality was 15% in the intervention group compared with 30% in the comparison group. These impressive results provide encouragement that age-related deterioration in well-being is not inevitable, and that psychosocial interventions might minimise some age-related changes (Rowe and Kahn, 1987).

The failure of interventions to influence *perceived* control is not uncommon. Wallston (1989) argues that this may be because the available measures of perceived control are insensitive. Alternatively, control in real life may not be something which is easily scaled. Assessment of behavioural utilisation of control (e.g. spontaneous requests or acts) might be a better index, and in *Langer and Rodin*'s study, there was behavioural evidence of greater interaction with staff. Despite this methodological problem, *Langer and Rodin*'s results were encouraging in terms of the benefits of decisional control. They have also been replicated in other nursing home studies (Baltes and Baltes, 1986). However, caution is required in extrapolating these results to other situations. The nursing home is a context in which control is comparatively easy to exert and response costs almost entirely absent. In some medical situations, the costs associated with the decision process may be high (i.e. the patient could take the *wrong* decision). Under those circumstances, patients may prefer to relinquish control to the professionals, as appears to be true for a significant minority of cancer patients (Sutherland *et al.*, 1989).

References

Andrew, J. M. (1970). Recovery from surgery, with and without preparatory instruction, for three coping styles. *Journal of Personality and Social Psychology*, **15**, 223–6.
Auerbach, S. M. (1989). Stress management and coping research in the health care setting: an overview and methodological commentary. *Journal of Consulting and Clinical Psychology*, **57**, 338–95.

Baltes, M. B. and Baltes, P. B. (eds.) (1986). *The Psychology of Control and Aging*. Hillsdale, NJ: Erlbaum.

Byrne, D. (1964). Repression–sensitization as a dimension of personality. In: *Progress in Experimental Personality Research*, B. A. Maher (ed.). New York: Academic Press.

Cassileth, B. R., Lusk, E. J., Miller, D. S., Brown, L. L. and Miller, C. (1985). Psychosocial correlates of survival in advanced malignant disease. *New England Journal of Medicine*, **312**, 1551–5.

Dean, C. and Surtees, P. G. (1989). Do psychological factors predict survival in breast cancer? *Journal of Psychosomatic Research*, **33**, 561–9.

Derogatis, L. R., Morrow, G. R., Fetting, J., Penman, D., Piasetsky, S., Schmale, A. G., Henrichs, M. and Carnicke, C. (1983). The prevalence of psychiatric disorders among cancer patients. *Journal of the American Medical Association*, **249**, 751–7.

Folkman, S. and Lazarus, R. S. (1980). An analysis of coping in a middle-aged community sample. *Journal of Health and Social Behavior*, **21**, 219–39.

Havik, O. E. and Maeland, J. G. (1988). Verbal denial and outcome in myocardial infarction patients. *Journal of Psychosomatic Research*, **32**, 145–57.

Holmes, J. A. and Stevenson, C. A. Z. (1990). Differential effects of avoidant and attentional coping strategies on adaptation to chronic and recent-onset pain. *Health Psychology*, **9**, 577–84.

Janis, I. L. (1958) *Psychological Stress: Psychoanalytic and Behavioral Studies of Surgical Patients*. New York: Wiley.

Johnson, J. E. and Leventhal, H. (1974). Effects of accurate expectations and behavioral instructions on reactions during a noxious medical examination. *Journal of Personality and Social Psychology*, **29**, 710–18.

Lazarus, R. S. and Folkman, S. (1984). *Stress, Appraisal and Coping*. New York: Springer.

Levenson, J. L., Mishra, A., Hamer, R. M. and Hastillo, A. (1989). Denial and medical outcome in unstable angina. *Psychosomatic Medicine*, **51**, 27–35.

Levine, J., Warrenberg, S., Kerns, R., Schwartz, G. E., Delaney, R., Fontana, A., Gradman, A., Smith, S., Allen, S. and Cascione, R. (1987). The role of denial in recovery from coronary heart disease. *Psychosomatic Medicine*, **49**, 109–17.

Levine, S. (1983). Coping: an overview. In: *Biological and Psychological Basis of Psychosomatic Disease*, pp. 15–26. H. Ursin and R. Murison (eds.). Oxford: Pergamon.

Linn, M. W., Linn, B. S. and Harris, R. (1982). Effects of counselling for late stage cancer patients. *Cancer*, **49**, 1048–55.

Ludwick-Rosenthal, R. and Neufeld, R. W. J. (1993). Preparation for undergoing an invasive medical procedure: interacting effects of information and coping style. *Journal of Consulting and Clinical Psychology*, **61**, 156–64.

Mathews, A. and Ridgeway, V. (1984). Psychological preparation for surgery. In: *Health Care and Human Behaviour*, pp. 231–59. A. Steptoe and A. Mathews (eds.). London: Academic Press.

Melamed, B. G. and Siegel, L. J. (1975). Reduction of anxiety in children facing hospitalization and surgery by use of filmed modelling. *Journal of Consulting and Clinical Psychology*, **43**, 511–21.

Miller, S. M. and Mangan, C. E. (1983). Interacting effects of information and coping style in adapting to gynecologic stress: should the doctor tell all? *Journal of Personality and Social Psychology*, **45**, 223–36.

Miller, S. M., Brody, D. S. and Summerton, J. (1988). Styles of coping with threat: implications for health. *Journal of Personality and Social Psychology*, **54**, 142–8.

Pettingale, K. W., Morris, T., Greer, H. S. and Haybittle, J. L. (1985). Mental attitudes to cancer: an additional prognostic factor. *Lancet*, **i**, 750.

Rodin, J. and Langer, E. J. (1977). Long-term effects of a control-relevant intervention with the institutionalized aged. *Journal of Personality and Social Psychology*, **35**, 897–902.

Rowe, J. W. and Kahn, R. L. (1987). Human aging: usual and successful. *Science*, **237**, 143–9.

Steptoe, A. (1991). Psychological coping, individual differences and physiological stress responses. In: *Personality and Stress: Individual Differences in the Stress Process*, pp. 205–33. C. L. Cooper and R. Payne (eds.). Chichester: John Wiley.

Steptoe, A. and Appels, A. (eds.) (1989). *Stress, Personal Control and Health*. Chichester: John Wiley.

Steptoe, A., Sutcliffe, I., Allen, B. and Coombes, C. (1991). Satisfaction with communication, medical knowledge, and coping style in patients with metastatic cancer. *Social Science and Medicine*, **32**, 627–32.

Suls, J. and Fletcher, B. (1985). The relative efficacy of avoidant and non-avoidant coping strategies: a meta-analysis. *Health Psychology*, **4**, 247–88.

Sutherland, H. J., Llewellyn-Thomas, H. A., Lockwood, G. A., Tritchler, D. L. and Till, J. E. (1989). Cancer patients: their desire for information and participation in treatment decisions. *Journal of the Royal Society of Medicine*, **82**, 260–3.

Vitaliano, D. P., Russo, J., Carr, J. E., Maiuro, R. D. and Becker, J. (1985). The Ways of Coping checklist: revision and psychometric properties. *Multivariate Behavioural Research*, **20**, 3–26.

Wallston, K. A. (1989). Assessment of control in health-care settings. In: *Stress, Personal Control and Health*, pp. 85–105. A. Steptoe and A. Appels (eds.) Chichester: John Wiley.

Wardle, J., Collins, W., Pernet, A., Bourne, T., Campbell, S. and Whitehead, M. (1993). The psychological impact of screening for familial ovarian cancer. *Journal of the National Cancer Institute*, **85**, 653–7.

Watson, M. and Ramirez, A. (1991). Psychological factors in cancer prognosis: In: *Cancer and Stress: Psychological, Biological and Coping Studies*, pp. 47–71. C. L. Cooper and M. Watson (eds.). Chichester: John Wiley.

Weinberger, D. A., Schwartz, G. E. and Davidson, J. R. (1979). Low anxious, high anxious and repressive coping styles: psychometric patterns and behavioral physiological responses to stress. *Journal of Abnormal Psychology*, **88**, 369–80.

Wiklund, I., Sanne, H., Vedin, A. and Wilhelmsson, C. (1984). Psychosocial outcome one year after a first myocardial infarction. *Journal of Psychosomatic Research*, **28**, 309–21.

Active coping processes, coping dispositions, and recovery from surgery

Frances Cohen, MA, and Richard S. Lazarus, PhD

From the Department of Psychology, University of California, Berkeley, USA

Abstract

Surgical patients with similar medical problems differ greatly in their rate of postoperative recovery. This study investigated the relationship between the mode of coping with preoperative stress and recovery from surgery. Sixty-one preoperative surgical patients were interviewed and classified into three groups based on whether they showed avoidance, vigilance, or both kinds of coping behavior, concerning their surgical problem. Coping dispositions referring to the same dimension, preoperative anxiety, and previous life stress were also measured. The five recovery variables included days in hospital, number of pain medications, minor medical complications, negative psychological reactions, and the sum of these. Results showed that the vigilant group had the most complicated postoperative recovery, although only two recovery variables (days in hospital and minor complications) were statistically significant. Coping dispositions, anxiety, and life stress showed no clear or consistent relationships with recovery. Ways in which mode of coping may have influenced recovery are discussed.

Clinical workers have long observed that surgical patients under roughly comparable medical conditions differ greatly in the course of postsurgical recovery. One of the psychological explanations of this variation is based on personality-related and hospital-induced differences in the modes of coping with stress (1–5). Questions about the role of coping have major theoretical as well as practical implications. From the practical standpoint, knowledge about the relevant coping processes, and the personality factors associated with them, could ultimately contribute greatly to improved patient care; for example, it may be possible to intervene selectively with suitable communications designed to facilitate coping.

From the theoretical standpoint, we must consider, among other things, the mechanisms by which coping styles and the course of recovery

Reprinted from Cohen, F. and Lazarus, R. S. Active coping processes, coping dispositions, and recovery from surgery. *Psychosomatic Medicine*, **35**, No. 5, 375–89, © American Psychosomatic Society, 1973.

from surgery might be linked. One such link is via the relations between coping and stress or emotion. Some types of coping activities reduce or short-circuit stress reactions by modifying stress-induced threat appraisals (6) (see also, Lazarus, Averill, and Opton (7) for a recent review), and others presumably provide an opportunity for anticipatory coping, that is, for working out prior to an impending crisis the harms and threats to be faced (1, 8). It is assumed in such analyses that the course of postsurgical recovery would be related to the increase or decrease of psychological stress during this period.

Evidence suggesting a possible physiological link between stress and bodily illness has been reported (9–13). Another possibility, more psychological in nature, is that the course of recovery is not only a matter of physical healing and the return of strength and energy, but involves a complex of behavioral events which could be influenced by coping styles, for example, complaints of pain, use of tranquilizers, use of pain medication, willingness to get out of bed and move around, response to the suggestion that the patient is ready to leave the hospital shortly, etc. The various elements of the recovery process have not been carefully analyzed and they probably include physiological, behavioral, and social events operating in a complex chain of causation.

The present study focused mainly on the relationship between individual differences in coping and the course of recovery. No plans were made to intervene experimentally in the patient's situation, although there has been evidence that such intervention can facilitate recovery (2, 3), depending on the patient's original coping dispositions (4, 5). Rather, we wanted to assess further the role of individual differences in coping and their importance in affecting surgical recovery. In particular, two approaches to coping activity were compared—dispositional measures and measures of ongoing coping activity.

Among the coping styles most commonly assessed by personality researchers is the dimension of repression-sensitization (14, 15), and the closely related concepts of repression-isolation (e.g., Ref. 16), and avoidance-coping (17). The latter dimension was employed, for example, in Andrew's (4) and DeLong's (5) research with surgical patients. Although these diverse assessment approaches to theoretically similar concepts have not been linked empirically (18), and may, therefore, represent different psychological processes (19), all three appear to deal with a general type of coping activity, avoidance versus vigilance, which could have an important bearing on the way a patient manages stressful events prior to and following surgery.

The above measures of coping style are all basically *dispositional*, that is, prior to a stressful event they assess the disposition or tendency in the person to use one or another coping process. Whether or not an avoider will actually display avoidance behavior in a given stress situation depends on the generality of the disposition and the relevance of that stress situation to the coping disposition (20). However, one can also study coping more directly in the very stress situation which calls for it. That is, by observing the person who is faced with stressful demands, measures can be obtained of the *active coping processes* being employed. It is of great theoretical and practical interest simultaneously to examine the patterns of relationship between such dispositional measures and measures of active coping obtained on the spot, as well as their relationship to recovery from surgery (or any other adaptive outcome). The central focus of this study of patient coping and recovery from surgery is, therefore, centered on comparisons of dispositional and active coping measures in such recovery.

Method

Subjects

Sixty-one surgical patients (22 male, 39 female) between the ages of 21 and 60 ($\bar{X}$ = 39.9, SD = 11.1) were studied.[1] They had entered the Kaiser Foundation Hospital in Hayward, California between November 5, 1968 and May 7, 1969 for elective operations for hernia (22), gall bladder (29), and thyroid (10) conditions. Patients who had previously had an operation of the same type were excluded from the sample.

In this sample, each of the 10 thyroid patients (age range 22–49, all female) had an admitting diagnosis of a nontoxic thyroid nodule. No cancer of the thyroid was present and final diagnoses included chronic thyroiditis, colloid adenoma with degeneration, involutionary nodule (4), thyroid adenoma, nodular colloid goiter, follicular adenoma, and para-thyroid cyst. Admitting and final diagnoses for the hernia patients were similar with one exception. Diagnoses included 18 patients with left or right inguinal hernia, left inguinal hernia with lipoma of the spermatic cord, or right femoral hernia (age range 27–58, 15 male, 3 female), 2 with bilateral inguinal hernia (age range 34–49, 1 male, 1 female), and one (age 40, male) with an admitting diagnosis of left inguinal hernia and a final diagnosis of sliding left inguinal hernia (with incarceration of sigmoid colon).

Admitting diagnoses for the gall bladder patients, excluding the 2 eliminated because of serious complications (as explained below), in-cluded 6 with cholecystitis (age range 26–52, 1 male, 5 female), 20 with cholelithiasis, cholelithiasis with cholecystitis, or cholecystitis with calculi (age range 22–56, 2 male, 18 female), one (age 21, female) with cholelithiasis (probably choledocholithiasis with obstructive jaundice), and one with hiatal hernia (age 32, male). The latter patient was included in the gall bladder category upon the advice of the physician, since the severity of the surgical procedure and the postoperative course were most comparable to that of a gall bladder operation. Diagnoses changed following surgery for 6 of the patients, resulting in one patient with a final diagnosis of cholecystitis (age 27, female), 24 with cholelithiasis, cholelithiasis with cholecystitis, or cholecystitis with calculi (2 male, 22 female), one with chronic cholecystitis, cholelithiasis, obstructive jaundice, one with chronic cholecystitis, cholelithiasis, choledocholithiasis, cholecystoduodenal fistula (age 44, male), and one with hiatal hernia (with hiatal hernioplasty, vagotomy, Finney pyloroplasty, and gastrostomy performed).

Procedure

Each patient in the sample was approached individually by the senior author, and asked if he or she would participate in a program of research.[2] All those accepting were interviewed in the hospital the afternoon or early evening of the day before their operation, approximately 1–3 hrs. after being admitted. In the interview (which was tape-recorded, and usually lasted 10–15 min.), questions were asked about the patient's emotional state, what he knew about his operation, what other information he wanted to know, etc., questions based on the procedures developed by Janis (1).

Following the interview, Andrew's (4) version of the Goldstein coper-avoider Sentence Completion Test (SCT) was administered, some general background questions were asked concerning education and occupation, and two pencil and paper tests were given, namely, the Epstein and Fenz (21) modified Repression-sensitization scale (modified R-S), and the Holmes and Rahe (22) Schedule of Recent Experiences (SRE). In a few instances where the experimenter felt it was in the patient's best interest to terminate the interview session (e.g., due to an excessively long interview that was interfering with the duties of the medical staff), the SRE was not given. Occasionally the patient terminated the interview session himself by refusing to continue to fill out questionnaires.[3] Thus, full questionnaire data were not obtained on every

[1] Patients over 60 years old were excluded because of the greater chance of complications due to age.

[2] Three subjects were lost by refusal. Two subjects were lost because their operations were cancelled for medical reasons. These subjects are not included in the totals listed above.

[3] Some patients rejected the SCT as being too personal, too difficult, too time-consuming, or as something they did not feel like answering. Although encouraged, patients were not forced to continue if they did not want to.

patient, and as a result, the N's vary slightly for different measures. While the patient was filling out the questionnaires, the interviewer took notes on the patient's behavior and general demeanor, and made two ratings, one on his use of avoidant and vigilant coping mechanisms, and another on anxiety, as explained later.

Control data were also obtained on a different sample of patients (N = 101) by examining the hospital records of the thyroid, gall bladder, and hernia operations performed by each of the four participating surgeons over the 6 months to 1 year prior to the start of the present research. These data were collected in order to test differences on several subsidiary variables, such as whether the surgeons as individuals contributed significantly to their patients' course of recovery. These control patients were not interviewed or tested; however, recovery measures were obtained for them as with the group that was interviewed and tested.

Recovery index

This index was devised using a modified version of the criteria employed by Andrew (4) in her study.[4] Four separate measures were obtained, namely, number of days in the hospital, number of pain medications, number of minor complications, and number of negative psychological reactions. They were also summed to give a fifth variable which is more or less equivalent to Andrew's recovery index. *Number of days in the hospital* requires no further explanatory comment. In the case of *pain medications*, analgesics and sedatives were both included. *Minor complications* included treatment for slight medical difficulties, such as fever and infection or bronchial spasms, and symptoms thought to be common manifestations of conversion reactions, such as nausea, inability to void, inability to move bowels, and headache (23). Anyone with serious complications, such as wound dehiscence (i.e. wound reopening),

---

[4] The minor complications category was greatly revised, omitting variables which did not reflect medical complications or which had no psychological implications (for example, the number of intravenous feedings), and weighting certain complications somewhat differently from Andrew. Minor complications were totalled as follows: inability to void, requires catheterization (2 points); inability to move bowels, enema given (2); nausea (1); nausea requiring medication (2); nausea plus vomiting plus medication (2); slight headache (1); severe headache, persistent (2); discomfort requiring hot water bottle (1); discomfort requiring ice pack (1); rectal tube for gas (1); routine postoperative antibiotics (1); antibiotics given to combat fever and infection (3); medication to prevent constipation or for urine stimulation (1); antacids given (1); medication given to counteract tetany (calcium gluconate) in thyroid operations (3); medication for diarrhea and/or gut irritability (1); medication (Aminophylline) for bronchial spasms (2); cough medication given when there was no fever (1); and nurse's observations that patient looked pale, dizzy, weak, etc. (1).

atelectasis (i.e. lung collapse), pneumonia, rehospitalization with high fever, and hypocalcemia (i.e. deficiency of calcium in the blood) after a thyroid operation, was excluded from the analysis, since the additional medical problem would interfere with a clear evaluation of the patient's recovery. The category of *negative psychological reactions* included such things as complaints by the patient and the number of tranquilizers given.

It should be be pointed out that the three types of operations used are heterogeneous—that is, the medical characteristics and severity of each varies. (Each has a differing course of recovery, with gall bladder patients, for example, staying more days in the hospital, etc.) On the other hand, the three operative groups did not differ to any significant extent in the proportion of patients in each of the 3 avoidant-vigilant groups. Due to the heterogeneity in the course of recovery for each operation, however, standard scores were employed as follows to equate for these differences.

Each patient's five recovery indexes were separately transformed for each operation into a T-score distribution with a mean of 50 and a standard deviation of 10, thereby transforming the range of scores within each type of operation to a common scale. Thus, a recovery score falling at the mean for the gall bladder patients and one at the mean for hernia patients will each be given a score of 50, regardless of the fact that gall bladder patients as a group take longer to recover. This statistical procedure, designed precisely for this sort of situation, allows us to talk in general about the effect of psychological coping activity on recovery from surgery without the results being distorted by the type of medical condition and the divergent surgical procedures.

Process ratings

These refer to several on-the-spot assessments of how the patient was coping with and reacting to the surgical threat. There were three such assessments: a rating of mode of coping, anxiety as judged by the interviewer, and anxiety as rated by the patient.

Mode of Coping

Avoidance and vigilance, as judged from the interview data, were treated as a dimension, and rated on a scale from 1 to 10, with high ratings (8–10) implying vigilant modes, low ratings implying avoidant modes (1–3), and a middle group (4–7) designed for patients emphasizing neither one nor the other. The rating was made by listening to tape recordings of the interviews, by the interviewer, as well as by an advanced clinical

graduate student,[5] so that reliability could be assessed. The
between the two sets of independent ratings was +0.878.
e and vigilance[6] were based on the following general charac-

Avoidance. The patient shows avoidance or denial of emotional or
threatening aspects of the upcoming medical experience, as indicated by
restriction of knowledge or awareness about the medical condition for
which surgery was recommended, the nature of the surgery, and the
postsurgical outlook, and by unwillingness to discuss thoughts about the
operation.

Vigilance. The patient is overly alert to emotional or threatening aspects
of the upcoming medical experience, as indicated by the seeking out of
knowledge about the medical condition, the nature of the surgery, and
the postsurgical outlook, and by the readiness to discuss thoughts about
the operation.

An example from a response considered avoidant is, "All I know is
that I have a hernia. . . . I just took it for granted . . . doesn't disturb me
one bit . . . . have no thoughts at all about it." An example from a
vigilant response is, "[after a detailed description of the medical problem
and the operation's procedure] . . . I have all the facts, my will is
prepared . . . . it is major surgery. . . . It's a body opening . . . you're
put out, you could be put out too deep, your heart could quit, you can
have a shock. . . . I go not in lightly."[7]

---

[5] Warren Gould, University of California, Berkeley.

[6] No distinction between the concepts of defense and coping was made (e.g., Ref. 24).

[7] Many detailed criteria were used in determining the process rating, and a clinical
judgment was made for each patient based on his total interview responses. For example,
knowledge of any of the following kinds of information put a person closer to the vigilant
end of the dimension: a description of the medical problem (including etiology), the risks if
surgery were not performed, the nature of the hospital experience, the operation's
procedure, medical problems which could occur during the operation, the expected general
course of postoperative recovery, possible postoperative complications, and the possibility
of recurrence of the medical condition. Patients who stated they had sought information
beyond what their doctor had told them were also placed toward the vigilant end.

Lack of knowledge about the medical condition put the person closer to the avoidance
end, as did statements that he had no thoughts at all about his operation and had not
discussed it with anyone, that he did not want to know anything about it, denial that an
operation was anything to be concerned about, and unusually positive statements ("having
an operation is like having a vacation").

The middle group were those who gave evidence of both avoidant and vigilant modes of coping.

The distribution of scores on this dimension of coping had a mean of 5.51, and a standard deviation of 2.22. Twenty-three percent of the patients (N = 14) were classed as avoiders, 16% as vigilant copers (N = 10), and 61% as falling in the middle group (N = 37). No strong differences were found among these coping groups with respect to the type of surgery they underwent, their sex, or social class as assessed by Warner's (25) revised scale for rating occupations.

Anxiety

The interviewer rated the amount of anxiety shown by the patient on a scale from 1–10, based on verbal and nonverbal cues such as jitteriness, nervous laughter, tremulousness, and rapid or impaired speech. It was impractical to obtain an independent set of ratings to check reliability, but these data are reported nonetheless. This distribution of anxiety ratings had a mean of 4.38 and a standard deviation of 2.23. On the basis of these scores, patients were divided into groups, with 51% (N = 31) classed as low anxiety, 13% (N = 8) as high anxiety, and 36% (N = 22) in the medium group.

In addition, a self-rating of anxiety was also obtained from each patient by having him respond to the following question as employed by Janis (1): "How worried or concerned about your operation are you? If I asked you to rate yourself on a 10-point scale, with 1 being not very worried or concerned at all and 10 being very worried or upset about your operation, where would you put yourself, from 1 to 10?" The resulting distribution of these self-ratings had a mean of 3.69, and a standard deviation of 2.76. Fifty-seven percent were classified as low anxiety (N = 35). 15% as high (N = 9) and 28% as medium (N = 17). The correlation between interviewer-rated anxiety and self-rated anxiety was +0.455 (p < 0.01).

[7]Contd.

   Categorizing patients as "vigilant" implies either that they sought out information about their operation or that they were sensitized (in terms of noting and remembering) to information when it was discussed, or both. It was difficult to separate out these two processes; from the interview data it appeared they usually occurred together, and our assumption is that they are related aspects of a vigilant mode. Similarly, we were not able to determine if those classed in the avoider group were unwilling to recall information, or to discuss it, or if they simply did not know certain things. Since all the surgeons had given information preoperatively as usual, we have assumed that there was avoidant activity in these patients, either in recall or in discussion.

Dispositional measures

These included a special form of the Goldstein Sentence-Completion Test of coping disposition (4), a modified version [by Epstein and Fenz (21)] of the Byrne scale of repression-sensitization, and the Schedule of Recent Experience as developed by Holmes and Rahe (22).

SCT coping disposition sources

This test consists of a series of sentence-completion stems, the responses to which are scored for "avoidance" if the emotional content of the stem is not acknowledged by the person, or for "coping" (sensitizing or vigilant modes) if the person accepts the emotional content, elaborates it and relates it to himself. Some examples of the items are: "My greatest fear is. . .", and "Sexual intercourse would be better if. . ." S's are divided into copying types depending on whether they display predominantly a "coping" or vigilant pattern of responses, an avoidant pattern, or fall in between the two extremes, thus being classed as "non-specific defenders."

In scoring this test, the method reported in Andrew (4) was followed. Dividing points (upper and lower 25%) for the three types of coping were determined separately for males and females, following Goldstein's (17) recommendations, since in his data and ours there was a difference between the distributions by sex. With a possible scoring range from 0 to 80, cutoff points were as follows: for females, 24–39 for avoiders, 42–50 for nonspecific defenders, and 53–64 for copers; for males, 15–30 for avoiders, 33–45 for nonspecific defenders, and 47–51 for copers. A second judge independently scored the SCT's, yielding a reliability of +0.926.

Modified R-S coping disposition scores

Epstein and Fenz developed a modification of the Byrne scale in order to eliminate some of the overlap between repression-sensitization and anxiety (e.g. Refs 26, 27). Byrne himself admits that the correlations between his MMPI-derived scale, the Taylor Scale of Manifest Anxiety, and the Edwards Social Desirability Scale are generally around +0.90 (15, 28). With the overlap with anxiety items eliminated, the Epstein and Fenz version should be more purely related to coping dispositions.

The R-S distributions for males and females were nearly identical, so separate cutoff points were not necessary as in the case of the SCT. The combined distribution had a mean of 13.21, and a standard deviation of 3.28. Selection of the upper and lower 25% required cutoff points as follows: 5–10 for repressors. 11–15 for middle group, and 16–20 for sensitizers. The possible range of scores is 0–30.

SRE-based life change units

This scale lists a number of life events which are either indicative of or require some change (positive or negative) in the ongoing life pattern of the individual. In our study this list was modified in a minor way to make it more personal and easy to understand. The subject indicated how many times in the preceding two-year period each of these life events had occurred. These events have been given life change unit (LCU) values by Holmes and Rahe (29), depending on how much social readjustment or coping was judged necessary to accommodate to each event. LCU values range from 11 (for the occurrence of minor violations of the law) to 100 (for the occurrence of the death of a spouse). Scoring was done by totaling the number of LCU's for each patient for the previous two years. This score was used in the analyses reported below. Patients were also divided into two groups, those who had LCU totals of 250 or more (N = 21), and those with totals of less than 250 (N = 31), according to the findings of Holmes and Rahe (30) concerning the likelihood of developing (or in a sense, disposition to develop) a stress-related illness.

Results

In the analysis of relationships among most preoperative variables, all 61 patients were used (except for 55 in the case of the SCT). Only 59 could be used in the analysis of the course of recovery since 2 patients who had severe complications had to be eliminated. Moreover, of these only 53 completed the SCT and 52 the SRE. In the control group, 99 out of the total of 101 patient records were used, since 2 had to be eliminated for major postsurgical complications.

The control data were analyzed for any differences in the recovery indexes on several subsidiary variables (including male–female, surgeon, previous surgical experience). No significant differences were found, so these variables were ignored in the analysis of the data in the patient group that had been interviewed and tested.

Relationships between recovery variables

Table 1 shows the correlations found between each of the recovery variables for the interviewed patient group.

Course of recovery and process ratings

Simple one-way analyses of variance were separately performed with each of the four indexes of recovery, and the sum of these making a fifth. Below are the findings for each.

Table 1. *Correlations among the recovery variables*

	Pain medications	Minor complications	Negative psychological reactions	Sum
Days in hospital	0.465^b	0.154	0.354^b	0.543^b
Pain medications		0.224	0.259^a	0.820^b
Minor complications			-0.133^b	0.662^b
Negative psychological reactions				0.345^b

Note—$N = 59$.
$^a p < 0.05$.
$^b p < 0.01$.

Avoidant vs. vigilant coping

The avoidant and middle groups of patients recovered somewhat faster from their operations than did vigilant patients. This trend could be observed in 4 recovery variables, but it was statistically significant only for days in the hospital ($F = 9.14$, $p < 0.01$), and minor complications ($F = 3.54$, $p < 0.05$). These relationships are diagramed in Figure 1.

Observer-rated anxiety

No significant relationships were found between anxiety, as rated by the interviewer, and any of the 5 recovery indexes.

Self-rated anxiety

These self-ratings were significantly related only to the incidence of negative postoperative psychological reactions ($F = 11.42$, $p < 0.001$), with patients high in self-reported anxiety showing more such reactions.

Course of recovery and dispositional measures

A simple one-way analysis of variance was employed to relate each of the coping dispositional measures to each of the indexes of recovery.

SCT coping disposition scores

Amount of pain medication was the only recovery index which showed a significant relationship with groups varying in the SCT measure of coping

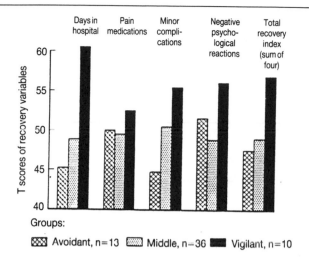

Fig. 1. Rate of recovery on 5 variables for groups differing in mode of active coping.

disposition (F = 4.20, p < 0.05). Patients classified as copers took significantly more pain medications than did the other two groups.

Modified R-S coping disposition scores

No significant differences were found between patient groups differentiated into repressors, sensitizers, or in-between, and any of the five recovery indexes.

SRE-based life change scores

Using a T-test analysis on each recovery index, no significant differences emerged between patients with high and low life change scores for the previous two years. Correlations between the total LCU score and each of the recovery indexes similarly showed no significant relationships.

Correlations among process ratings and dispositional measures

Table 2 reveals a few small, but significant, relationships. Two dispositional measures (SCT and modified R-S) showed a correlation of +0.369 (p < 0.01) with each other. The modified R-S showed a low but significant correlation (i.e. r = +0.268, p < 0.05) with the process rating of coping, but the SCT did not show any significant relationship to this process rating. The correlations between the dispositional measures and the process ratings of anxiety showed no significant relationships.

Table 2. *Correlations of dispositional measures and process ratings*

	Anxiety	Self-rating of Anxiety	SCT	Modified R-S
Active coping process rating	0.283^b	0.481^c	0.082^a	0.268^b
Anxiety rating		0.455^c	0.220^a	0.247
Self-rating of anxiety			0.056^a	0.216
SCT				$0.369^{a,c}$

^{a}N = 55. N = 61 for other variables.
^{b}p < 0.05
^{c}p < 0.01

Other findings

Low, insignificant correlations were found between age and social class, and the recovery variables. Years of schooling showed a significant relationship with two recovery variables, days in hospital (r = +0.276, p < 0.05) and number of negative psychological reactions (r = +0.278, p < 0.05).

A one-way analysis of variance showed no significant differences between coping groups on how anxious they were rated by the observer. Further, a discrepancy score was obtained by subtracting the self-rated anxiety score from the anxiety score given by the interviewer. A one-way analysis of variance showed there were no significant differences in this discrepancy among the three process-rated coping groups.

A one-way analysis of variance of LCU scores for the process-rated coping groups revealed no significant differences between groups on their total life-stress score.

It is quite possible that intervention of any sort, even an interview before surgery, may affect the recovery process by singling out the patient and thereby implicitly expressing concern for him. This possibility was examined by comparing the recovery pattern of a control group not so interviewed and the interviewed group. However, T-tests revealed no significant differences between the control (N = 99) and interviewed (N = 59) groups on any of the 5 recovery variables, showing that the interview itself did not affect the patients' recovery.

The correlation of +0.481 (p < 0.01) between the process rating of coping and the self-reported anxiety rating, reported in Table 2, suggests that the latter was confounded somewhat with the ratings of coping behavior. To eliminate this confounding, a one-way analysis of covariance was done on each of the 4 recovery variables (omitting the sum), thus partialing out the rating of self-reported anxiety. The results showed slightly reduced statistical significance, but remained essentially the same. Days in the hospital remained significantly related to process ratings of coping beyond the 0.01 level (F = 6.45), but the relationship between minor complications and coping was reduced to just below statistical significance at the 0.05 level (F = 3.11). Negative psychological reactions continued to show a trend in the same direction.

Discussion

The main positive finding of this study was that inferences made just before surgery about whether patients coped with the threat by avoidance or vigilance were significantly related to various indexes of postsurgical recovery. Patients using vigilant modes of coping generally showed a slower course of recovery in 4 of the 5 recovery variables—number of days in the hospital, frequency of minor complications, and a combined index created by summing the other four variables. Although this trend was found for 4 of the 5 indexes of recovery, it was strongest for number of days in the hospital and frequency of minor complications, reaching statistical significance in these instances. Patients using avoidant modes of coping generally did best in recovery, although their recovery measures were not significantly different from those of the middle group. Overall these findings should be considered suggestive, rather than definitive, considering the fact that many statistical analyses were performed, thereby increasing the possibility of obtaining significant relationships by chance. However, there do seem to be indications of a clear trend.

It is important to note that there are many factors of a medical and clinical nature which could have a bearing on both a patient's attitude toward his operation and his subsequent recovery from surgery. The procedure, discussed earlier, of obtaining separate standard score distributions for each type of operation adequately takes care of this heterogeneity across operations, but it does not control for heterogeneity within operative groups. For example, one type of gall bladder condition could be far more serious than another. And although in this study we did not try to investigate the influence of individual differences in medical condition, since [we] were oriented toward investigating more general factors—coping activity and recovery variables—it is possible that such influence could have occurred and could, in part, account for our results. For example, a patient who discovers he has a more severe condition could become more vigilant about his operation than the patient with a routine medical problem; in addition, since the disorder is more serious, he may take longer to recover postoperatively.

In effect, if seriousness of medical condition is a prime factor in affecting recovery and it also affects how much information the patient is told or seeks out, any relationship between the patient's knowledge of his medical problem and recovery would, in fact, be controlled by a third factor, namely the seriousness of the medical condition. It is, therefore of some interest to explore this possibility, in order to clarify the relationship we observed between psychological coping and recovery from surgery.

Due to the small number of subjects and the lack of a wide variety of clinical diagnoses for which the operations were performed, it was not possible to determine the extent of this relationship statistically. Scatter plots of the 2 recovery variables that showed significant results—days and minor complications—were made separately for each operative group. Diagnoses for each operation (e.g. gall bladder) were divided into least, middle, and most serious types, and the recovery variables were plotted for each type. In addition, scatter plots relating the seriousness of the medical condition and the avoidance-vigilance grouping were made. These plots revealed no relationship between seriousness of medical condition within each type of operation and either the recovery variables for that operation, or the avoidance-vigilance classification.

If, however, those patients with the 4 most serious medical conditions contained in the sample are examined, there appears to be some indication that seriousness of medical condition may have some bearing on coping classification and possibly on recovery. Concerning mode of coping, 3 of these 4 patients were classified as vigilant, and 1 was classified in the middle group. On both the days and minor complications recovery variables, 2 (both vigilant) of the 4 patients had scores greater than one standard deviation above the mean, and the other 2 had scores close to the mean. These data are suggestive, but are not sufficient to explain the significant relationships found between coping activity and recovery. Further research using a larger sample and detailed clinical examinations and ratings of seriousness of medical condition might be desirable to determine the way individual medical factors could affect both recovery from surgery and mode of coping with its threats.

Contrary to anything we expected from past research, those who knew the most about their operation—the vigilant group—showed the most complicated recovery from surgery. One possible interpretation is that the vigilant copers are more demanding patients—who act in such a way that doctors keep them in the hospital longer, etc. However, this interpretation does not seem plausible, since this group did not show significantly higher use of pain medications. This variable was the one most under their control, because in this hospital patients must ask for pain medications to get them.

It is possible that the vigilant group was actually more anxious postoperatively, but then we might have expected increased use of pain medications (31), which was not found. The possibility that the vigilant group was more "stressed," and thus more vulnerable, was also not substantiated, since there were no differences among coping groups on the total SRE-based life stress scores. Thus, an explanation based simply on anxiety or stress does not especially fit our data.

Another possible interpretation can be offered if we view vigilant copers as individuals who were using a strategy of actively trying to master the world by seeking information and trying to learn everything about their operation. In the postoperative hospital context, however, with its incapacitation and pain, they cannot "master" the situation actively as they would wish, but are forced to be dependent and passive. This could produce lowered self-esteem and an increased sense of vulnerability, which could conceivably impede the patient's recovery. This hypothesis is consistent with the findings that the vigilant group did not show increased use of pain medications, which their strategy of coping might lead them to reject as a solution. It is important to note, too, that vigilant patients not only had more detailed medical information but usually were also aware of possible negative complications. Perhaps knowledge of these threatening possibilities, obtained and remembered in their search for information, helped create their more complicated recovery, though we have no clear idea of the processes involved.

It is not appropriate to compare these findings with those of Andrew (4) and DeLong (5) since both these researchers used only a dispositional measure of coping. Moreover, even Andrew's and DeLong's findings are not entirely consistent with each other in the obtained pattern of relationship between coping disposition and recovery from surgery. Nonetheless, our findings are also not in accord with other studies that have suggested that the avoidant patient should show the poorest course of recovery, since this form of coping prevents the working through of the threat (1, 8, 32). However, it should be pointed out that Janis' work (1), which has never been replicated, dealt only with relationships between pre- and postoperative emotional reactions, and did not examine modes of coping separately or look at medical recovery variables, as we did.

The inconsistencies among studies do suggest, however, the possibility that given coping processes may be more useful for certain stressful situations than for others, or in particular periods of a prolonged crisis yet not in others. Thus, for example, many parents of children dying of leukemia profited from avoidant-denial defenses prior to the child's death (33) but suffered more afterwards (32). It is possible that surgery is one of those stressful occurrences that can be more effectively dealt with by avoidant-denial forms of coping than by vigilant ones, since although many threats exist in the surgical context, few actually materialize. This is consistent with Hackett and Weisman's (34) observations that patients can benefit more from denial if there is the possibility of a positive outcome (as in coronary infarction, for example, as opposed to terminal cancer). This possibility needs to be tested. In any case, our data do provide some support for the idea that individual differences in active coping may have an important bearing on the course of recovery from surgery.

A second major finding is that measures of dispositional coping, as distinguished from active coping processes, do not appear to be clearly or consistently associated with the course of recovery, or even strongly correlated with active coping processes, although one might have assumed they should be. It is becoming increasingly clear that behavior is determined by many factors, including situational ones to which the person must accommodate (35, 36), as well as factors within the individual. Research in this area has not yet determined how specific situational demands interact with coping dispositions.

There is another negative finding that bears comment, especially in the light of the great current interest in the relationship between life changes and susceptibility to illness. One might have anticipated from the research of Holmes and Rahe and their associates that patients with high life change scores should have fared worse in recovery from surgery than those with low life change scores. Our data did not bear out this expectation although the approach used here (assessing recovery from surgery) is quite different from theirs (predicting the development of illness), making comparisons with their findings somewhat tenuous. Different factors may be operating in these two processes, or, as Spilken and Jacobs (37) have recently suggested, it may be that life stress (or perhaps the perception or judgment of life stress) increases treatment-seeking behavior, rather than illness. If so, a simple relationship to recovery would not be expected.

A final comment is also in order about the indexes of recovery. There is a sense in which it is arbitrary to say that the course of recovery is better or worse insofar as the patient goes home sooner, takes less pain medication, has fewer minor complications, and exhibits fewer complaints. Such allegations adopt a particular set of values, largely behavioral in sphere, generated in part by practical considerations within the hospital setting. However, nothing seems to be known about the determinants of each of these indexes, and the decision process related to discharging a patient, giving tranquilizers, etc. Nor do we have a calculus of the importance of these recovery variables in reflecting the patient's return to health. We have kept the indexes separate, as well as combining them in order to keep better track of the contribution of coping style to each.

From a practical point of view, clinical workers look toward the possibilities of using knowledge about individual differences in coping to understand the process of recovery from illness, as well as to develop methods of intervention to speed recovery, or make its course more favorable in other ways. Effective intervention will ultimately depend on what we can learn about the factors influencing recovery, especially those related to coping. This study also raises many questions concerning whether and when avoidance or vigilance as styles of coping are effective in helping people to adapt to inevitable life stresses. Research to date has not provided the answers, but has strongly suggested the fruitfulness of the questions.

Summary

Surgical patients with similar medical problems often differ greatly in their course of postoperative recovery. This study investigated the relationship between mode of coping with preoperative stress—using both measures of ongoing coping activity and dispositional coping—and recovery from surgery.

Sixty-one preoperative surgical patients were interviewed and classified into avoidant, vigilant, or middle groups based on whether their interview responses showed avoidance of or vigilance toward information about their operations, or both kinds of behaviour. Coping dispositions or traits referring to the same type of dimension were also measured using two different personality tests. Self-report and observer ratings of preoperative anxiety were made, and a measure of previous life stress was obtained. The five recovery measures included days in hospital, number of pain medications, minor medical complications, negative psychological reactions, and the sum of these four.

Results showed that the vigilant group—those who knew the most about their operation—had a more complicated recovery than did the other two groups on 4 of the 5 recovery measures, although only two (days in hospital, and minor complications) were statistically significant. The dispositional tests were not clearly or consistently associated with the course of recovery, nor correlated with the active coping processes. No significant relationships were found between observer ratings of preoperative anxiety, previous life stress, and any of the 5 recovery variables. Self-reported anxiety showed a significant relationship with only one recovery measure (negative psychological reactions).

Ways in which the mode of coping may have influenced recovery measures were discussed. These findings raise the possibility that knowledge of threatening aspects of surgery, if untempered by denial, could result in a more complicated postoperative recovery, and that an avoidant orientation may be an effective mode of coping in a medical situation where the likelihood of threats occurring is small.

Acknowledgements

The authors greatly appreciate the assistance of Norman T. Walter, M.D., Surgery Department, Kaiser Foundation Hospital, Hayward, California, who was instrumental in arranging for permission for this study to be done, and who willingly gave his time and expertise to advise and answer questions. We are also grateful to the administrator of Kaiser Hospital for approving this study, to the medical and nonmedical staff for their cooperation, and to Edward M. Opton, Ph.D., for his efforts during the preliminary stages of this study.

The research reported here was supported in part by a research grant (MH-2136) from the National Institute of Mental Health. Financial support for the senior author was provided by a predoctoral traineeship from the Rehabilitation Services Administration (Grant No. RH4), and to the junior author through a Miller Professorship at the University of California, Berkeley.

Part of this research was presented at the Western Psychological Association Convention, Los Angeles, California, April, 1970.

References

1. Janis I: Psychological Stress, New York, Wiley, 1958.
2. Egbert LD, Battit BE, Welch CE, Bartlett MK: Reduction of postoperative pain by encouragement and instruction of patients. N Engl J Med 270: 825–827, 1964
3. Healy KM: Does preoperative instruction make a difference? Am J Nurs 68:62–67, 1968
4. Andrew JM: Coping styles, stress-relevant learning and recovery from surgery. Unpublished doctoral dissertation, University of California, Los Angeles, 1967
5. DeLong DR: Individual differences in patterns of anxiety arousal, stress-relevant information and recovery from surgery. Unpublished doctoral dissertation, University of California, Los Angeles, 1970. (Referenced in Goldstein MJ: Individual differences in responses to stress. Paper given at conference entitled "Stress: Its Impact on Thought and Emotion," University of California Medical Center, San Francisco, June 2–3, 1972)
6. Lazarus RS: Psychological Stress and the Coping Process. New York, McGraw Hill, 1966
7. Lazarus RS, Averill JR, Opton EM: Towards a cognitive theory of emotion, Feelings and Emotions (Edited by MB Arnold), New York, Academic Press, 1970, pp 207–232
8. Golstein MJ, Jones RB, Clemens TL, Flagg G, Alexander F: Coping style as a factor in psychophysiological response to a tension-arousing film. J Pers Soc Psychol 1:290–302, 1965
9. Rahe RH, Meyer M, Smith M, Kjaer G, Holmes TH: Social stress and illness onset. J. Psychosom Res 8:35–44, 1964
10. Rahe RH, McKean JD, Arthur RJ: a longitudinal study of life change and illness patterns, J Psychosom Res 10:355–366, 1967

11. Wyler AR, Masuda M, Holmes TH: Magnitude of life events and seriousness of illness. Psychosom Med 33:115–122, 1971

12. Jacobs MH, Spilken A, Norman M: Relationship of life change, maladaptive aggression, and upper respiratory infection in male college students. Psychosom Med 31:31–44, 1969

13. Querido A: Forecast and followup: an investigation into the clinical, social, and mental factors determining the results of hospital treatment. Br J Prev Soc Med 13:33–49, 1959

14. Byrne D: The Repression-sensitization scale: rationale, reliability, and validity. J Pers 29:334–349, 1961

15. Byrne D: Repression-sensitization as a dimension of personality, Progress in Experimental Personality Research, Vol 1 (Edited by BA Maher), New York, Academic Press, 1964, pp 170–220

16. Gardner RW, Holzman PS, Klein GS, Linton HB, Spense DP: Cognitive control: a study of individual consistencies in cognitive behavior. Psychol Issues 1:No. 4, 1959

17. Goldstein MJ: The relationship between coping and avoiding behavior and response to fear-arousing propaganda. J Abnorm Soc Psychol 58:247–252, 1959

18. Levine M, Spivack G: The Rorschach Index of Repressive Style. Springfield, Ill. Charles C. Thomas, 1964

19. Lazarus RS, Averill JR, Opton EM: The psychology of coping: issues of research and assessment. Paper given at conference entitled "Coping and Adaptation," Stanford University Department of Psychiatry, Standford, California, March 20–22, 1969

20. Averill JR, Opton EM: Psychophysiological assessment: rationale and problems, Advances in Psychological Assessment. Vol 1 (Edited by P McReynolds), Palo Alto, Cal. Science and Behavior Books, 1968, pp. 265–288

21. Epstein S, Fenz WD: The detection of areas of emotional stress through variations in perceptual threshold and physiological arousal. J Exp Res Pers 2:191–199, 1967

22. Holmes TH, Rahe RH: Schedule of Recent Experiences. Seattle, University of Washington School of Medicine, 1967.

23. Engel GL: Psychological Development in Health and Disease. Philadelphia, WB Saunders Company, 1962

24. Haan N: A tripartite model of ego functioning: Values and clinical research applications. J Nerv Ment Dis 148:14–30, 1969

25. Warner WL (with Meeker M, Feels K): Social Class in America. New York, Harper & Row, 1960

26. Golin S, Herron EW, Lakota R, Raineck L: Factor analytic study of the Manifest Anxiety, Extraversion, and Repression-sensitization scales. J Consult Psychol 31:564–569, 1967

27. Lefcourt HM: Repression-sensitization: a measure of the evaluation of emotional expression. J Consult Psychol 30:444–449, 1966

28. Schwartz M, Krupp N, Byrne D: Repression-sensitization and medical diagnosis. J Abnorm Psychol 78:286–291, 1971

29. Holmes TH, Rahe RH: The social readjustment rating scale. J Psychosom Res 11:213–218, 1967

30. Holmes TH, Rahe RH: Life crisis and disease onset: II. Qualitative and

quantitative definition of the life crisis and its association with health change, Seattle, University of Washington School of Medicine, unpublished paper

31. Drew FL, Moriarty RW, Shapiro AP: An approach to the measurement of the pain and anxiety responses of surgical patients, Psychosom Med 30:826–836, 1968

32. Chodoff P, Friedman SB, Hamburg DA: Stress, defenses and coping behavior: observations in parents of children with malignant disease. Am J Psychiatry 120:743–749, 1964

33. Wolff CT, Friedman SB, Hofer MA, Mason JW: Relationship between psychological defenses and mean urinary 17-hydroxycorticosteroid excretion rates: I. A predictive study of parents of fatally ill children. Psychosom Med 26:576–591, 1964

34. Hackett TP, Weisman AD: Reactions to the imminence of death, The Threat of Impending Disaster. (Edited by GH Grosser, H Wechsler, M Greenblatt), Cambridge, Massachusetts, MIT Press, 1964, pp. 300–311

35. Wicker AW: Attitudes versus actions: the relationship of verbal and overt behavioral responses to attitude objects. J Soc Issues 25:41–78, 1969

36. Brigham JC: Racial stereotypes, attitudes, and evaluations of and behavioral intentions toward Negroes and whites. Sociometry 34:360–380, 1971

37. Spilken AZ, Jacobs MA: Predictions of illness behavior from measures of life crisis, manifest distress, and maladaptive coping. Psychosom Med 33:251–264, 1971

The impact of denial and repressive style on information gain and rehabilitation outcomes in myocardial infarction patients

Richard E. Shaw, MA, Frances Cohen, PhD,
Brigid Doyle, RN, MS, and Judith Palesky, RN, BSN

From the Health Psychology Program, School of Medicine, University of California, San Francisco and the Pacific Medical Center, San Francisco, USA

Abstract

The impact of denial, repressive style, and social desirability on information gained during hospitalization and their effects on recovery were studied in 30 patients with documented myocardial infarction (MI). Using three scores of cardiac knowledge as dependent variables, three significant findings emerged: 1) patients who denied more gained less information about heart anatomy and physiology; 2) patients who scored high on social desirability gained less information about systems indicating heart problems and activities appropriate for recovery; and 3) patients who were repressors gained less information about heart disease risk factors. Twenty-four of the 30 patients completed a survey of functioning 6 months after discharge. Dividing patients into four groups representing a match or mismatch between repressive style and information level, it was found that 1) repressors with high risk factor information reported more complications and poorer psychomedical functioning, and 2) sensitizers with low risk factor information reported poorer social functioning.

Introduction

Cardiac rehabilitation in the form of patient education has become an integral part of treatment during hospitalization for patients recovering from a heart attack. Although it is well established that cardiac education

Reprinted from Shaw, R. E., Cohen, F., Coyle, B. and Palesky, J. The impact of denial and repressive style on information gain and rehabilitation outcomes in myocardial infarction patients. *Psychosomatic Medicine*, **47**, No. 3, 262–73, © American Psychosomatic Society, 1985.

369

programs lead to significant gain in knowledge about rehabilitation (1–3), the impact of information gained on subsequent recovery from myocardial infarction (MI) remains unclear. Some studies have demonstrated that higher levels of information lead to minimal or even negative effects on the recovery process (4–6), whereas others have shown that the amount of information gained during cardiac education is positively related to compliance with diet and drug regimens, reduced readmission to the hospital (7), and increased return to work and decreased smoking (8). The findings of one study suggest that the crucial factor is not merely the level of information, but rather the combination of information and other rehabilitation factors. Cromwell et al. (6) randomly assigned patients admitted to the Coronary Care Unit into groups in which the amount of information, the level of outside stimulation, and the extent to which patients were allowed to participate in their own treatment were all experimentally controlled. They found that patients who experienced high levels of information and were allowed to engage in activities to help themselves but who also had low levels of stimulation and diversion spent the fewest days in the CCU and had the shortest total hospital stay. Patients with high levels of .information who were not allowed to participate in their treatment and had more diversion did much worse than patients who were in conditions of low information.

Denial

The use of denial by patients who have had heart attacks has been the subject of numerous investigations. Although it is widely accepted that denial can influence recovery, its impact on all aspects of the recovery process is not completely understood. Studies of denial before hospitalization have demonstrated that high levels of denial can have negative effects by leading to a delay in seeking treatment (9), whereas denial may be beneficial during hospitalization (6, 10, 11), resulting in reduced morbidity and mortality in the CCU. Studies of the effects of denial on physiologic and psychologic outcomes after hospital discharge have produced inconsistent findings. One study supported a negative relationship between denial and compliance with medical regimens (12), whereas another found no relationship (13). Other studies have shown that deniers have a higher rate of return to work and show less anxiety, depression, mood disturbance and physical disability than non-deniers (14, 15).

The diversity of these findings may reflect differences in the definitions of denial and the measures that have evolved from these definitions. Some researchers studying denial in MI patients have followed a conceptualization that reflects the classical definition of denial as an unconscious process used to negate unpleasant reality, measured either through inference (see ref. 10), or in response to direct questions to the patient about whether an MI has occurred (12). Hackett and Cassem have defined denial in broader terms, including both conscious and unconscious activities associated with denial processes. They refer to this as a "multifaceted behavioral complex" (16, p. 95) that has the goal of allaying the anxiety and fear associated with the occurrence of an MI. The measure they developed taps present and past situations, including assessment of content found both in direct statements and indirect manifestations of denial (e.g., minimization of symptoms, regularly debunking worry, and using cliches when asked about death). This measure has been criticized by coping theorists for lumping together a variety of "denial-like" coping mechanisms without making sharp distinctions between denial and other similar concepts, such as avoidance (18, 19). We chose to use the Hackett and Cassem measure because it is the most commonly used measure of denial in heart disease patients (see refs. 13, 14), has been validated with clinical ratings (17), and provides the most detailed, structured, and quantitative method for assessing denial.

Repressive style

Repression–sensitization is a somewhat similar psychologic construct that has received less attention than denial in cardiac rehabilitation literature. Whereas denial is the negation of an unpleasant external reality, repression is remaining unaware of internal impulses or feelings. Rather than studying the direct use of the mechanism of repression, most studies of this concept utilize a trait measure, thought to represent one's general tendency to use repression as a defense. One study of MI patients examined the effect of the combination of repression–sensitization status and information level on outcomes (6). The authors speculated that because of their respective styles, repressors should be more comfortable in a low information setting, whereas sensitizers should do better in a high information situation. The analyses revealed that repressors in high information conditions and sensitizers in low information conditions had more heart monitor alarms and were less cooperative with staff.

Of the numerous methods used to measure repression–sensitization (20, 21), the most commonly used measure is the Byrne Repression–Sensitization (R-S) scale, which measures one's tendency to use repression or sensitization (22). Although this measure has been used extensively, it has been criticized on both psychometric and theoretic grounds (23). It appears that there is not a unidimensional continuum between repressors and sensitizers (24). Further, there is a high, positive correlation (about 0.9) between the Byrne scale and the Taylor Manifest Anxiety scale (25). It is questionable whether this scale is tapping repressive style or merely manifest anxiety. An alternate method for measuring repressive style was developed by Weinberger, Schwartz, and Davidson (26) utilizing both the Taylor Manifest Anxiety Scale (27) and the Marlowe-Crowne Social Desirability Scale (28). Weinberger et al. (26) wanted to differentiate those people who report no emotional upset in a stressful situation because they are experiencing low levels of anxiety from those who are actually repressing anxious feelings. True repressors, it was felt, would report very little upset while actually experiencing high levels of anxiety. Either the Taylor Manifest Anxiety scale or the R-S scale would classify both the low anxious and the true repressor groups as repressors. To differentiate these two different groups, Weinberger et al. used both the Taylor Manifest Anxiety Scale and the Marlowe–Crowne Social Desirability Scale. The Taylor Manifest Anxiety Scale (TMAS) was chosen because of its brevity and its 0.91 correlation with the Byrne scale (25, 29).

The Weinberger group hypothesized that the truly "low-anxious" people (those subjects with both low scores on the TMAS and social desirability) would perform well on behavioral and cognitive tasks because they would not be experiencing much anxiety. The true repressors (low on the TMAS but high on social desirability) would strive to "look good" and tend to underreport their level of anxiety, which would nonetheless result in poor performance on cognitive and behavioral tasks. They found significant differences between these two groups on self-report, physiologic, and behavioral measures, with true repressors showing poorer performance on cognitive tasks and greater discrepancy between physiologic reactions to stress and report of emotional disturbance. They concluded that this alternate measure tapped repressive style without being influenced by the reporting tendencies of the subject. A recent study replicated these findings, demonstrating that "true repressors" had more discrepancy between self-reported anxiety, heart rate, and facial anxiety, with self-reports indicating that they were experiencing little anxiety, whereas physiologic measures reflected a high state of arousal (30). The construct validity of this measure of repressive style, however, has not been solidly established.

Social desirability

Social desirability is in itself an important construct that may be related to rehabilitation outcomes. Although several studies have demonstrated that subjects high on social desirability tend to make and accept significantly more favorable responses about themselves than subjects low on social desirability, they also accept significantly fewer unfavorable interpretations (31). This finding suggests that information that threatens the self-esteem of these subjects may be denied in some way. In a study by Lefcourt (32), subjects who were high on social desirability perceived fewer human movement responses in a projective ink-blot test, indicating less imagination, expressiveness, and intellectual effort. In addition, the subjects who were both high on social desirability and were also low in the R-S scale [a group similar to the Weinberger et al. (26) true repressors] reported the fewest movements of all subjects. Another study found that children, especially boys, who were high in social desirability showed poorer discrimination learning, responded impulsively, and had higher heart rates than those low on this dimension (33). The authors speculated that these learning situations may produce apprehension, which, in children who are especially concerned about performance outcome, leads to an arousal state that may impair stimulus input and processing. Although it might be predicted that those who are high on social desirability would perform better in their attempt to "look good," this concern for approval linked with material that is arousing may disrupt thinking and problem solving, or even lead to attempts at avoiding information (34). These findings suggest that high social desirability tendencies may have negative outcomes on information gain in cardiac rehabilitation, where the context of the information may induce high arousal.

This review of the literature suggests that there is a need to further explore the impact of denial, repressive style, and social desirability on information outcomes in heart attack patients, and to examine the effects of these factors and information on posthospital outcomes. Based on this literature, the authors hypothesized that there would be a negative correlation between the level of denial measured in MI patients going through cardiac rehabilitation and the amount of cardiac information they gain. To assess this relationship, it would be necessary first to control for the effects of intelligence and age of the patient. In addition, the authors speculated that patients who were more repressed and had higher scores on social desirability would gain less information in the cardiac knowledge areas, but that denial would explain a greater amount of the variance. Although the authors thought that greater information might lead to better rehabilitation outcomes after hospital discharge, the Cromwell et al. study (6) suggests that repressors with knowledge scores above the mean and sensitizers with knowledge scores below the mean might have poorer rehabilitation outcomes at 6 months. Both of these points of view were examined in our data analysis.

Methods

Subjects

The 30 subjects (26 males, 4 females) involved in this study were patients admitted to the coronary care units (CCU) of Moffitt Hospital at the University of California, San Francisco, Medical Center, and Pacific Medical Center in San Francisco. The patients who were included were English-speaking males and females, between the ages 30 and 75, who had been admitted to the CCU for treatment of myocardial infarction. The diagnosis of each patient was confirmed through a combination of ECG, blood enzymes, and/or pyrophosphate nuclear imaging. Patients who met the above criteria and were judged to be candidates for cardiac rehabilitation by the attending cardiologist were approached after their condition had stabilized by a nurse[1] who specializes in cardiac rehabilitation. Patients who agreed to participate signed a consent form and then were given the pretest materials. Only one patient refused to participate in this study on grounds that he had been a subject in another study in which he had received unexpected questionnaires after the study had supposedly ended. One other patient was dropped during the study because her diagnosis was changed based on more extensive testing. All other exclusions occurred before patients entered the study based on the above criteria of age and documentation of an MI.

Psychologic measures

Denial was measured using a structured interview based on the work by Hackett and Weisman (35) and Hackett and Cassem (16). For the present study, the authors[2] developed a structured interview, which was sent to Hackett and Cassem for their approval. The authors used the scoring scheme published by Hackett and Cassem (16), but systematized it by providing a more elaborate description of how situations would be coded. This detailed scoring manual enabled us to achieve a high reliability of coding between raters. However, the tapes of our interviews, the detailed scoring manual, and the final scores for our patients were not reviewed by Hackett and Cassem to determine reliability between our raters and theirs.

The R-S (22) and Weinberger (26) measures were used to tap repressive style. The Weinberger measure is constructed by dividing the TMAS and the Marlowe–Crowne Social Desirability Scale at the means,

---

[1] B.D. or J.P.
[2] R.E.S. and F.C.

and combining high and low scores to form four groups. The "true repressors" have low scores on the TMAS and high scores on social desirability.

To rule out of the effects of IQ on information gain, the 40-word vocabulary subscale of the Wechsler Adult Intelligence Scale (WAIS) was used. The vocabulary subtest was chosen because it is easily administered and reliability studies have shown correlations of 0.85 to 0.91 between this subtest and the IQ score obtained from administration of the entire (WAIS) (36). These correlations are higher than for any other subtests in the scale.

Cardiac information measures

Cardiac information was measured using the Cardiac Knowledge Test (CKT), which consists of 23 interview questions, including open ended, multiple choice, and true–false questions. The test was constructed by clinical specialists at the University of California, San Francisco. Three scores can be derived from the CKT: 1) knowledge about heart anatomy and physiology; 2) knowledge about risk factors that may predispose a person to heart disease and also inhibit recovery from a heart attack; and 3) knowledge about symptoms indicating heart problems and activity and dietary regimens beneficial to heart functioning. Detailed criteria were developed to score this measure.

Six-month behavioral follow-up

A self-report measure of functioning developed by Soloff (13) was used as the 6-month follow-up measure. This measure consists of a total functioning score, and three subscales that describe the patients' compliance with medical regimens, psychomedical functioning (sleep disturbance, depression, tension), and level of social functioning (work level, and recreational and social participation). Patients also reported whether their physicians had indicated that they had experienced any medical complications such as arrhythmias, fluid retention, and the like over the 6-month period.

Procedure

Patients judged to be medically stable and appropriate for the interview were approached by the cardiac nurse. Initially, alternative items from the information subscale of the WAIS were given at pre- and posttest time points to determine if the cognitive functioning of the patient might have been suppressed at the pretest, which could explain the gain of information in cardiac rehabilitation knowledge. Since no significant differences were found between the two testing times for the first 12 patients, this measure was not used for the remaining patients in the study. After signing appropriate consent forms, the patient was given the cardiac knowledge test (CKT).

Assessment of the level of denial occurred after patients had been moved from the CCU to the special floor designated for heart patients. The subjects remained in the CCU an average of 3.5 days. Once the patients arrived on the cardiac floor, a comprehensive rehabilitation program was begun for each patient, involving verbal, written, and audiovisual materials. The information was given by the nursing staff, physical therapists, and dietary personnel. The nurse at each site who performed the CKT pretest did not participate in these rehabilitation efforts and had no contact with the patient until discharge from the hospital. The interview to assess denial was done by the first author on either the second or third day after the patient was moved from the CCU. The interview was tape recorded and lasted between 45 and 60 min. After the denial assessment, each patient completed the vocabulary subscale of the WAIS. Each patient was then given a 208-item questionnaire to complete at his or her leisure over the following few days. The questionnaire contained the Byrne R-S Scale, the TMAS, and the short version of the Marlowe–Crowne Social Desirability Scale (37).

On the day before discharge, the nurse who had done the pre-CKT interviewed the patient again, using the alternate form of the CKT. On the average, patients spent 14.5 days in the hospital, with a range of between 8 and 25 days. Results from medical tests done upon discharge (submaximal treadmill test and 24-hr Holter monitor), other tests during hospitalization (cardiac angiography, heart wall motion studies, and echocardiograms), and information about the patient's course of treatment during hospitalization were compiled from the hospital chart and used by the chief cardiologist to rate the severity of illness for each patient.[3] This scale included three levels, ranging from not very serious to very serious illness. To ensure objectivity, the cardiologist was blind to the identity of the patients when he made the severity ratings. This severity rating and the length of the patient's hospital stay were related to the pre- and post-cardiac information scores to determine if either illness severity or length of time in the hospital systematically altered the information outcomes.

Six months after discharge from the hospital, patients were sent the

---

[3] This rating was performed by Thomas Ports, M.D., Assistant Professor of Medicine and Director of Cardiology, University of California, San Francisco.

behavioral follow-up questionnaire to complete. Patients who did not return the survey were sent another, and, if necessary, this was followed by a phone contact with the patient.

Preliminary analyses

The CKT pre- and posttests were scored by the cardiac nurse interviewers (B.D. and J.P.) after scoring procedures were established and training completed. Content validity, criterion validity and test–retest reliability for the CKT were found to be adequate and are available from the authors upon request. The first two authors (R.E.S. and F.C.) constructed an 18-page coding manual that elaborated upon the descriptions presented by Hackett and Cassem (16) and was used to score the structured denial interview. Each denial interview was transcribed and scored by the first author using both the tape recording and transcript. A coder was trained to use this scoring procedure. A reliability analysis was performed using 7 of the 30 cases, with each case coded independently by the first author and the trained coder.[4]

Complete data were obtained for each variable on all patients. Although the two hospital sites had been chosen because of the similarity of their cardiac rehabilitation programs, it was important to test the equivalence of the patient groups. This was done using Students t test to determine if there were any site differences on the major variables. No significant differences were found between the two samples on the continuous variables of age, intelligence, education, pre- and post-CKT subscores, pre- and post-Total CKT score, Hackett–Cassem denial score, and length of hospital stay. Chi-square analysis of the discrete variables of socioeconomic status, ethnic background and severity of illness revealed no differences between the sites. Based on these analyses, the two groups were assumed to be equivalent and the data pooled from each site in subsequent analyses.

To determine if severity of disease and length of hospital stay systematically influenced information scores, Pearson correlation analysis was used. No significant relationships were found between the rating of severity of illness, length of hospital stay, and the pre- and post-cardiac test scores, suggesting that differences in information outcome could not be attributed to disease severity or length of time in the hospital.

A reliability analysis was performed on the scores obtained by the author and those of the trained coder for Hackett–Cassem denial scale. Using 7 of the 30 cases, a reliability correlation of 0.82 was achieved,

---

[4] Coding done by Lynda LaMontagne, D.S.N., Assistant Professor of Nursing, Arizona State University.

suggesting that the scoring procedure was producing reliable scores for denial. In a reliability analysis using 30% of the CKT tests, correlations between the two nurse raters ranged from between 0.85 to 0.94 for the four CKT scores.

Major data analyses

Since one goal of this research was to determine the unique relationship of the psychologic variables to information outcomes, over and above any variance attributable to other variables such as IQ, age, and level of information upon entry into the hospital, a multiple regression correlation (MRC) approach was used. Such an approach allowed a predetermined, hierarchic entry of variables so that the unique effects of each of the variables could be assessed and then those effects removed so that the unique contribution of the next variable set could be determined. In addition, since it has been demonstrated that using simple change scores between pre- and posttest situations is less desirable because it assumes a perfect correlation between the scores (38), an MRC approach permits the use of pretest scores as covariates, which results in a more accurate and powerful statistical test. In this study, MRC analyses were performed using each of the CKT posttest scores as the major dependent variable, and the IQ, age, and the pretest score corresponding to the dependent variable used were entered as a set of covariates. The psychologic variables of denial, repressive style, social desirability, depression, and anxiety were entered next in the analysis, followed by interaction terms among all the independent variables. Chi-square analyses and one-way ANOVAs were used to examine the relationships between psychologic variables, information level at discharge, and the 6-month outcomes.

Results

Findings during hospitalization

As was expected, in all of the MRC analyses the correlation between the covariate set and the dependent variable was significant, with higher CKT pretest scores related to higher posttest knowledge scores, higher IQ related to higher information posttest scores, and increasing age related to lower information posttest scores (see Table 1).

Next the psychologic variables were entered to determine the amount of variance they could explain over and above that explained by the covariate set. For the analysis in which the Anatomy/Physiology posttest score was used as the dependent variable, the denial scale was significantly negatively correlated with it ($F = 7.295$; $p < 0.01$; sr $= -0.45$). In this

Table 1. *Semipartial correlations and percent variance explained in the dependent variables by the covariate set*

Variables in covariate set	Dependent variables		
	Post Anatomy Physiology	Post Symptom Activity	Post Risk Factors
Corresponding pretest	0.65	0.39	0.56
IQ	0.50	0.32	0.08
Age	−0.32	−0.30	−0.41
Percent variance explained by covariate set	54%	22%	35%

regression analysis, denial accounted for 10% of the total variance explained. This finding suggests that patients with higher levels of denial gain significantly less Anatomy/Physiology information and confirms part of the original hypothesis about the relationship between denial and reduced information gain.

Using the Symptoms/Activity posttest score as the major dependent variable, there was a significant negative relationship found between the social desirability measure and information gain ($F = 3.159$; $p < 0.05$; sr $= -0.52$), with social desirability accounting for 21% of the total variance explained. This suggests that patients who attempt to "look good" gain significantly less information about Symptoms/Activities. Although it was originally hypothesized that social desirability might be related to lower information gain, the magnitude of this relationship was not anticipated.

Using the Risk Factors posttest score as the major dependent variable, again there was a significant relationship between social desirability and information gain ($F = 3.028$; $p < 0.05$; sr $= -0.50$): in addition, however, an interaction was found between the social desirability measure and the Byrne R-S scale that was significantly and negatively related to the information posttest score ($F = 3.158$; $p < 0.05$; sr $= -0.41$). Social desirability alone accounted for 18% of the variance in the information outcome, whereas the interaction between social desirability and the Byrne R-S scale explained another 16% of the total variance. To understand the interaction and main effects, the mean post-Risk Factor scores were calculated for low and high scores on the Byrne R-S scale, and low and high scores on Marlowe–Crowne social desirability, and the results were plotted (Fig. 1).

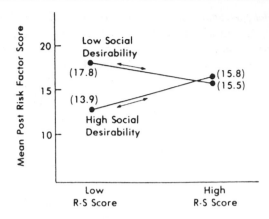

Fig. 1. Plot of the main and interaction effects for Repression–Sensitization (R-S) and Social Desirability on Risk Factor Information Scores.

Figure 1 demonstrates that the main effect of social desirability occurs for low values of the Byrne R-S scale (i.e., repressors), whereas there is no significant main effect of social desirability for high R-S scores (i.e., sensitizers). The group with the lowest mean post-Risk Factor score (low R-S, high social desirability) is similar to the group described by Weinberger et al. (26) as "true repressors," the Lefcourt group (32) who reported the fewest human movements, and the discrepant repressors of Asendorpf and Scherer (30). The pattern of our findings corresponds to that found in all of these studies in that true repressors are demonstrating poorer performance (in this case gaining less information), whereas the group that has low scores on the R-S scale and low scores on social desirability (called "low anxious") have significantly better information outcomes.

Six-month findings

In examining the psychologic variables, information level at discharge, and 6-month rehabilitation outcomes, no relationships were found between severity of illness and reported complications or any of the behavioral functioning scores. Similar analyses revealed no significant relationships between any of the psychologic variables and reported complications or behavioral functioning scores. The level of knowledge patients had upon discharge in the cardiac knowledge areas was not related to any of the 6-month outcomes. The sample was then divided to form the "match" groups (repressors with low information levels and sensitizers with high information levels) and "mismatch" groups (repressors with high information and sensitizers with low information) similar to those used in the Cromwell et al. (6) study. Significant differences were found between the match/mismatch groups, with the mismatch group reporting more complications ($\chi^2 = 9.05$; $p < 0.01$). By partitioning between the subgroups in these analyses, it was found that this difference was due exclusively to the subgroup of repressors with high risk knowledge. In analyses of the behavioral functioning scores, one-way ANOVA demonstrated that mismatch patients reported lower total rehabilitation success ($F = 7.8$; $p < 0.01$), lower psychomedical functioning ($F = 4.1$; $p < 0.05$), and lower social functioning ($F = 4.1$; $p < 0.05$) than the match group. To understand the contribution of each of the subgroups to this relationship, further one-way ANOVA analyses were performed and revealed that the repressor–high-risk knowledge subgroup accounted for the differences in psychomedical functioning, whereas the sensitizer–low-risk knowledge subgroup accounted for the differences in social functioning. The same results were found in these analyses using either the Byrne R-S measure or the Weinberger *et al.* measure to assess repressive style.

Discussion

The results of this study suggest that psychologic factors and level of cardiac information are important variables that may affect the amount of information MI patients gain during hospitalization and influence the success of their recovery after discharge. The effects of the psychologic factors on information gain in the hospital are significant even when other factors that affect information, such as intelligence and age, have been controlled. It is possible to speculate why the psychologic variables were related differentially to specific areas of cardiac knowledge. It is not surprising that our measure of denial, which is basically a state measure, and our measures of repressive style, both trait measures, were related to different information outcomes. This pattern has been found in other studies that demonstrate that state and trait measures predict different health outcomes (18, 39). Additional explanations for our results become clear when the meaning and implications associated with each type of information are taken into account. For example, the type of information conveyed in the Anatomy/Physiology area may challenge patients to accept the fact that actual physical damage has occurred to them. This type of information may be very threatening to patients; those who utilize high levels of denial may be less able to assimilate it. On the other hand, information about symptoms of heart problems and effects of activities on heart function is future oriented and requires that patients attend to very detailed information, such as the amount of weight one may carry at various stages in recovery. Perhaps patients trying to "look good" may fail to ask important questions that may help them clarify problem areas and to assimilate this type of information, or they may be less open to the idea of monitoring their body's response to events because it might interfere with activities seen as socially desirable. The Risk Factor information deals with life-style factors that may have led to the heart attack and may complicate recovery. Those who characteristically repress may filter information about life-style changes to avoid the increase in anxiety that may accompany consideration of the need for life-style changes.

The 6-month findings suggest that for repressors, even the filtering process that occurs as part of their style may not screen out enough of the risk information to prevent their being overloaded. Sensitizers who leave the hospital with little risk factor knowledge may be in a position in which they do not adequately understand the recommendations they have been given and overreact to situations by unnecessarily curtailing their social functions. These interpretations coincide with empirical research that suggests that a mismatch between repressive style and information is associated with poor recovery outcomes (40, 41).

From the standpoint of cardiac rehabilitation, differential treatment of patients who are denying the significance of their heart attack may not be useful, since the relationship of denial to knowledge about anatomy and physiology may reflect a healthy reaction in that the patient is not ready to accept the full impact of this traumatic event. Our 6-month analyses revealed no differences in outcome for patients with high and low levels of denial. It may be more important, however, to identify those patients with strong social desirability tendencies and those who are repressors. Our findings suggest that patients high on social desirability may gain less information not from a need to avoid anxiety directly but from a need to appear capable of understanding and assimilating rehabilitation information that may in fact be very confusing and overwhelming to them. Thus, it may be beneficial to adopt teaching strategies that probe their level of cardiac knowledge and do not depend on patients asking questions about information that is confusing to them. It may be beneficial to reassess the understanding these patients have about rehabilitation concepts and information at several stages during the recovery process.

In conclusion, the results from this study demonstrate that denial, social desirability, and repressive style are important predictors of the specific information gained by patients going through cardiac rehabilitation during hospitalization. Higher levels of denial predicted less information gain about anatomy and physiology of the heart, higher levels of social desirability predicted lower information scores on activity and symptoms, and repressive style predicted less information gain in the area of cardiac risk factors. Six-month data revealed that repressors who leave the hospital with risk information levels above the average are more likely to have complications and poorer psychomedical functioning, whereas sensitizers who leave the hospital with lower than average levels of risk factor information are more likely to experience decreased social functioning. These findings suggest that psychologic and information factors need to be considered in evaluating and tailoring cardiac programs designed to convey rehabilitation information to the heart attack patient.

Acknowledgements

The authors wish to thank the cardiology departments and staff members of Moffitt Hospital at the University of California, San Francisco, and Pacific Medical Center in San Francisco, and the patients who participated in this study. This work was supported in part by IUC funds from the University of California Computer Center.

References

1. Barbarowicz P, Nelson M, DeBusk RF, Haskell WL: A comparison of in-hospital education approaches for coronary bypass patients. Heart Lung 9:127–133, 1980
2. Guzetta CE: Relationship between stress and learning, Adv Nurs Sci 1:35–50, 1979
3. Murdaugh C: Using research in practice. Focus Am Assoc Crit Care Nurses 11–14, June/July 1982
4. Bille DA: A study of patients' knowledge in relation to teaching format and compliance. Supervisor Nurse 55–62, March 1977
5. Scalzi C, Burke LE, Greenland S: Evaluation of an inpatient educational program for coronary patients and families. Heart Lung 9:854–865, 1980.
6. Cromwell RL, Butterfield EC, Brayfield FM, Curry JJ: Acute Myocardial Infarction: Reaction and Recovery. St Louis, Mosby, 1977
7. Rosenberg SC: Patient education leads to better care for heart attack patients. HSMHA Health Rep 86:793–802, 1971
8. Pozen MW, Stechmiller JA, Harris W, Smith S, Fried DD, Voigt GC: A nurse rehabilitator's impact on patients with myocardial infarction. Med Care 15:830–837, 1977
9. Gentry WD: Prehospital behavior after a heart attack. Psychiatr Ann 8:2–30, 1978
10. Gentry WD, Foster S, Haney T: Denial as a determinant of anxiety and perceived health status in the coronary care unit. Psychosom Med 34:39–44, 1972
11. Hackett TP, Cassem NH, Wishnie HA: The coronary-care unit: an appraisal of its psychologic hazards. N Engl J Med 279:1365–1370, 1968
12. Croog SH, Shapiro DS, Levine S: Denial among male heart patients. Psychosom Med 33:385–397, 1971

13. Soloff PH: Effects of denial on mood, compliance, and quality of functioning after cardiovascular rehabilitation. Gen Hosp Psychiatry 2:134–140, 1980
14. Stern MJ, Pascale L, Ackerman A: Life adjustment post myocardial infarction: determining predictive variables. Arch Intern Med 137:1680–1685, 1977
15. Stern MJ, Pascale L, McLoone JB: Psychological adaptation following an acute myocardial infarction. J Chronic Dis 29:513–526, 1976
16. Hackett TP, Cassem NH: Development of a quantitative rating scale to assess denial. J Psychosom Res 18:93–100. 1974
17. Froese AP, Vasquez E., Cassem NH, Hackett TP: Validation of anxiety, depression and denial scales in a coronary care unit. J Psychosom Res 18:137–141, 1973
18. Cohen F, Lazarus RS: Coping with the stresses of illness. In Stone GC, Cohen F, Adler NE, et al. (ed), Health Psychology—A Handbook. San Francisco, Jossey–Bass, 1979, pp 217–254
19. Lazarus RS: The costs and benefits of denial. In Breznitz S (ed), Denial of Stress. New York International University Press, 1983, pp 1–30.
20. Gardner RW, Holzman PS, Klein GS, Linton HB, Spence DP: Cognitive control: a study of individual consistencies in cognitive behavior. Psychol Issues 1:165–172, 1959
21. Levine M, Spivack G: The Rorschach Index of Repressive Style. Springfield, IL, Thomas, 1964
22. Byrne D, Barry J, Nelson D: Relation of the revised repression–sensitization scale to measures of self description. Psychol Rep 61:67–72, 1963
23. Lazarus RS, Averill JR, Opton EM: The psychology of coping: issues of research and assessment. In Coelho GV, Hamburg DA, Adams JE (eds), Coping and Adaptation, New York, Basic Books, 1974, pp 249–315
24. Carlson RW: Dimensionality of the repression–sensitization scale. J Clin Pyschol 35:78–84, 1979
25. Dahlstrom W, Grant GS, Dahlstrom LE: An MMPI Handbook. volume II: Research Applications: Minneapolis, MN, University of Minnesota Press, 1975
26. Weinberger DA, Schwartz GE, Davidson JR: Low anxious, high anxious and repressive coping styles: psychometric patterns and behavioral physiological responses to stress. J Abnorm Psychol 88:369–380, 1979
27. Taylor JA: A personality scale of manifest anxiety. J Abnorm Soc Psychol 48:285–290, 1953
28. Crowne DP, Marlowe D: A new scale of social desirability independent of psychopathology. J Consult Psychol 24:349–354, 1960
29. Joy VL: Repression-sensitization and interpersonal behavior. Paper presented at the American Psychological Association Convention, Philadelphia, August, 1963
30. Asendorpf JB, Scherer KR: The discrepant repressor: differentiation between low anxiety, high anxiety, and repression of anxiety by autonomic–facial–verbal patterns of behavior. J Pers Soc Psychol 45:1334–1346
31. Mosher DL: Approval motive and acceptance of "fake" personality test interpretations which differ in favorability. Psychol Rep 17:395–402, 1965
32. Lefcourt HM: Need for approval and threatened negative evaluation as determinants of expressiveness in a projective test. J Consult Clin Psych 33:96–102, 1969

33. Crowne DP, Holland CH. Conn LK: Personality factors in discrimination learning in children. J Person Soc Psychol 10:420–430, 1968
34. Crowne DP: The Experimental Study of Personality, New York, Wiley, 1979, pp 153–183
35. Hackett TP, Weisman AD: Denial as a factor in patients with heart disease and cancer. Ann NY Acad Sci 164:802–817, 1969
36. Wechsler D: Wechsler Adult Intelligence Scale – Revised Manual. New York, Harcourt Bracc Jovanovich, 1981, pp. 46–49
37. Strahan R, Gerbasi KC: Short, homogeneous versions of the Marlowe–Crowne social desirability scale. J Clin Psychol 28:191–193, 1972
38. Cohen J, Cohen P: Applied Multiple Regression/Correlation Analysis for the Behavioral Sciences, New York, Wiley, 1975
39. Cohen F, Lazarus RS: Active coping processes, coping dispositions, and recovery from surgery. Psychosom Med 35:375–389, 1973
40. Andrew JM: Recovery from surgery, with and without preparatory instruction, for three coping styles. J Pers Soc Psychol 15:223–226, 1970
41. DeLong DR: Individual differences in patterns of anxiety arousal, stress-relevant information, and recovery from surgery. Unpublished doctoral dissertation, University of California, Los Angeles, 1970

Reduction of postoperative pain by encouragement and instruction of patients: a study of doctor–patient rapport

Lawrence D. Egbert, MD, George E. Battit, MD, Claude E. Welch, MD, and Marshall K. Bartlett, MD

From the departments of Anesthesia and Surgery, Massachusetts General Hospital and Harvard Medical School, USA

Many reports have discussed the treatment of patients suffering after operation. Narcotics are not without danger; they also vary considerably in effectiveness. Hypnosis will reduce pain but is difficult to achieve and requires special training for the operator. Despite considerable effort the problems of treating postoperative pain remain.

Janis[1] has shown that patients who were told about their operations before the procedure remembered the operation and its sequelae more favorably than those who were not well informed. We have determined the effects of instruction, suggestion and encouragement upon the severity of post operative pain.

Method

We studied 97 patients after elective intra-abdominal operations (Table 1). All patients were visited the night before operation by the anesthetist, who told them about the preparation for anesthesia, as well as the time and approximate duration of the operation, and warned them that they would wake up in the recovery room. Preanesthetic medication, consisting of pentobarbital sodium, 2 mg. per kilogram of body weight, and atropine, 0.6 mg., was administered intramuscularly approximately one hour before operation. Induction of anesthesia was accomplished with thiopental sodium; intubation of the trachea was performed on all

Reprinted from Egbert, L. D., Battit, G. E., Welch, C. E. and Bartlett, M. K. Reduction of postoperative pain by encouragement and instruction of patients: a study of doctor–patient rapport. *New England Journal of Medicine*, **270**, 825–7, 1964.

patients. Anesthesia was maintained with ether and cyclopropane or nitrous oxide and curare.

The patients were divided into two groups by random order; 51 patients (control group) were not told about postoperative pain by the anesthetist. The "special-care" group consisted of 46 patients who were told about postoperative pain. They were informed where they would feel pain, how severe it would be and how long it would last and reassured that having pain was normal after abdominal operations. As soon as the patients appeared aware of the nature of the suffering that would begin on the following day, they were told what would be done about the pain. They were advised that pain is caused by spasm of the muscles under the incision and that they could relieve most of the pain themselves by relaxing these muscles. They could achieve relaxation by slowly taking a deep breath and consciously allowing the abdominal wall to relax. Also, they were shown the use of a trapeze that was hanging over the middle of the bed (control patients also had the trapeze but were not instructed by the anesthetist). Special-care patients were taught how to turn onto one side by using their arms and legs while relaxing their abdominal muscles. Finally, they were told that at first they would find it difficult to relax completely. If they could not achieve a reasonable level of comfort, they should request medication. The presentation was given in a manner of enthusiasm and confidence; the patients were not informed that we were conducting a study. The surgeons, not knowing which patients were receiving special care, continued their practices as usual.

After the operations, narcotics were ordered by the surgical residents; these were later administered by the ward nurses, who were also unaware that we were studying these patients. After the patients were discharged we tabulated the total dose of morphine in milligrams for the first five twenty-four-hour periods after the operation. When meperidine had been administered, we assumed 100 mg. of meperidine to be equal to 10 mg. of morphine (Lasagna and Beecher[2] indicated that "meperdine, in parenteral doses of 50 to 100 mg., was at least as good as 10 mg. of morphine in incidence and duration of pain relief"); 60 mg. of codeine was assumed to be nearly equal to 10 mg. of morphine.[2]

During the afternoon after operation (day zero) the anesthetist visited his patients receiving special care. He reiterated what he had taught the patients the night before and reassured them that the pain they were experiencing was normal; they were again told to request pain medication whenever they could not make themselves tolerably comfortable. The anesthetist listened to their breathing and encouraged them to take a deep breath and relax. All this was repeated on the morning after operation and once or twice a day until they had no further need of narcotics.

Table 1. *Types of operations and anesthetics**

Procedure	Control Group no. of patients	Special-Care Group no. of patients
Operation:		
Cholecystectomy	15	17
Hiatus hernia	4	1
Gastrectomy	9	8
Bowel resection	9	6
Colectomy	6	9
Hysterectomy	6	4
Ventral hernia	2	1
Totals	51	46
Anesthesia:		
Cyclopropane & ether	31	27
Nitrous oxide & curare	20	19

*Differences not statistically significant.

On the first and second postoperative days 57 of the patients were visited by an anesthetist whom the patients had not met and who was not aware of the type of treatment being received. This independent observer attempted to record without bias the patients' evaluations about their pain as well as his own impressions from this appearance.

Comparisons of differences between the two groups were made with the use of the t test.

Results

Table 1 shows the types of operations done and the anesthetics given. The average age of the patients in the control group was fifty-two and two-tenths years; in the special-care group the average age of the patients was fifty-two years. There were 17 men in each group. Randomization in the selection of patients seems to have been satisfactory.

Figure 1 compares the narcotic requirements of the patients. On the day of operation the difference was not statistically significant. For the next five days, however, patients receiving special care requested less narcotics (p less than 0.01).

All the suggestions given the special-care patients favored a reduction in postoperative narcotics. Table 2 shows that these patients did not suffer through the postoperative course just to please the doctor. The

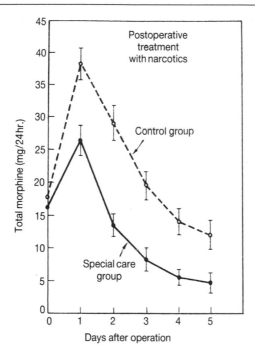

Figure 1. Postoperative treatment with narcotics (means for each day ± standard error of the mean).

independent observer recorded that the special-care patients appeared to be more comfortable and in better physical and emotional condition than the control group. This was emphasized by the surgeons, who, although unaware of the care each patient received, sent the special-care patients home an average of two and seven-tenths days earlier than the control group (p less than 0.01).

Discussion

Approximately 9 out of every 10 patients will respond at some time to placebo therapy for postoperative pain[3]; this time of emotional stress is readily modified by psychotherapy.[1,4,5] Placebo effect may be defined as one that is not attributable to a specific pharmacologic property of the treatment[5]; the effects of placebos are readily modified by suggestion[4,5] and depend upon the symbolic implications of the physician and his ministrations.[5] We believe that our discussions with patients have changed the meaning of the postoperative situation for these patients. By utilizing an active placebo action, we have been able to reduce their postoperative pain.

Table 2. *Pain on the first and second days after operation (averages ± standard errors)*

	Severity of Pain*	
Postoperative Day	Control Group (30 patients)	Special-Care Group (27 patients)
1st:		
Subjective report	1.768 ± 0.200	1.594 ± 0.205
Objective report	1.735 ± 0.191	1.187 ± 0.192†
2nd:		
Subjective report	1.333 ± 0.188	0.966 ± 0.195
Objective report	1.333 ± 0.216	0.827 ± 0.172‡

*Pain graded as follows: severe, +++; moderate, ++; mild, +; & almost none, 0.
†Difference statistically significant (p < 0.05).
‡Approaches significance (p < 0.1).

Others have shown that talking out anxieties and understanding the source of anxiety helps patients.[1] Our data demonstrate that anesthetists, untrained in hypnotism or formal psychiatry, may nevertheless have a very powerful effect on their patients. We have previously shown[7] that this reassurance (we call it "superficial psychotherapy") can be started during the preoperative visit; it should be continued into the postoperative period.

It should be pointed out that a great deal more work is involved in this practice of anesthesia than in the customary practice of anesthesia. We found that our methods of talking to patients changed during the study – for example, 1 of our early patients became hysterical during the discussion about postoperative pain, and we now know it is wise to build up the discussion slowly in patients who become too frightened. Nevertheless, retreating from the frightened patient before operation exposes that patient to greater psychic stress during the postoperative period.[1] The patient who persistently avoids discussing these problems before he is operated on is a particularly troublesome patient later. Another error was of interest: 1 patient was seen before operation and anesthetized, and then the anesthetist went on vacation without notifying the patient or surgeon. Upon seeing the patient five days later, the anesthetist was greeted with great annoyance ("Where the hell have you been?") by the patient. To balance these errors, we found that almost none of the patients in the special care group had the complaint, "Why didn't you tell me it was going to be like this?" – which was not uncommon in the control group. Each patient has his own personal psychologic makeup; each patient needs "special" treatment, tailored to meet his own particular psychologic needs.

The specialty of anesthesia has been criticized sharply as lacking in involvement with patient care and responsibility.[8] Our data show that an anesthetist is able to establish rapport with surgical patients and that a useful purpose is served by this contact. Since the sole purpose of the anesthetist in administering anesthesia is to reduce pain associated with operations, it appears reasonable for him to consider the whole job. The anesthetist who understands his patient and who believes that each patient is "his" patient ceases to be merely a clever technician in the operating room.

Summary and conclusions

The effect of encouragement and education on 97 surgical patients was studied. "Special-care" patients were told what to expect during the postoperative period; they were then taught how to relax, how to take deep breaths and how to move so that they would remain more comfortable after operation. Comparing these patients with a control group of patients, we were able to reduce the postoperative narcotic requirements by half. Patients who were encouraged during the immediate postoperative period by their anesthetists were considered by their surgeons ready for discharge from the hospital two and seven-tenths days before the control patients. We believe that if an anesthetist considers himself a doctor who alleviates pain associated with operations, he must realize that only part of his work is in the operating rooms; the patients need ward care by their anesthetists as well.

Acknowledgements
This study was supported in part by a grant (MH 00987-09) from the United States Public Health Service.

References
1. Janis, I. L. *Psychological Stress: Psychoanalytic and behavioral studies of surgical patients.* 439 pp. New York: Wiley, 1958.
2. Lasagna, L., and Beecher, H. K. Analgesic effectiveness of codeine and meperidine (Demerol). *J. Pharmacol. & Exper. Therap.* **112**:306–311, 1954.
3. Houde, R. W., Wallenstein, S. L., and Rogers, A. Clinical pharmacology of analgesics. 1. Method of assaying analgesic effect. *Clin. Pharmacol. & Therap.* **1**:163–174, 1960.

4. Keats, A. S. Postoperative pain: research and treatment. *J. Chronic Dis.* **4**:72–83, 1956.
5. Modell, W., and Houde, R. W. Factors influencing clinical evaluation of drugs; with special reference to double-blind technique. *J.A.M.A.* **167**:2190–2199, 1958.
6. Wolf, S. Pharmacology of placebos. *Pharmacol. Rev.* **11**:689–704, 1959.
7. Egbert, L. D., Battit, G. E., Turndorf, H., and Beecher, H. K. Value of preoperative visit by anesthetist: study of doctor-patient rapport, *J.A.M.A.* **185**:553–555, 1963.
8. Dripps, R. D., et al. Special report to American Society of Anesthesiologists. *A.S.A. Newsletter*, August, 1963.

Psychological response to breast cancer: effect on outcome

S. Greer, T. Morris and K. W. Pettingale

Faith Courtauld Unit for Human Studies in Cancer, King's College Hospital Medical School, London SE5, UK

Summary

A prospective, multidisciplinary, 5-year study of 69 consecutive female patients with early ($T_{0,1}$ $N_{0,1}$ M_0) breast cancer was conducted. Patients' psychological responses to the diagnosis of cancer were assessed 3 months postoperatively. These responses were related to outcome 5 years after operation. Recurrence-free survival was significantly common among patients who had initially reacted to cancer by denial or who had a fighting spirit than among patients who had responded with stoic acceptance or feelings of helplessness and hopelessness.

Introduction

When faced with a diagnosis of cancer, individuals respond psychologically in several different ways. According to some clinicians, the particular coping responses adopted by cancer patients may influence prognosis.[1-3] That opinion is based upon isolated clinical observations which, though stimulating and valuable, require verification. The few published studies have been succinctly summarised.[4] It is clear that systematic, long-term follow-up studies are needed, and that these studies should focus on patients with early, as opposed to advanced cancer in order to obviate (as far as possible) the effect of the disease process itself on psychological responses. We report here the results of one such study.

Patients and methods

A consecutive series of women admitted to King's College Hospital with breast cancer were studied, the criteria for inclusion being age under 70, no previous history of malignant disease, a breast lump less than 5 cm in diameter with or without palpable ipsilateral axillary glands, no deep

Reprinted from Greer, S., Morris, T. and Pettingale, K. W. Psychological response to breast cancer: effect on outcome. *Lancet*, ii, 785–7, 1979.

attachment of the lump, and no distant metastases. Consequently, all patients fell within the Manchester classifications[5] of stage I or II or $T_{0,1}$ $N_{0,1}$ M_0. No patients had occult metastases as shown by routine chest X-ray, skeletal survey, full blood count, and serum chemistry (bilirubin, alkaline phosphatase, aspartate transaminase and hydroxybutyrate dehydrogenase, calcium, phosphate, uric acid, sodium, potassium, and urea).

Patients were treated by simple mastectomy; in addition 25 randomly selected patients also received a routine course of prophylactic postoperative radiotherapy to ipsilateral axillary nodes as part of the King's/ Cambridge Breast Trial.[6]

Both clinical and psychological assessments were carried out preoperatively, 3 and 12 months postoperatively, and then annually for a further 4 years.

Clinical assessment

At each follow-up, patients were given a complete physical examination, and information about relevant investigations was obtained from their case notes. Additional investigations were carried out if patients had symptoms or signs suggestive of recurrence. A system of quantifying approximate tumour mass was devised to produce a numerical score, and it was based on all available clinical, radiological, and pathological data. The patient's score was derived from (i) the diameter of the breast tumour measured after removal; (ii) histological evidence of spread of the tumour to involve skin, pectoral muscles, or lymph nodes; (iii) postoperative recurrence of the tumour in the scar or lymph nodes; (iv) the development of any metastatic lesion confirmed by biopsy or X-ray; and (v) the development of suspected metastases—e.g., positive bone scan, raised alkaline phosphatase. Equal weighting was given to proven metastases, irrespective of site, so that successive scores reflected the overall increases or decreases in the tumour mass. This scoring system has been fully described.[7]

Psychological assessment

Patients were interviewed with a structured interview schedule, and they completed standard psychological tests. Where possible, husbands or close relatives were interviewed separately to verify information elicited from patients. As well as standard demographic data, information was obtained about initial reactions on discovering the breast lump, whether there was delay of more than 3 months between first sign of breast lump and first medical attendance, characteristic response to stressful events, ability to express anger and other feelings, and occurrence of depressive illness or psychological stress—including loss of a significant person—during the five years before appearance of the breast lump. Rating scales were devised to measure social adjustment[8] with regard to marital, sexual, and interpersonal relationships and work record. Depression was measured by means of the Hamilton rating scale,[9] hostility by the Caine and Foulds hostility and direction of hostility questionnaire (HDHQ),[10] and extraversion and neuroticism by the Eysenck personality inventory (EPI);[11] the Mill Hill vocabulary scale[12] was used to estimate intelligence. These data were obtained before operation. At follow-up examination, ratings of social adjustment and of depression were repeated; in addition, patients' psychological responses to the diagnosis of cancer were assessed.

Psychological response to breast cancer

This was assessed 3 months after operation by asking patients how they perceived the nature and seriousness of their disease and how their lives had been affected by it. The psychological response was categorised according to patients' verbatim statements and accompanying mood. A pilot survey showed that it was possible to group the psychological responses in four mutually exclusive categories and that independent ratings by two observers produced a high level of agreement. The categories were:

Denial.—Apparent active rejection of any evidence about their diagnosis which might have been offered, including the evidence of breast removal, such as "it wasn't serious, they just took off my breast as a precaution". Such patients were usually extremely guarded in their replies and restricted discussion of the subject. They neither showed nor reported any emotional distress.

Fighting spirit.—A highly optimistic attitude, accompanied by a search for greater information about breast cancer. Such patients had usually asked a doctor in some detail about their chances and had read or asked friends about the disease. They planned to do everything in their power to "conquer" cancer. "I can fight it and defeat it" was a characteristic comment. No distress was reported or evident at interview.

Stoic acceptance.—Acknowledgement of the diagnosis without inquiry for further information unless new symptoms developed. Such patients ignored the illness and any symptoms as far as possible and carried on normal life: "I know what it is, I know it's cancer, but I've just got to carry on as normal." The recognition that they had breast cancer was emotionally distressing at first, but the stoic attitude which they adopted had gradually alleviated their distress during the 3 months following operation.

Feelings of helplessness/hopelessness.—Complete engulfment by knowledge of the diagnosis. These patients regarded themselves as gravely ill and sometimes as actually dying. Their lives were frequently disrupted by recurring preoccupations with cancer and impending death. They were devoid of hope: "There is nothing they can do—I'm finished". Patients with this psychological response showed obvious emotional distress which had been present since operation.

Results

69 consecutive female patients with breast cancer were studied. All were traced at 5-year follow-up. 2 had died from disorders other than cancer (1 suicide, 1 myocardial infarct) and were excluded from subsequent analysis. Psychological assessment of patients' responses to the diagnosis of cancer was conducted 3 months postoperatively on only 57 patients; however, the 10 missing patients closely resembled the other patients (see below) in respect of outcome at 5 years: 5 were alive and well, 3 were alive with metastases, and 2 had died.

Outcome at 5 years

Of the 67 patients in the original sample, 33 (49%) were alive and well with no sign of recurrence, 16 (24%) were alive but had had metastases (there were no patients with only local recurrence), and 18 (27%) had died of breast cancer.

Psychological response to cancer and tumour mass

There was no relationship between psychological response to the diagnosis of cancer and approximate tumour mass at 3 months after operation. A patient with direct clinical evidence of metastases had died by this date.

Radiotherapy, psychological response, and outcome

Statistical comparisons between the 25 patients who received radiotherapy and those who did not revealed no significant differences either in psychological response 3 months after operation or in outcome at 5 years.

Initial psychological responses to cancer by 5-year outcome

Psychological response 3 months after operation	Outcome at 5 years			
	Alive with no recurrence (n = 28)	Alive with metastases (n = 13)	Dead (n = 16)	Total (n = 57)
Denial	7	2	1	10
Fighting spirit	8	1	1	10
Stoic acceptance	12	10	10	32
Helplessness/ hopelessness	1	. . .	4	5

Comparing recurrence-free survival (n = 28) with metastatic disease alive or dead (n = 29): χ^2 = 9.0, d.f.3, p < 0.03.

Psychosocial factors and outcome

There were no significant associations between 5-year outcome and the following variables: age, social class, reaction on first discovering the breast lump, delay in seeking medical advice, habitual reaction to stressful events, expression/suppression of anger, depression scores on the Hamilton scale,[9] hostility scores on the HDHQ,[10] depressive illness during previous 5 years, psychological stress including loss of a significant person during previous 5 years, sexual adjustment, interpersonal relationships and work record, extraversion and neuroticism scores on the EPI,[11] and scores of verbal intelligence.[12]

There was a tendency for patients who were unmarried (not cohabiting) or who reported poor marital relationships at the time of diagnosis to have a less favourable outcome (χ^2 = 6.53, p < 0.09; and χ^2 = 7.00, p < 0.08, respectively).

Psychological response to cancer and outcome

There was a statistically significant association between patients' initial psychological responses to the diagnosis of cancer (as assessed 3 months after operation) and outcome at 5 years (table). A favourable outcome was more frequent in patients whose responses were categorised as denial or fighting spirit (15/20, 75%) than in patients who showed either stoic acceptance or a helpless/hopeless response (13/37, 35%). The relationship between psychological response to the diagnosis of cancer and subsequent outcome can also be seen clearly when extremes of outcome are compared, i.e., death versus recurrence-free survival. Of the women who subsequently died, 88% (14/16) initially reacted with stoic acceptance or helplessness/hopelessness whereas only 46% (13/28) of the women who remained alive and well had demonstrated these reactions ($\chi^2 = 9.35$, d.f. 1, $p < 0.025$).

Discussion

In this prospective study, a statistically significant association has been demonstrated between psychological response of women 3 months after confirmation of diagnosis of breast cancer and outcome 5 years later. Statistical associations, however, cannot be taken ipso facto as causal associations. Other possible explanations for our results must be considered.

The first possibility is that the particular psychological responses associated with subsequent unfavourable outcome were themselves the result of occult metastatic disease. The possibility that undiscovered malignant disease affected psychological responses cannot be excluded, although what evidence we have lends no support to this hypothesis, since psychological responses to the diagnosis of cancer 3 months after operation were not related to measures of approximate tumour mass[7] at that time. Moreover, studies of psychological effects of malignant diseases[13,14] suggest that only advanced cancers are likely to have a direct effect on psychological functions. Consequently, this explanation seems implausible.

A second and, in our view, more likely explanation for our result is that the kind of psychological response adopted by patients affected their outcome. Presumably, any such effect is mediated through biological mechanisms—possibly neuroendocrine or immune pathways. It should be noted, however, that the number of women we studied was small, and so similar studies of other patient populations are required before any generalisations can be made. Such studies, besides verifying present results, should attempt to refine and test the reliability and validity of our broad categories of psychological response, to identify the major determinants of these responses, and to search for associated biological changes. Our findings, if confirmed, have important implications, not least for the clinical management of patients with breast cancer.

Acknowledgements

We thank Mrs F. Scott Elliot for generous research funds, Prof. R. Cawley for valuable criticism, the consultant surgeons at King's College Hospital who allowed us to study their patients, and the patients themselves for forbearance and willing cooperation.

References

1. Southam CM. Emotions, immunology and cancer: how might the psyche influence neoplasia? *Ann NY Acad Sci* 1969; **164**: 473–75.
2. Laxenaire M, Chardot C, Bentz L. Quelques aspects psychologiques du malade cancereux. *La Presse Medicale*, 1971; **79**: 2497–500.
3. Meares A. Regression of osteogenic sarcoma metastases associated with intensive meditation. *Med J Aust* 1978; **ii**: 433.
4. Anonymous. Mind and cancer. *Lancet* 1979; **i**: 706–07.
5. Wise L, Mason AY, Ackerman LV. Local excision and irradiation: an alternative method for the treatment of early mammary cancer. *Ann Surg* 1971; **174**: 393–99.
6. Baum M, Edwards MH, Magarey CJ. Organisation of clinical trial on national scale: management of early cancer of the breast. *Br Med J* 1972; **iv**: 476–78.
7. Pettingale KW, Merrett TG, Tee DEH. Prognostic value of serum levels of immunoglobulins (IgG, IgA, IgM and IgE) in breast cancer: a preliminary study. *Br J Cancer* 1977; **36**: 550–57.
8. Morris, T. Greer HS, White P. Psychological and social adjustment to mastectomy, *Cancer* 1977; **40**: 2381–87.
9. Hamilton M. Development of a rating scale for primary depressive illness. *Br J Soc Clin Psychol* 1967; **6**: 278–96.
10. Caine TM, Foulds GA. Personality questionnaire (HDHQ). London: University of London Press, 1967.
11. Eysenck HJ, Eysenck SBG. Manual of the Eysenck personality inventory. London: University of London Press, 1964.
12. Raven JC. The Mill Hill vocabulary scale. London: HK Lewis, 1958.
13. Davies RK, Quinlan DM, McKegney FP, Kimball CP. Organic factors and psychological adjustment in advanced cancer patients. *Psychosom Med* 1973; **35**: 464–71.
14. Plumb MM, Holland J. Comparative studies of psychological function in patients with advanced cancer. 1. Self-reported depressive symptoms. *Psychosom Med* 1977; **39**: 264–76.

The effects of choice and enhanced personal responsibility for the aged: a field experiment in an institutional setting

Ellen J. Langer and Judith Rodin

Graduate Center, City University of New York, USA; Yale University, USA

Abstract

A field experiment was conducted to assess the effects of enhanced personal responsibility and choice on a group of nursing home residents. It was expected that the debilitated condition of many of the aged residing in institutional settings is, at least in part, a result of living in a virtually decision-free environment and consequently is potentially reversible. Residents who were in the experimental group were given a communication emphasizing their responsibility for themselves, whereas the communication given to a second group stressed the staff's responsibility for them. In addition, to bolster the communication, the former group was given the freedom to make choices and the responsibility of caring for a plant rather than having decisions made and the plant taken care of for them by the staff, as was the case for the latter group. Questionnaire ratings and behavioral measures showed a significant improvement for the experimental group over the comparison group on alertness, active participation, and a general sense of well-being.

The transition from adulthood to old age is often perceived as a process of loss, physiologically and psychologically (Birren, 1958; Gould, 1972). However, it is as yet unclear just how much of this change is biologically determined and how much is a function of the environment. The ability to sustain a sense of personal control in old age may be greatly influenced by societal factors, and this in turn may affect one's physical well-being.

Typically the life situation does change in old age. There is some loss of roles, norms, and reference groups, events that negatively influence one's

Langer, E. J. and Rodin, J. The effects of choice and enhanced personal responsibility for the aged: a field experiment in an institutional setting. *Journal of Personality and Social Psychology*, **34**, 191–8. Copyright (1976) by the American Psychological Association. Reprinted by permission.

perceived competence and feeling of responsibility (Bengston, 1973). Perception of these changes in addition to actual physical decrements may enhance a sense of aging and lower self-esteem (Lehr & Puschner, Note 1). In response to internal developmental changes, the aging individual may come to see himself in a position of lessened mastery relative to the rest of the world, as a passive object manipulated by the environment (Neugarten & Gutman, 1958). Questioning whether these factors can be counteracted, some studies have suggested that more successful aging—measured by decreased mortality, morbidity, and psychological disability—occurs when an individual feels a sense of usefulness and purpose (Bengston, 1973; Butler, 1967; Leaf, 1973; Lieberman, 1965).

The notion of competence is indeed central to much of human behavior. Adler (1930) has described the need to control one's personal environment as "an intrinsic necessity of life itself" (p. 398). deCharms (1968) has stated that "man's primary motivation propensity is to be effective in producing changes in his environment. Man strives to be a causal agent, to be the primary locus of, causation for, or the origin of, his behavior; he strives for personal causation" (p. 269).

Several laboratory studies have demonstrated that reduced control over aversive outcomes increases physiological distress and anxiety (Geer, Davison, & Gatchel, 1970; Pervin, 1963) and even a nonveridical perception of control over an impending event reduces the aversiveness of that event (Bowers, 1968; Glass & Singer, 1972; Kanfer & Seidner, 1973). Langer, Janis, and Wolfer (1975) found that by inducing the perception of control over stress in hospital patients by means of a communication that emphasized potential cognitive control, subjects requested fewer pain relievers and sedatives and were seen by nurses as evidencing less anxiety.

Choice is also a crucial variable in enhancing an induced sense of control. Stotland and Blumenthal (1964) studied the effects of choice on anxiety reduction. They told subjects that they were going to take a number of important ability tests. Half of the subjects were allowed to choose the order in which they wanted to take the tests, and half were told that the order was fixed. All subjects were informed that the order of the tests would have no bearing on their scores. They found that subjects not given the choice were more anxious, as measured by palmar sweating. In another study of the effects of choice, Corah and Boffa (1970) told their subjects that there were two conditions in the experiment, each of which would be signaled by a different light. In one condition they were given the choice of whether or not to press a button to escape from an aversive noise, and in the other one they were not given the option of escaping. They found that the choice instructions decreased the aversiveness of the threatening stimulus, apparently by increasing perceived control. Although using a very different paradigm, Langer (1975) also demonstrated the importance of choice. In that study it was found that the exercise of choice in a chance situation, where choice was objectively inconsequential, nevertheless had psychological consequences manifested in increased confidence and risk taking.

Lefcourt (1973) best summed up the essence of this research in a brief review article dealing with the perception of control in man and animals when he concluded that "the sense of control, the illusion that one can exercise personal choice, has a definite and a positive role in sustaining life" (p. 424). It is not surprising, then, that these important psychological factors should be linked to health and survival. In a series of retrospective studies, Schmale and his associates (Adamson & Schmale, 1965; Schmale, 1958; Schmale & Iker, 1966) found that ulcerative colitis, leukemia, cervical cancer, and heart disease were linked with a feeling of helplessness and loss of hope experienced by the patient prior to the onset of the disease. Seligman and his co-workers have systematically investigated the learning of helplessness and related it to the clinical syndrome of depression (see Seligman, 1975). Even death is apparently related to control-relevant variables. McMahon and Rhudick (1964) found a relationship between depression or hopelessness and death. The most graphic description of this association comes from Bettelheim (1943), who in his analysis of the "Muselmanner," the walking corpses in the concentration camps, described them as:

Prisoners who came to believe the repeated statements of the guards—that there was no hope for them, that they would never leave the camp except as a corpse—who came to feel that their environment was one over which they could exercise no influence whatsoever. . . . Once his own life and the environment were viewed as totally beyond his ability to influence them, the only logical conclusion was to pay no attention to them whatsoever. Only then, all conscious awareness of stimuli coming from the outside was blocked out, and with it all response to anything but inner stimuli.

Death swiftly followed and, according to Bettelheim,

[survival] depended on one's ability to arrange to preserve some areas of independent action, to keep control of some important aspects of one's life despite an environment that seemed overwhelming and total.

Bettelheim's description reminds us of Richter's (1957) rats, who also "gave up hope" of controlling their environment and subsequently died.

The implications of these studies for research in the area of aging are clear. Objective helplessness as well as feelings of helplessness and hopelessness—both enhanced by the environment and by intrinsic changes that occur with increasing old age—may contribute to psychological withdrawal, physical disease, and death. In contrast, objective control and feelings of mastery may very well contribute to physical health and personal efficacy.

In a study conceived to explore the effects of dissonance, Ferrare (1962; cited in Seligman, 1975; Zimbardo & Ruch, 1975) presented data concerning the effects of the ability of geriatric patients to control their place of residence. Of 17 subjects who answered that they did not have any other alternative but to move to a specific old age home, 8 died after 4 weeks of residence and 16 after 10 weeks of residence. By comparison, among the residents who died during the initial period, only one person had answered that she had the freedom to choose other alternatives. All of these deaths were classified as unexpected because "not even insignificant disturbances had actually given warning of the impending disaster."

As Zimbardo (Zimbardo & Ruch, 1975) suggested, the implications of Ferrare's data are striking and merit further study of old age home settings. There is already evidence that perceived personal control in one's residential environment is important for younger and noninstitutional populations. Rodin (in press), using children as subjects, demonstrated that diminished feelings of control produced by chronic crowding at home led to fewer attempts to control self-reinforcement in the laboratory and to greater likelihood of giving up in the face of failure.

The present study attempted to assess directly the effects of enhanced personal responsibility and choice in a group of nursing home patients. In addition to examining previous results from the control-helplessness literature in a field setting, the present study extended the domain of this conception by considering new response variables. Specifically, if increased control has generalized beneficial effects, then physical and mental atertness, activity, general level of satisfaction, and sociability should all be affected. Also, the manipulation of the independent variables, assigning greater responsibility and decision freedom for relevant behavior, allowed subjects real choices that were not directed toward a single behavior or stimulus condition. This manipulation tested the ability of the subjects to generalize from specific choices enumerated for them to other aspects of their lives, and thus tested the generalizability of the feelings of control over certain elements of the situation to more broadly based behavior and attitudes.

Method

Subjects

The study was conducted in a nursing home, which was rated by the state of Connecticut as being among the finest care units and offering quality medical, recreational, and residential facilities. The home was large and modern in design, appearing cheerful and comfortable as well as clean and efficient. Of the four floors in the home, two were selected for study because of similarity in the residents' physical and psychological health and prior socioeconomic status, as determined from evaluations made by the home's director, head nurses, and social worker. Residents were assigned to a particular floor and room simply on the basis of availability, and on the average, residents on the two floors had been at the home about the same length of time. Rather than randomly assigning subjects to experimental treatment, a different floor was randomly selected for each treatment. Since there was not a great deal of communication between floors, this procedure was followed in order to decrease the likelihood that the treatment effects would be contaminated. There were 8 males and 39 females in the responsibility-induced condition (all fourth-floor residents) and 9 males and 35 females in the comparison group (all second-floor residents). Residents who were either completely bedridden or judged by the nursing home staff to be completely noncommunicative (11 on the experimental floor and 9 on the comparison floor) were omitted from the sample. Also omitted was one woman on each floor, one 40 years old and the other 26 years old, due to their age. Thus 91, ambulatory adults, ranging in age from 65 to 90, served as subjects.

Procedure

To introduce the experimental treatment, the nursing home administrator, an outgoing and friendly 33-year-old male who interacts with the residents daily, called a meeting in the lounge of each floor. He delivered one of the following two communications at that time:

[*Responsibility-induced group*]   I brought you together today to give you some information about Arden House, I was surprised to learn that many of you don't know about the things that are available to you and more important, that many of you don't realize the influence you have over your own lives here. Take a minute to think of the decisions you can and should be making. For example, you have the responsibility of caring for yourselves, of deciding whether or not you want to make this a home you can be proud of and happy in. You should be deciding how you want your rooms to be arranged—whether you want it to be as it is or whether you want the staff to help you rearrange the furniture. You should be deciding how you want to spend your time, for example, whether you want to be visiting your friends who live on this floor or on other floors, whether you want to visit in your room or your friends' room, in the lounge, the dining room, etc., or whether you want to be watching television, listening to the radio, writing, reading, or planning social events. In other words, it's your life and you can make of it whatever you want.
    This brings me to another point. If you are unsatisfied with anything here, you

have the influence to change it. It's your responsibility to make your complaints known, to tell us what you would like to change, to tell us what you would like. These are just a few of the things you could and should be deciding and thinking about now and from time to time everyday. You made these decisions before you came here and you can and should be making them now.

We're thinking of instituting some way for airing complaints, suggestions, etc. Let [nurse's name] know if you think this is a good idea and how you think we should go about doing it. In any case let her know what your complaints or suggestions are.

Also, I wanted to take this opportunity to give you each a present from the Arden House. [A box of small plants was passed around, and patients were given two decisions to make: first, whether or not they wanted a plant at all, and second, to choose which one they wanted. All residents did select a plant.] The plants are yours to keep and take care of as you'd like.

One last thing, I wanted to tell you that we're showing a movie two nights next week, Thursday and Friday. You should decide which night you'd like to go, if you choose to see it at all.

[*Comparison group*] I brought you together today to give you some information about the Arden House. I was surprised to learn that many of you don't know about the things that are available to you; that many of you don't realize all you're allowed to do here. Take a minute to think of all the options that we've provided for you in order for your life to be fuller and more interesting. For example, you're permitted to visit people on the other floors and to use the lounge on this floor for visiting as well as the dining room or your own rooms. We want your rooms to be as nice as they can be, and we've tried to make them that way for you. We want you to be happy here. We feel that it's our responsibility to make this a home you can be proud of and happy in, and we want to do all we can to help you.

This brings me to another point. If you have any complaints or suggestions about anything, let [nurse's name] know what they are. Let us know how we can best help you. You should feel that you have free access to anyone on the staff, and we will do the best we can to provide individualized attention and time for you.

Also, I wanted to take this opportunity to give you each a present from the Arden House. [The nurse walked around with a box of plants and each patient was handed one.] The plants are yours to keep. The nurses will water and care for them for you.

One last thing, I wanted to tell you that we're showing a movie next week on Thursday and Friday. We'll let you know later which day you're scheduled to see it.

The major difference between the two communications was that on one floor, the emphasis was on the residents' responsibility for themselves, whereas on the other floor, the communication stressed the staff's responsibility for them. In addition, several other differences bolstered this treatment: Residents in the responsibility-induced group were asked to give their opinion of the means by which complaints were handled rather than just being told that any complaints would be handled by staff members; they were given the opportunity to select their own plant and to care for it themselves, rather than being given a plant to be taken care of by someone else; and they were given their choice of a movie night, rather than being assigned a particular night, as was typically the case in the old age home. However, there was no difference in the amount of attention paid to the two groups.

Three days after these communications had been delivered, the director visited all of the residents in their rooms or in the corridor and reiterated part of the previous message. To those in the responsibility-induced group he said, "Remember what I said last Thursday. We want you to be happy. Treat this like your own home and make all the decisions you used to make. How's your plant coming along?" To the residents of the comparison floor, he said the same thing omitting the statement about decision making.

Dependent variables

Questionnaires

Two types of questionnaires were designed to assess the effects of induced responsibility. Each was administered 1 week prior to and 3 weeks after the communication. The first was administered directly to the residents by a female research assistant who was unaware of the experimental hypotheses or of the specific experimental treatment. The questions dealt with how much control they felt over general events in their lives and how happy and active they felt. Questions were responded to along 8-point scales ranging from 0 (none) to 8 (total). After completing each interview, the research assistant rated the resident on an 8-point scale for alertness.

The second questionnaire was responded to by the nurses, who staffed the experimental and comparison floors and who were unaware of the experimental treatments. Nurses on two different shifts completed the questionnaires in order to obtain two ratings for each subject. There were nine 10-point scales that asked for ratings of how happy, alert, dependent, sociable, and active the residents were as well as questions about their eating and sleeping habits. There were also questions evaluating the proportion of weekly time the patient spent engaged in a variety of activities. These included reading, watching television, visiting other patients, visiting outside guests, watching the staff, talking to the staff, sitting alone doing nothing, and others.

Behavioral measures

Since perceived personal control is enhanced by a sense of choice over relevant behaviors, the option to choose which night the experimental group wished to see the movie was expected to have measurable effects on active participation. Attendance records were kept by the occupational therapist, who was unaware that an experiment was being conducted.

Another measure of involvement was obtained by holding a competition in which all participants had to guess the number of jelly beans in a large jar. Each patient wishing to enter the contest simply wrote his or her name and estimate on a piece of paper and deposited it in a box that was next to the jar.[1]

Finally, an unobtrusive measure of activity was taken. The tenth night after the experimental treatment, the right wheels of the wheelchairs belonging to a randomly selected subsample of each patient group were covered with 2 inches (.05 m) of white adhesive tape. The following night, the tape was removed from the chairs and placed on index cards for later evaluation of amount of activity, as indicated by the amount of discoloration.

Results

Questionnaires

Before examining whether or not the experimental treatment was effective, the pretest ratings made by the subjects, the nurses, and the interviewer were compared for both groups. None of the differences approached significance, which indicates comparability between groups prior to the start of the investigation.

The means for responses to the various questionnaires are summarized in Table 1. Statistical tests compared the posttest minus pretest scores of the experimental and comparison groups.

In response to direct questions about how happy they currently were, residents in the responsibility-induced group reported significantly greater increases in happiness after the experimental treatment than did the comparison group, $t(43) = 1.96$, $p < .05$.[2] Although the comparison

---

[1] We also intended to measure the number of complaints that patients voiced. Since one often does not complain after becoming psychologically helpless, complaints in this context were expected to be a positive indication of perceived personal control. This measure was discarded, however, since the nurses failed to keep a systematic written record.

[2] All of the statistics for the self-report data and the interviewers' ratings are based on 45 subjects (25 in the responsibility-induced group and 20 in the comparison group), since these were the only subjects available at the time of the interview.

Table 1. *Mean scores for self-report, interviewer ratings, and nurses' ratings for experimental and comparison groups*

Questionnaire responses	Responsibility induced (n = 24)			Comparison (n = 28)			Comparison of change scores (p<)
	Pre	Post	Change: Post–Pre	Pre	Post	Change: Post–Pre	
Self-report							
Happy	5.16	5.44	.28	4.90	4.78	−.12	.05
Active	4.07	4.27	.20	3.90	2.62	−1.28	.01
Perceived Control							
Have	3.26	3.42	.16	3.62	4.03	.41	—
Want	3.85	3.80	−.05	4.40	4.57	.17	—
Interviewer rating							
Alertness	5.02	5.31	.29	5.75	5.38	−.37	.025
Nurses' ratings							
General improvement	41.67	45.64	3.97	42.69	40.32	−2.39	.005
Time spent							
Visiting patients	13.03	19.81	6.78	7.94	4.65	−3.30	.005
Visiting others	11.50	13.75	2.14	12.38	8.21	−4.16	.05
Talking to staff	8.21	16.43	8.21	9.11	10.71	1.61	.01
Watching staff	6.78	4.64	−2.14	6.96	11.60	4.64	.05

group heard a communication that had specifically stressed the home's commitment to making them happy, only 25% of them reported feeling happier by the time of the second interview, whereas 48% of the experimental group did so.

The responsibility-induced group reported themselves to be significantly more active on the second interview than the comparison group, $t(43) = 2.67$, $p < .01$. The interviewer's ratings of alertness also showed significantly greater increase for the experimental group, $t(43) = 2.40$, $p < .025$. However, the questions that were relevant to perceived control showed no significant changes for the experimental group. Since over 20% of the patients indicated that they were unable to understand what we meant by control, these questions were obviously not adequate to discriminate between groups.

The second questionnaire measured nurses' ratings of each patient. The correlation between the two nurses' ratings of the same patient was .68 and .61 ($ps < .005$) on the comparison and responsibility-induced floors, respectively.[3] For each patient, a score was calculated by averaging the two nurses' ratings for each question, summing across questions, and subtracting the total pretreatment score from the total posttreatment score.[4] This yielded a positive average total change score of 3.97 for the responsibility-induced group as compared with an average negative total change of −2.37 for the comparison group. The difference between these means is highly significant, $t(50) = 5.18$, $p < .005$. If one looks at the percentage of people who were judged improved rather than at the amount of judged improvement, the same pattern emerges: 93% of the experimental group (all but one subject) were considered improved, whereas only 21% (six subjects) of the comparison group showed this positive change ($\chi^2 = 19.23$, $p < .005$).

The nurses' evaluation of the proportion of time subjects spent engaged in various interactive and noninteractive activities was analyzed by comparing the average change scores (post–precommunication) for all of the nurses for both groups of subjects on each activity. Several significant differences were found. The experimental group showed increases in the proportion of time spent visiting with other patients (for the experimental group, $X = 12.86$ vs. −6.61 for the comparison group), $t(50) = 3.83$, $p < .005$; visiting people from outside of the nursing home (for the experimental group, $X = 4.28$ vs. −7.61 for the comparison group, $t(50) = 2.30$, $p < .05$; and talking to the staff (for the experimental group, $X = 8.21$ vs. 1.61 for the comparison group), $t(50) = 2.98$, $p < .05$.[5] In addition, they spent less time passively watching the staff (for the experimental group, $X = −4.28$ vs. 9.68 for the comparison group), $t(50) = 2.60$, $p < .05$. Thus, it appears that the treatment increased active, interpersonal activity but not passive activity such as watching television or reading.

Behavioral measures

As in the case of the questionnaires, the behavioral measures showed a pattern of differences between groups that was generally consistent with the predicted effects of increased responsibility. The movie attendance was significantly higher in the responsibility-induced group than in the

[3] There was also significant agreement between the interviewer's and nurses' ratings of alertness ($r = .65$).

[4] Since one nurse on the day shift and one nurse on the night shift gave the ratings, responses to the questions regarding sleeping and eating habits were not included in the total score. Also, in order to reduce rater bias, patients for whom there were ratings by a nurse on only one shift were excluded from this calculation. This left 24 residents from the experimental group and 28 from the comparison group.

[5] This statistic is based only on the responses of nurse on duty in the evening.

control group after the experimental treatment ($z = 1.71$, $p < .05$, one-tailed), although a similar attendance check taken one month before the communications revealed no group differences.[6]

In the jelly-bean-guessing contest, 10 subjects (21%) in the responsibility-induced group and only 1 subject (2%) from the comparison group participated ($\chi^2 = 7.72$, $p < .01$). Finally, very little dirt was found on the tape taken from any of the patients' wheelchairs, and there was no significant difference between the two groups.

Discussion

It appears that inducing a greater sense of personal responsibility in people who may have virtually relinquished decision making, either by choice or necessity, produces improvement. In the present investigation, patients in the comparison group were given a communication stressing the staff's desire to make them happy and were otherwise treated in the sympathetic manner characteristic of this high-quality nursing home. Despite the care provided for these people, 71% were rated as having become more debilitated over a period of time as short as 3 weeks. In contrast with this group, 93% of the people who were encouraged to make decisions for themselves, given decisions to make, and given responsibility for something outside of themselves, actually showed overall improvement. Based on their own judgments and by the judgments of the nurses with whom they interacted on a daily basis, they became more active and felt happier. Perhaps more important was the judged improvement in their mental alertness and increased behavioral involvement in many different kinds of activities.

The behavioral measures showed greater active participation and involvement for the experimental group. Whether this directly resulted from an increase in perceived choice and decision-making responsibility or from the increase in general activity and happiness occurring after the treatment cannot be assessed from the present results. It should also be clearly noted that although there were significant differences in active involvement, the overall level of participation in the activities that comprised the behavioral measures was low. Perhaps a much more powerful treatment would be one that is individually administered and repeated on several occasions. That so weak a manipulation had any effect suggests how important increased control is for these people, for whom decision making is virtually nonexistent.

The practical implications of this experimental demonstration are straightforward. Mechanisms can and should be established for changing

---

[6] Frequencies were transformed into arc sines and analyzed using the method that is essentially the same as that described by Langer and Abelson (1972).

situational factors that reduce real or perceived responsibility in the elderly. Furthermore, this study adds to the body of literature (Bengston, 1973; Butler, 1967; Leaf, 1973; Lieberman, 1965) suggesting that senility and diminished alertness are not an almost inevitable result of aging. In fact, it suggests that some of the negative consequences of aging may be retarded, reversed, or possibly prevented by returning to the aged the right to make decisions and a feeling of competence.

Acknowledgements

The authors would like to express sincere thanks to Thomas Tolisano and the members of his staff at the Arden House in Hamden, Connecticut, for their thoughtful assistance in conducting this research

Reference note

1. Lehr, K., & Puschner, I. *Studies in the awareness of aging*. Paper presented at the 6th International Congress on Gerontology, Copenhagen, 1963.

References

Adamson, J., & Schmale, A. Object loss, giving up, and the onset of psychiatric disease. *Psychosomatic Medicine*, 1965, *27*, 557–576.

Adler, A. Individual psychology. In C. Murchinson (Ed.), *Psychologies of 1930*. Worcester, Mass.: Clark University Press, 1930.

Bengston, V. L. Self determination: A social and psychological perspective on helping the aged. *Geriatrics*, 1973.

Bettelheim, B. Individual and mass behavior in extreme situations. *Journal of Abnormal and Social Psychology*, 1943, *38*, 417–452.

Birren, J. Aging and psychological adjustment. *Review of Educational Research*, 1958, *28*, 475–490.

Bowers, K. Pain, anxiety, and perceived control. *Journal of Consulting and Clinical Psychology*, 1968, *32*, 596–602.

Butler, R. Aspects of survival and adaptation in human aging. *American Journal of Psychiatry*, 1967, *123*, 1233–1243.

Corah, N., & Boffa, J. Perceived control, self-observation, and response to aversive stimulation. *Journal of Personality and Social Psychology*, 1970, *16*, 1–4.

deCharms, R. *Personal causation*. New York: Academic Press, 1968.

Geer, J., Davison, G., & Gatchel, R. Reduction of stress in humans through nonveridical perceived control of aversive stimulation. *Journal of Personality and Social Psychology*, 1970, *16*, 731–738.

Glass, D., & Singer J. *Urban stress*. New York: Academic Press, 1972.

Gould, R. The phases of adult life: A study in developmental psychology, *American Journal of Psychiatry*, 1972, *129*, 521–531.

Kanfer, R., & Seidner, M. Self-Control: Factors enhancing tolerance of noxious stimulation. *Journal of Personality and Social Psychology*, 1973, *25*, 381–389.

Langer, E. J. The illusion of control. *Journal of Personality and Social Psychology*, 1975, *32*, 311–328.

Langer, E. J., & Abelson, R. P. The semantics of asking a favor: How to succeed in getting help without really dying. *Journal of Personality and Social Psychology*, 1972, *24*, 26–32.

Langer, E. J., Janis, I. L., & Wolfer, J. A. Reduction of psychological stress in surgical patients. *Journal of Experimental Social Psychology*, 1975, *11*, 155–165.

Leaf, A. Threescore and forty. *Hospital Practice*, 1973, *34*, 70–71.

Lefcourt, H. The function of the illusion of control and freedom. *American Psychologist*, 1973, *28*, 417–425.

Lieberman, M. Psychological correlates of impending death: Some preliminary observations. *Journal of Gerontology*, 1965, *20*, 181–190.

McMahon, A., & Rhudick, P. Reminiscing, adaptational significance in the aged. *Archives of General Psychiatry*, 1964, *10*, 292–298.

Neugarten, B., & Gutman, D. Age-sex roles and personality in middle age: a thematic apperception study. *Psychological Monographs*, 1958, *72*(17, Whole No. 470).

Pervin, L. The need to predict and control under conditions of threat. *Journal of Personality*, 1963, *31*, 570–585.

Richter, C. On the phenomenon of sudden death in animals and man. *Psychosomatic Medicine*, 1957, *19*, 191–198.

Rodin, J. Crowding, perceived choice, and response to controllable and uncontrollable outcomes. *Journal of Experimental Social Psychology*, in press.

Schmale, A. Relationships of separation and depression to disease. I.: A report on a hospitalized medical population. *Psychosomatic Medicine*, 1958, *20*, 259–277.

Schmale, A., & Iker, H. The psychological setting of uterine cervical cancer. *Annals of the New York Academy of Sciences*, 1966, *125*, 807–813.

Seligman, M. E. P. *Helplessness*. San Francisco: Freeman, 1975.

Stotland, E., & Blumenthal, A. The reduction of anxiety as a result of the expectation of making a choice. *Canadian Review of Psychology*, 1964, *18*, 139–145.

Zimbardo, P. G., & Ruch, F. L. *Psychology and life* (9th ed.). Glenview, Ill.: Scott, Foresman, 1975.

Section 6

Behavioural interventions in medicine

Readings

Randomised controlled trial of nicotine chewing-gum.
  M. J. Jarvis, M. Raw, M. A. H. Russell and C. Feyerabend. *British Medical Journal*, **285**, 537–40, 1982.

Conditioned side effects induced by cancer chemotherapy: prevention through behavioral treatment.
  T. G. Burish, M. P. Carey, M. G. Krozely and F. A. Greco. *Journal of Consulting and Clinical Psychology*, **55**, 42–8, 1987.

Improvement of medication compliance in uncontrolled hypertension.
  R. B. Haynes, D. L. Sackett, E. S. Gibson, D. W. Taylor, B. C. Hackett, R. S. Roberts and A. L. Johnson. *Lancet*, **i**, 1265–8, 1976.

Effect of psychosocial treatment on survival of patients with metastatic breast cancer.
  D. Spiegel, J. R. Bloom, H. C. Kraemer and E. Gottheil. *Lancet*, **ii**, 888–91, 1989.

Alteration of type A behavior and its effect on cardiac recurrences in post myocardial infarction patients: summary results of the recurrent coronary prevention project.
  M. Friedman, C. E. Thoresen, J. J. Gill, D. Ulmer, L. H. Powell, V. A. Price, B. Brown, L. Thompson, D. D. Rabin, W. S. Breall, E. Bourg, R. Levy and T. Dixon. *American Heart Journal*, **112**, 653–65, 1986.

Can lifestyle changes reverse coronary heart disease? The Lifestyle Heart Trial.
  D. Ornish, S. E. Brown, L. W. Scherwitz, J. H. Billings, W. T. Armstrong, T. A. Ports, S. M. McLanahan, R. L. Kirkeeide, R. J. Brand and K. L. Gould. *Lancet*, **336**, 129–33, 1990.

Introduction

The recognition that behavioural scientists have a contribution to make to treatment outside the psychiatric arena was first widely acknowledged at a conference on behavioural medicine held in Yale, USA, in 1977 (Schwartz and Weiss, 1977). Since that time, the range of treatments which have been used, and target conditions to which psychological treatments have been applied, has expanded enormously. A growing number of specialist journals and handbooks are now available and illustrate the expansion in research in the area. The involvement of health psychologists in clinical settings has also increased, allowing research developments to be put into practice (Pearce and Wardle, 1989). The readings in this section have been selected to illustrate the range of psychological interventions which have proved effective in clinical settings.

Behavioural interventions have developed from two main sources. Psychophysiology has contributed methods such as biofeedback which have been applied to the management of musculoskeletal disorders and to the control of stress responses (Gatchel and Price, 1979). Clinical psychology has contributed techniques such as counselling, relaxation, stress management and self-control which have been applied to the management of emotional and behavioural reactions to illnesses and to the modification of risk factors (Kaptein *et al.*, 1990). These interventions have developed against the background of psychosomatic medicine, with its emphasis on the individual's psychological makeup as a determinant of responses to illness and treatment (Lipowski, 1977).

Behavioural treatments have been applied at many stages in the disease process from risk factor modification to terminal care and many of these are illustrated in the readings in this section. The modification of risk behaviors such as food choice, exercise, or smoking (*Jarvis et al.*) is a key feature of many current public health approaches and is targeted in governmental publications such as *The Health of the Nation* (Department of Health, 1992), in the UK, or *Healthy People 2000* (US Department of Health and Human Services, 1990) in the USA (see Section 4). Secondary prevention, targeting future episodes of morbidity and mortality in people with established disease states, is another important aspect of psychological intervention which has been developed most fully in the area of cardiovascular disease, where modification of lifestyle in post-coronary patients has been shown to have a significant impact on survival (*Friedman et al.*). The management of the emotional consequences of serious or life-threatening illness is a well-established application of psychological treatment (*Burish et al.*; *Spiegel et al.*) Interventions directed towards helping patients to cope better with their illness can both improve their quality of life and may even influence the progression of the disease process (see Section 5). Direct treatment of the disease process is probably one of the most controversial aspects of psychological intervention. However, the early biofeedback research laid the groundwork for subsequent psychological interventions, and a range of disorders have been found to be susceptible to direct intervention (*Ornish et al.*). Finally, psychological research has played an important part in understanding issues of treatment adherence (*Haynes et al.*), since incomplete adherence to advice and medication poses a continuing challenge to therapeutics.

Primary prevention through smoking cessation

Of all the lifestyle risk factors, smoking poses the most serious threat to health. Estimates of premature deaths attributable to smoking have increased alarmingly in the developed world, and are set to rise in the same way in the developing countries in which the population is only just now taking up the smoking habit. In response to the range of health promotion initiatives, price controls, and anti-smoking legislation, smoking levels have fallen in most western countries since the peaks of a few decades ago. Nevertheless, recruitment to smoking continues steadily among teenagers, and although the majority of adult smokers say that they wish to quit, only a minority succeeds. Reducing recruitment to smoking among adolescents offers one approach to the control of smoking and has been discussed in Section 4 (*Walter et al.*). Unfortunately, despite the force of the health message, it has not always proved easy to dissuade young people from taking up smoking. The influence of adult smoking 'models' may well encourage young people to take up smoking. This suggests that helping adult smokers to quit must remain an essential part of the process of health promotion.

Smoking cessation treatments can be divided into two kinds: intensive interventions designed to achieve maximum impact on selected groups of smokers – for example in specialist smoking cessation clinics – and lower intensity interventions designed to be applied on a population-wide basis, albeit with a smaller impact. One example of the latter approach was Russell *et al.*'s (1979) study in which all smokers who visited their general practitioner (GP) during a two-week period were randomised to control (no intervention) or were simply advised to stop smoking. Although the overall quit rates were very low, nevertheless those who were given GP advice were significantly more likely to be continuously abstinent over the next year. In this study, the impact of GP advice was least among the heaviest smokers, among whom stopping smoking appeared to be hampered by the difficulty of withdrawing from nicotine.

The fact that nicotine-dependence is one of the principal barriers to quitting for many smokers has encouraged the development of treatment methods which might minimise withdrawal effects. One such technique is the use of adjunctive replacement nicotine during the period that the patient first gives up smoking. The reading by *Jarvis, Raw, Russell and Feyerabend* describes one of the first controlled trials to evaluate the addition of nicotine replacement to group-based clinic counselling. Smokers referred to a specialist smokers' clinic entered a six-week group treatment programme incorporating advice and support on giving up smoking. Patients also received chewing gum which they were told contained nicotine and which they were instructed to use in situations where withdrawal symptoms or craving were a problem. For half the treatment groups, the gum contained 2 mg of buffered nicotine, which when chewed vigorously can produce blood nicotine levels comparable to smoking a single cigarette. For the other group, the gum contained 1 mg of unbuffered nicotine, thus tasting similar, but produced a much smaller blood nicotine rise. Subjects in the nicotine replacement group had fewer withdrawal symptoms, and a biochemically validated abstinence rate which was twice as high as those who received the placebo gum. A similar doubling of abstinence rates has been reported in a GP-based study using nictone patches (ICRF General Practice Research Group, 1993), suggesting that nicotine replacement also has a role to play in the less-intensive treatment environment. The use of a combined psychological and drug treatment to enhance behaviour change is part of a growing interest in combining pharmacotherapy with psychological treatment. Craighead and Agras (1991), for example, suggested that long-term combined treatment offers a viable option for some obese patients.

Prevention of treatment side-effects

Few effective medical treatments are entirely free from unwanted effects, and in some cases the impact of side effects on quality of life can be so severe that patients may reject the treatment altogether. This problem has been especially severe in relation to the use of cytotoxic drugs for the treatment of cancer. A spectrum of side effects from hair loss, fatigue, mouth ulceration, increased susceptibility to infection, and nausea and vomiting, are common in the short term. The nausea and vomiting have attracted particular attention from psychologists following the observation that after several treatment cycles they may start to appear *before* the administration of chemotherapy. In one series, almost 20% of patients had anticipatory nausea or vomiting (ANV), developing after the sixth session of treatment and beginning up to five hours before subsequent sessions (Nicholas, 1982). Other studies have produced even higher figures for the level of ANV (Leventhal *et al.*, 1988). It has been argued that nausea and vomiting are initially direct drug-effects, which can become conditioned to other features of the treatment environment, such as the smells, tastes, or even thoughts associated with the treatment (Morrow and Morrell, 1982). Once conditioning has occurred, the symptoms may appear as soon as the patient arrives for treatment or even before, and they may generalise outside the treatment environment to the hospital and beyond.

The possibility of using psychological procedures to minimise ANV has been considered for some time. A number of forms of psychological treatment have been shown to reduce the severity of the side effects, including relaxation training (Lyles *et al.*, 1982) and distraction (Redd *et al.*, 1987). The reading by *Burish, Carey, Krozely and Greco* considers the application of psychological strategies to *prevent* the development of ANV. In a randomised, controlled study the experimental patients were given training in relaxation and guided imagery before chemotherapy began, with further training in the first three chemotherapy sessions. For subsequent sessions they were encouraged to apply the methods themselves. Measures of anxiety and nausea were obtained from patients and nurses after each session. Patients in the control group were encouraged to relax themselves during each session. Anxiety was reduced markedly in the experimental patients during the three treatment sessions with changes persisting into the follow-up sessions. Nausea stayed at low levels in the treated group but increased over time in the control group. Anxiety, nausea and vomiting were also lower in the 72 hours post-treatment in the treated group, and emotional distress was lower in anticipation of chemotherapy in the treated group. These very encouraging results add to a substantial literature which demonstrates the efficacy of psychological treatment of ANV. The high proportions of treated patients who had no nausea at the fifth session (90% vs. 46%) is a strong endorsement of the benefits of starting the psychological intervention early in the chemotherapy process.

Increasing medication compliance

The problems of treatment compliance are not limited to difficult lifestyle change, but extend across the full spectrum of therapeutic advice. Estimates of non-adherence across different treatment regimens have ranged from 35–60% (Sackett and Snow, 1979) with even higher levels when adherence is defined strictly. Apart from the therapeutic costs of non-compliance with treatment, there are also financial costs in terms of wasted drugs and the subsequent medical complications arising from non-compliance.

One important line of research has been to investigate what factors are associated with poor compliance. There is a widely held view that some patients are 'good', and therefore compliant, and others are not. However, the evidence for any particular personality type being less compliant has not been forthcoming (Ley, 1988). Similarly, aspects of social background such as income or education have not been shown to be strongly related to adherence (Haynes, 1976; Sherbourne *et al.*, 1992). By contrast, patients' understanding of their condition and its treatment, or their satisfaction with their medical care, have proved to be more significant predictors of compliance. Francis *et al.* (1969) found that mothers who were satisfied with their consultation with the paediatrician were many times more likely to be compliant than mothers who were dissatisfied. As discussed in Section 4, beliefs and expectations about illness are also consistently found to be associated with compliance across a range of behaviours. In a recent large-scale study of compliance (the Medical Outcomes Study), a range of predictors were investigated in a multivariate analysis to evaluate their relationship with adherence (Sherbourne *et al.*, 1992). The pattern of results confirmed that satisfaction with care and social support were predictors. Coping style also proved important, with avoidant coping being linked to non-compliance.

There have been several studies in which aspects of the medical encounter or the treatment regimen have been modified in an attempt to maximise the probability of following advice. In the reading by *Haynes and his colleagues* the modification of non-compliance is approached by targeting it in a programme of treatment for hypertension. The subjects were drawn from a workplace study of detection and treatment of hypertension (Sackett *et al.*, 1975) and 39 men who had failed to follow the anti-hypertensive treatment advice took part. They were allocated to experimental or control groups through a matching procedure. The experimental treatment was based on behavioural strategies of self-monitoring, tailoring of instructions, increased supervision and reinforcement both of compliance and outcome (reduced blood pressure). This represented a treatment package incorporating almost the full spectrum of behavioural principles. The effects of the treatment were impressive, with compliance increasing by over 20% in the intervention group compared with the pre-treatment phase, while compliance was slightly reduced in the controls. The efficacy of the intervention was also supported by changes in the target symptoms, with a significant drop in diastolic blood pressure in the experimental group. These are encouraging results, especially in view of the fact that this was a group that had already showed themselves to be resistant to advice, and they set a target for future investigations. Similar techniques have been applied to cholesterol-lowering advice in a series of pilot studies, and again the results support the view that frequent feedback, tailored programmes, adherence recording, and reinforcements, are among the factors which produce improved compliance and a better treatment outcome (Southard *et al.*, 1992).

Psychosocial interventions in cancer

Over the past few decades, there has been increasing recognition that the treatment of cancer patients must also encompass the emotional distress which is often associated with the disease (Fallowfield, 1991). The term psychosocial oncology has been coined to describe this field of work. The distress associated with the diagnosis and progression of cancer, both for the patient and the family, have encouraged the development of techniques for ameliorating emotional reactions. These range from ways of communicating the diagnosis which might minimise the trauma of the 'bad news' to elaborate cognitive-behavioural treatments designed to help patients to adjust to the disease and the threat to survival.

There is a strong body of evidence that psychological treatments can improve psychological well-being for cancer patients. Individual psychotherapy has been shown to reduce emotional distress in patients undergoing radiotherapy (Forester *et al.*, 1985). Moorey and Greer (1989) have developed a form of cognitive-behavioural therapy – adjuvant psychological therapy – which is directed towards reducing anxiety and depression and inducing a more positive attitude to cancer. Case studies and an uncontrolled case series of cancer patients have provided evidence for the clinical effectiveness of this treatment (Moorey, 1991). Group-based therapies have also been associated with a better psychological outcome (Telch and Telch, 1986).

Whether psychological interventions might influence not only emotional reactions to cancer, but also its progression, is attracting increasing attention. The 'healing power of the mind' has long been promoted in the popular press (Simonton et al., 1978; Cousins, 1989). The reading by *Spiegel, Bloom, Kraemer and Gottheil* is one of the few controlled evaluations of the effect of group therapy on cancer survival, although extending life had not been the original intent of the intervention. The group treatment programme was designed particularly to help women to cope with the trauma of metastatic breast cancer. Women who were prepared to take part in a group treatment programme were randomised to group therapy or to a usual care control group and the first report showed significant positive effects of the treatment on quality of life (Spiegel *et al.*, 1981). The present paper describes the survival of the patients at a 10-year follow-up. Over the initial intervention year there had been slightly (but non-significantly) more deaths in the intervention group. However, over the entire 10-year follow-up period, patients in the intervention group survived almost twice as long as those in the control group.

One concern about these results is that the patients in the intervention group may have had a less advanced stage of cancer at the start of the intervention. However, *Spiegel et al.* reanalysed their data controlling for the initial stage of the cancer and found that the group differences in survival time remained significant. Similar results were reported by Richardson *et al.* (1990) with a much less intensive intervention, again not intended to promote survival, but found to be a significant predictor of survival. Linn *et al.* (1982), in a study of male late-stage cancer patients, used an individually based counselling treatment with demonstrable benefits on quality of life, but found no effects on survival. However, the follow-up period for this sample was only 12 months, by which time fewer than 20% of the sample had survived.

Although there is still a long way to go, there appears to be a consensus that psychological factors may have some influence on the progression of cancer and a number of possible mechanisms have been considered. In the study by Richardson *et al.* (1990) the primary target of the intervention was treatment compliance, which was significantly increased in the intervention group. However, the intervention appeared to have effects on survival which were independent of compliance, so other processes must have contributed to the survival effect. In a shorter-term study of patients with malignant melanomas, Fawzy *et al.* (1990) used a group-based psychiatric intervention which was shown both to improve psychological well-being and to influence natural killer cell levels and activity. The exciting possibility that the psychoneuroimmune axis provides the intermediary stages whereby stress might influence the progression of cancer is discussed in Section 2.

Reducing recurrence of cardiac events

The associations between Type A behavior and coronary heart disease identified in population studies were described in Section 3. Irrespective of the consistency of the epidemiological evidence, the causal significance of a putative pathogenic agent like Type A behaviour is best established through a randomised controlled trial. The modification of Type A behaviour might be carried out on healthy populations in a primary prevention trial, but this presents difficulties. Motivating people to change even circumscribed aspects of lifestyle (such as physical inactivity) is not easy, and these difficulties are compounded with a broad construct such as Type A that touches on so many aspects of behaviour and emotional life. Prohibitively large cohorts would be required to identify changes in disease incidence within a reasonable time period. Attempts to modify Type A behaviour in healthy populations have therefore been small scale, aiming to demonstrate that changes can be made rather than documenting reductions in disease incidence (Roskies *et al.*, 1986).

The reading by *Friedman and his colleagues* describes the alternative strategy of modifying Type A behaviour in people who have already suffered a myocardial infarction. Such people are at high risk for cardiac recurrences, so might be positively motivated to make efforts to reduce risk. The aim of the Recurrent Coronary Prevention Project was to assess whether Type A behaviour could be modified in a randomised controlled trial, and to discover whether changes in behaviour would reduce recurrence of cardiac events such as myocardial infarction or cardiac death. In order for the study to have sufficient statistical power to show differences in recurrence, large numbers of patients were enrolled, and the study is impressive logistically as well as scientifically.

The basic design was a comparison between 'cardiac counselling' and cardiac counselling plus a Type A intervention programme. It is important to note that participants were not selected for their interest and knowledge in type A behaviour, so the implications of the results are not confined to specifically motivated groups. The cardiac counselling was substantial, involving more than 30 one-and-a-half-hour sessions of advice and education over four-and-a-half years, far more than a typical post-infarction patient might experience. Patients in the Type A condition had the opportunity to participate in 62 sessions over this period, although the average number attended was rather fewer. The complex programme used to modify Type A behaviour is not described in detail in this paper, but mobilised the full panoply of psychological methods including relaxation training, behaviour modification, cognitive restructuring and modelling, attitude change and social support. Interestingly, most patients persevered with the programme, although 6.8% proved so intractable in their Type A behaviour that they were withdrawn. The results described in this paper indicate that Type A behaviour was reduced to a greater extent in the experimental intervention than cardiac counselling conditions. The two groups also differed in cardiac recurrences, with a cumulative rate over four-and-a-half years of 12.9% in the Type A and 21.2% in the cardiac counselling subjects. The recurrence rate in the cardiac counselling group was comparable with that reported in other US samples. The attribution of this effect to Type A modification is strengthened by the observation that recurrence was less common among patients in the intervention condition who displayed objective evidence of behaviour change than in those whose Type A behaviour was not reduced. Moreover, a subsequent paper has reported that when Type A counselling was offered to participants in the control group, they too showed a reduction in Type A behaviour and reduced recurrence (Friedman *et al.*, 1987).

It is not known whether all the components of this complex and lengthy treatment programme are needed, since there is some evidence that less intensive psychological interventions may reduce mortality (Frasure-Smith and Prince, 1989). An independent study has shown that the treatment package is effective in reducing Type A behaviour, this time in middle-aged cardiac patients from Sweden, and that the change is accompanied by modifications in psychophysiological activity (Burell *et al.*, 1994). Other forms of psychological intervention following infarction have been primarily concerned with reducing psychological distress and improving quality of life (Langosch, 1989; Lewin *et al.*, 1992). Nonetheless, the Recurrent Coronary Prevention Project provides powerful evidence for Type A being a causal factor in heart disease, and for the effectiveness of behavioural interventions in prolonging active life.

Reversing chronic disease processes

The previous two readings have suggested that psychological methods may reduce morbidity and retard the progression towards death from serious chronic illness. The final reading from *Ornish and co-workers* demonstrates that lifestyle modifications may actually reverse the disease process in the case of coronary atherosclerosis, the disorder underlying coronary artery disease. Such a possibility has been virtually impossible to study until recently, since methods for quantifying coronary stenosis (or blockage) were poorly developed. *Ornish et al.* were able to take advantage of sophisticated imaging techniques to assess the degree of coronary artery occlusion before and after treatment. Their Lifestyle Heart Trial involved intensive investigation of a small group of patients with advanced disease in a randomised controlled trial. The multifactorial experimental intervention programme included a low-fat vegetarian diet, regular exercise, stress management techniques such as relaxation and imagery, together with regular group counselling sessions. It was introduced during a one-week residential induction course, followed by meetings for four hours per week. The group meetings were designed to establish social support and to help to maintain adherence to the demanding intervention.

Significant changes were recorded over one year in lifestyle, lipid levels and angina symptoms in the experimental group. These effects were greater than those recorded in the control group, some of whom may have modified their lifestyles on their own account without any support. More impressively, coronary lesions regressed to a small but significant extent in the experimental group, compared with some progression in controls. Over the year, the analyses of lesions involving more than 50% blockage of arteries showed a substantial regression in the experimental group, compared with an increase in the control group.

As in the case of the Recurrent Coronary Prevention Project, it is not certain whether some or all the components of this treatment programme were necessary to produce the favourable effects. Regression or slowing of the coronary lesion development has been reported with low-fat diets (Watts *et al.*, 1992) or diet combined with regular exercise (Schuler *et al.*, 1992) in the absence of any attempts at stress management. However, subsequent analyses of the Lifestyle Heart Trial have shown that regression was correlated with adherence to the lifestyle change programme, but not with changes in blood pressure, cholesterol or lipid fractions (Ornish *et al.*, 1992). This suggests that changes in conventional risk factors are not entirely responsible for the positive effects on coronary lesions. *Ornish et al.* do not consider that their programme is necessarily practical as a general clinical technique. However, the documentation of changes at the level of structural pathology is important, since it indicates that lifestyle modifications do not operate simply in terms of clinical presentation. As such, the paper reaffirms the importance of the integrated perspective on human health and illness that is at the heart of this set of readings.

References

Burell, G., Öhman, A., Sundin, Ö., Ström, G., Ramund, B., Cullhed, I. and Thoresen, C. E. (1994). Modification of the Type A behavior pattern in post-myocardial infarction patients: a route to cardiac rehabilitation. *International Journal of Behavioral Medicine*, **1**, 32–54.

Cousins, N. (1989). *Head First: The Biology of Hope and the Healing Power of the Human Spirit*. New York; Penguin.

Craighead, L. W. and Agras, W. S. (1991). Mechanisms of action in cognitive-behavioral and pharmacological interventions for obesity and bulimia nervosa. *Journal of Consulting and Clinical Psychology*, **59**, 115–25.

Department of Health (1992). *The Health of The Nation*, London: HMSO.

Fallowfield, L. (1991). Counselling patients with cancer. In: *Counselling and Communication in Health Care*, pp. 253–69. H. Davis and L. Fallowfield (eds.). Chichester: John Wiley.

Fawzy, I., Kemeny, M. E., Fawzy, R. N., Elashoff, R., Morton, D., Cousins, N. and Fahey, J. L. (1990). A structured psychiatric intervention for cancer patients. II. Changes over time in immunological measures. *Archives of General Psychiatry*, **47**, 729–35.

Forester, B., Kornfeld, D. and Fleiss, J. (1985). Psychotherapy during radiotherapy: effects on emotional and physical distress. *American Journal of Psychiatry*, **142**, 22–7.

Francis, V., Korsch, B. M. and Morris, J. (1969). Gaps in doctor–patient communication. *New England Journal of Medicine*, **280**, 535–40.

Frasure-Smith, N. and Prince, R. (1989). Long-term follow-up of the Ischaemic Heart Disease Life-Stress Monitoring Program. *Psychosomatic Medicine*, **51**, 485–513.

Friedman, M., Powell, L. H., Thoresen, C. E., Ulmer, D., Price, V., Gill, J. J., Thompson, L., Rabin, D. D., Brown, B., Breall, W. S., Levy, R. and Bourg, E. (1987). Effect of discontinuance of Type A behavioral counselling on Type A behavior and cardiac recurrence rate of post myocardial infarction patients. *American Heart Journal*, **114**, 483–90.

Gatchel, R. J. and Price, K. P. (eds.). (1979). *Clinical Biofeedback: Appraisal and Status*. New York, Pergamon.

Haynes, R. B. (1976). A critical review of the 'determinants' of patient compliance with therapeutic regimens. In: *Compliance with Therapeutic Regimens*, pp. 49–62. D. L. Sackett and R. B. Haynes (eds.). Baltimore: Johns Hopkins University Press.

ICRF General Practice Research Group (1993). Effectiveness of a nicotine patch in helping people stop smoking: results of a randomised trial in general practice. *British Medical Journal*, **306**, 1304–8.

Kaptein, A. A., van der Ploeg, H. M., Garssen, B., Schreurs, P. J. G. and Beunderman, R. (eds.) (1990). *Behavioural Medicine: Psychological Treatment of Somatic Disorders*. Chichester: John Wiley.

Langosch, W. (1989). Cardiac rehabilitation. In: *The Practice of Behavioural Medicine*, pp. 27–49. S. Pearce and J. Wardle (eds.). Oxford: Oxford University Press.

Leventhal, H., Easterling, D. V., Nerenz, D. R. and Love, R. R. (1988). The role of motion sickness in predicting anticipatory nausea. *Journal of Behavioral Medicine*, **11**, 117–30.

Lewin, B., Robertson, I. H., Cay, E. L., Irving, J. V. and Campbell, M. (1992). Effects of self-help post-myocardial infarction rehabilitation on psychological adjustment and use of health services. *Lancet*, **339**, 1036–40.

Ley, P. (1988). *Communicating with Patients*. London: Croom Helm.

Linn, M. W., Linn, B. S. and Harris, R. (1982). Effects of counselling for late stage cancer patients. *Cancer*, **49**, 1048–55.

Lipowski, Z. J. (1977). Psychosomatic medicine in the seventies: an overview. *American Journal of Psychiatry*, **134**, 223–5.

Lyles, J. N., Burish, T. G., Krozely, M. G. and Oldham, R. K. (1982). Efficacy of relaxation training and guided imagery in reducing the aversiveness of cancer chemotherapy. *Journal of Consulting and Clinical Psychology*, **50**, 509–29.

Moorey, S. (1991). Adjuvant psychological therapy for anxiety and depression. In: *Cancer Patient Care: Psychosocial Treatment Methods*, pp. 94–110. M. Watson (ed.). Cambridge: Cambridge University Press.

Moorey, S. and Greer, S. (1989). *Psychological Therapy for Patients with Cancer: A New Approach*. Oxford: Heinemann Medical.

Morrow, G. R. and Morrell, C. (1982). Behavioral treatment for anticipatory nausea and vomiting induced by cancer chemotherapy. *New England Journal of Medicine*, **307**, 1476–80.

Nicholas, D. R. (1982). Prevalence of anticipatory nausea and emesis in cancer chemotherapy patients. *Journal of Behavioral Medicine*, **5**, 461–3.

Ornish, D., Brown, S. E., Scherwitz, L. W., Billings, J. H., Armstrong, W. T., Ports, T. A., Kirkeeide, R. L., Gould, K. L., Brand, R. J. and Gould, K. L. (1992). Influences of behavioral and medical factors on regression and progression of coronary artery disease. *Abstracts of 2nd International Congress of Behavioral Medicine*, p. 8.

Pearce, S. and Wardle, J. (eds.). (1989). *The Practice of Behavioural Medicine*. Oxford: Oxford University Press.

Redd, W. H., Jacobsen, P. B. Die-Trill, M., Dermatis, H., McEvoy, M. and Holland, J. (1987). Cognitive/attentional distraction in the control of conditioned nausea in pediatric cancer patients receiving chemotherapy. *Journal of Consulting and Clinical Psychology*, **55**, 391–5.

Richardson, J. L., Shelton, D. R., Krailo, M. and Levine, A. M. (1990). The effects of compliance with treatment on survival among patients with hematologic malignancies. *Journal of Clinical Oncology*, **8**, 356–64.

Roskies, E., Seraganian, P., Oseasohn, R., Hanley, J. A., Collu, R., Martin, N. and Smilga, C. (1986). The Montreal Type A Intervention Project: major findings. *Health Psychology*, **5**, 45–69.

Russell, M. A. H., Wilson, C., Taylor, C. and Baker, C. D. (1979). Effect of general practitioners advice against smoking. *British Medical Journal*, **2**, 231–5.

Sackett, D. L. and Snow, J. C. (1979). The magnitude of compliance and noncompliance. In: *Compliance in Health Care*, pp. 11–22. R. B. Haynes, D. W. Taylor and D. L. Sackett (eds.). Baltimore: Johns Hopkins University Press.

Sackett, D. L., Haynes, R. B. and Gibson, E. S. (1975). Randomised clinical trial of strategies for improving medication compliance in primary hypertension. *Lancet*, 1205–7.

Schuler, G., Hambrecht, R., Schlierf, G., Niebauer, J., Houer, K., Neumann, J., Hoberg, E., Drinkmann, A., Bacher, F., Grunze, M. and Kübler, W. (1992). Regular physical exercise and low-fat diet: effects on progression of coronary artery disease. *Circulation*, **86**, 1–11.

Schwartz, G. E. and Weiss, S. (1977). What is behavioral medicine? *Psychosomatic Medicine*, **36**, 377–81.

Sherbourne, C. D., Hays, R. D., Ordway, L., DiMatteo, M. and Kravitz, R. (1992). Antecedents of adherence to medical recommendations: results from the Medical Outcomes Study. *Journal of Behavioral Medicine*, **15**, 447–65.

Simonton, D. C., Matthews-Simonton, S., Creighton, J. L. (1978). *Getting Well*

Again. Los Angeles: Tacher-St Martins.

Southard, D. R., Winett, R. A., Walberg-Rankin, J. L., Neubauer, T. E., Donckers-Roseveare, K., Burkett, P. A., Gould, R. A., Lombard, D. and Moore, J. F. (1992). Increasing the effectiveness of the National Cholesterol Education Program: dietary and behavioral interventions for clinical settings. *Annals of Behavioral Medicine*, **14**, 21–30.

Spiegel, D., Bloom, J. and Yalom, I. D. (1981). Group support for patients with metastic breast cancer. *Archives of General Psychiatry*, **38**, 527–33.

Telch, C. F. and Telch, M. J. (1986). Group coping skills instruction and supportive group therapy for cancer patients: a comparison of strategies. *Journal of Consulting and Clinical Psychology*, **54**, 802–8.

US Department of Health and Human Services (1990). *Healthy People 2000*. Washington DC: USDHHS.

Watts, G. F., Lewis, B., Brunt, J. N. H., Lewis, E. S., Coltart, D. J., Smith, L. D. R., Mann, J. I. and Swan, A. V. (1992). Effects on coronary artery disease of lipid-lowering diet or diet plus cholestyramine in the St Thomas's Atherosclerosis Regression Study (STARS). *Lancet*, **339**, 563–9.

Randomised controlled trial of nicotine chewing-gum

M. J. Jarvis, Martin Raw, M. A. H. Russell and C. Feyerabend

Addiction Research Unit, Institute of Psychiatry, Maudsley Hospital, London SE5, UK; Poisons Unit, New Cross Hospital, London SE14, UK

Abstract

The effectiveness of 2 mg nicotine chewing-gum as an aid to stopping smoking was compared with a placebo containing 1 mg nicotine, but unbuffered, in a double-blind randomised trial. Of 58 subjects given the active gum, 27 (47%) were not smoking at one-year follow-up compared with 12 (21%) of the 58 subjects treated with placebo (p < 0·025). By the most stringent criterion of outcome, 18 (31%) subjects in the active treatment group and eight (14%) in the placebo group had not smoked at all from the start of treatment to follow-up at one year (p < 0·05).

Subjects receiving the active gum experienced less severe withdrawal symptoms and rated their gum as more helpful than did the placebo group. Minor side effects were common but only gastric symptoms were more frequent with the active gum. Subjects receiving active gum used it for longer than those receiving placebo but most stopped using it within six months and only four (7%) developed longer-term dependence. The number of gums used daily correlated significantly with pretreatment blood nicotine concentrations in the active treatment group and with pretreatment cigarette consumption in the placebo group. A lower pretreatment blood nicotine value was the best predictor of success at one year (p < 0·001) but there was no significant relation to cigarette consumption, sex, and social class.

The results clearly confirm the usefulness of nicotine chewing-gum as an aid to stopping smoking and imply a definite role for nicotine in cigarette dependence and withdrawal. Successful use of the gum requires careful attention to subjects' expectations and clear instructions on how to use it.

Introduction

Many smokers give up smoking without any special help or treatment, but others have great difficulty and fail many times. The first smoking-

Reprinted from Jarvis, M. J., Raw, M., Russell, M. A. H. and Feyerabend, C. Randomised controlled trial of nicotine chewing-gum. *British Medical Journal*, **285**, 537–40, 1982.

cessation clinic was started in Stockholm in 1955.[1] Since then there has been an intensive search for an effective treatment for dependent smokers. Simple support and encouragement, given individually or in groups, has a success rate of around 15–25% abstinent at one-year follow-up.[2] Numerous other methods have been tried, including tranquillisers,[3] lobeline,[4] electric aversion therapy,[5] rapid smoking,[6] hypnosis,[7] and, more recently, acupuncture.[8] None of these methods, however, has been found to have a specific effect over and above the attention-placebo element inherent in any treatment.

We have reported encouraging results from the use of nicotine chewing-gum (Nicorette) in our smokers' clinic. In a comparative study the success rate of smokers who received the gum was 38% abstinent at one year of follow-up compared with only 14% of those who had had intensive psychological treatment.[9] We now report the results of a randomised double-blind placebo-controlled trial of the gum with one-year follow-up and biochemical validation of reported abstinence from smoking.

Subjects and methods

The active gum contained 2 mg nicotine and was identical with the commercially available preparation. The placebo gum contained 1 mg nicotine and its biological availability was reduced by the lack of an alkaline buffer to promote absorption through the buccal mucosa. The placebo was designed in this way to mimic the nicotine taste of the active gum without providing an effective pharmacological dose. In pretrial tests the placebo gum did produce appreciable plasma nicotine concentrations with excessive chewing (117 nmol/l (19 ng/ml) when chewed half-hourly for four hours). This suggests that anyone chewing 20 or more placebo gums a day would get a pharmacologically effective dose. The study could therefore be described as a dose-response study. Whatever terminology is preferred, there is no doubt that the "placebo" provided a fairly stringent test of the pharmacological role of nicotine in the efficacy of the active gum. Both active and placebo gums were packed identically and labelled as 2 mg Nicorette.

A total of 116 subjects were entered into the trial. All were cigarette smokers who attended the Maudsley Hospital smokers' clinic for treatment between November 1979 and October 1980 and who agreed to participate in a trial of nicotine chewing-gum. They were treated in groups of about 10, taken in order from the waiting list, each group being allocated at random to receive either the active or placebo gum. There were 12 groups in all, with each of two therapists treating three active-treatment and three placebo groups. Fifty-eight subjects were

Table I. *Comparison of demographic and pretreatment smoking characteristics of subjects receiving active gum and placebo*

	Active gum (n = 58)	Placebo gum (n = 58)
Mean age (years)	41.0	38.4
No (%) of men in group	29 (50.0)	23 (39.7)
No (%) of subjects in social classes I and II	33 (56.9)	29 (50.0)
Mean No of cigarettes smoked daily	30.9	26.5*
Mean plasma nicotine concentration (nmol/l)	199.1	220.7
Mean carboxyhaemoglobin value (%)	7.2	7.0

*$p < 0.05$. (No other differences statistically significant.)
Conversion: SI to traditional units Nicotine: $1 \text{ nmol/l} \approx 0.16 \text{ ng/ml}$.

assigned to the active gum and 58 to the placebo. Therapists and subjects were blind to the allocation.

Before treatment all subjects completed questionnaires about their smoking and attended an assessment interview at which a blood sample was taken two minutes after finishing a cigarette to determine their baseline smoking values of plasma nicotine.[10] Expired-air carbon monoxide[11] or carboxyhaemoglobin[12] values were also measured. Subjects assigned to the two treatments were well matched in demographic characteristics and pretreatment smoking habits, with the exception that those assigned to the active gum tended to be the heavier smokers ($t = 2.1$: $p < 0.05$; table I).

All subjects were given the same instructions about the gum. They were told that it contained nicotine which would be absorbed through the lining of the mouth as it was chewed, and that it would reduce the craving for cigarettes and help to relieve other withdrawal symptoms. They were warned that it might take a few days to get used to the taste, and that they should not expect it to be a miracle cure that removed the necessity for them to work very hard at stopping. They were encouraged to stop smoking completely on the first day of treatment and told to chew a piece of gum whenever the desire to smoke was particularly strong. No restrictions were placed on the number of gums to be chewed each day. It was recommended that they should use the gum for at least three months before attempting to do without it.

Group meetings were held weekly for one hour for the first six weeks. Attendance was similar in those receiving the active and placebo gums, with 28 and 29 subjects respectively attending three or more meetings. Thereafter subjects attended as needed to collect gum and for follow-up

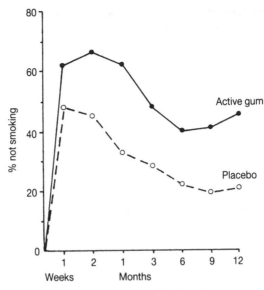

Success rates during treatment and at up to one-year follow-up for subjects receiving active and placebo gums. Percentages based on 58 subjects in each group. Difference at one week not statistically significant; by two weeks significant at 5% level; at one year significant at 1% level.

at three months, six months, and one year. At the one-year follow-up claims of abstinence were validated by measurement of expired air carbon monoxide concentrations. There were no cases of deception. In six subjects assigned to active gum and six assigned to placebo biochemical validation was not done but confirmatory reports were obtained from friends or relatives.

At each attendance subjects completed ratings of withdrawal symptoms, acceptability of their gum, and a check list of potential side effects. They were also given cards to record daily consumption of gum and cigarettes.

Statistical analyses were based on the binomial test, χ^2 test, and t test. Two-sided tests were used except for the analysis of outcome, where the one-sided hypothesis that the active gum was superior to the placebo was tested.

Results

Outcome

The figure shows the success rates of the active and placebo gums. A significant advantage for the active gum emerged as early as two weeks after the start of treatment, when 39 subjects assigned to the active gum were not smoking as compared with only 26 assigned to the placebo ($Z = 2 \cdot 24; p < 0 \cdot 025$). At one year 27 (47%) of those given the active gum were abstinent as compared with 12 (21%) of those given the placebo (see Table II).

The results were unusual in that there were more subjects abstinent in the active-treatment group at one year than at six months, indicating that several subjects who had relapsed at the earlier point stopped smoking again before one year. Table II therefore gives the result of applying more stringent criteria of success to supplement the conventional analysis. Whichever criterion of success was applied the active gum was clearly more effective than the placebo.

Of those abstinent at the one-year follow-up, six in the active-treatment group and two in the placebo group were still using the gum. When for the sake of extreme stringency these subjects were excluded from the one-year abstainers, the active gum retained its clear-cut advantage over placebo with 21 (36%) abstinent at one year compared with 10 (17%) of the placebo group ($Z = 2 \cdot 10$; $p < 0 \cdot 05$). At a mean of 22 months after starting treatment, five of the six subjects given the active gum were still abstinent and three were still using the gum. Both subjects given the placebo had relapsed to smoking.

The figure shows that the main effect of the active gum was to enable more subjects to stop smoking initially. There were also fewer relapses in the active-treatment group, although this failed to reach statistical significance. In the active-treatment group 12 of the 39 subjects abstinent at two weeks had relapsed to smoking at one year, compared with 14 of the 26 in the placebo group ($\chi^2 = 2 \cdot 57$; df = 1; NS).

Quantity and duration of gum use

Use of the active gum was greater than the placebo at every stage of treatment and follow-up both in terms of the proportion of subjects who were using it and the number of pieces they were chewing a day. The differences, however, were statistically significant only at three and six months (table III). Of the seven subjects using active gum and three using placebo gum at the one-year follow-up, only four, all in the active group, had used it continuously throughout the year. The incidence of dependence on the active gum was therefore 7%, and there were no such cases in the placebo group.

Among those who were not smoking at one month there was a significant correlation between the number of gums used daily at that time and the pretreatment blood nicotine concentration in those assigned to the active gum ($r = 0 \cdot 48$; n = 31; $p < 0 \cdot 01$) but not in those assigned

Table II. *Success rates at one-year follow-up according to three different criteria.*
(Figures are numbers (%) of successful subjects)

Criterion of success	Active gum (n = 58)	Placebo gum (n = 58)	Binomial test (Z)	*t* (10 df)*
Abstinent at one year	27 (47)	12 (21)	2.75; $p < 0.01$	2.31; $p < 0.025$
Abstinent at end of initial treatment and at six months and one year	22 (38)	9 (16)	2.52; $p < 0.01$	2.38; $p < 0.025$
No smoking at all from first week of treatment to one year of follow-up	18 (31)	8 (14)	2.00; $p < 0.025$	1.92; $p < 0.05$

Note: One subject receiving active gum was lost to follow-up and classified as a failure despite being abstinent from start of treatment to last contact at five months.
*Since treatment was randomised over groups, not individual subjects, group effects could exist which would invalidate use of binomial test. The more conservative *t* test allows for this possibility. *t* value derived from analysis of variance of angular transformation of group success rates.

Table III. *Comparison of gum use at various times after start of treatment*

Time from start of treatment	No (%) of subjects using gum		Mean No of gums/day†	
	Active gum (n = 58)	Placebo gum (n = 58)	Active gum (n = 58)	Placebo gum (n = 58)
1 week	47 (81)	39 (67)	7.9	6.1
2 weeks	40 (69)	36 (62)	8.1	6.5
1 month	33 (57)	29 (50)	7.5	5.7
3 months	24 (41)	8 (14*)	6.0	3.9
6 months	12 (21)	1 (2*)	6.0	2.0
9 months	5 (9)	1 (2)	7.3	4.0
1 year	7 (12)	3 (5)	5.7	3.7

*$p < 0.005$. (No other differences between active and placebo groups statistically significant.)
†Number of gums daily are averages for those who were using it.

to placebo (r = 0·17; NS). Conversely, pretreatment daily cigarette consumption correlated significantly with daily gum use at one month in those receiving the placebo (r = 0·47; n = 19; p < 0·05) but not in those receiving the active gum (r = 0·11; NS). Correlations with duration of gum use did not reach statistical significance in either group, though similar trends were evident.

There was a positive relation between duration of gum use and success rate at the one-year follow-up which was evident in both the active-treatment and placebo groups. Of 24 subjects in the active group who chewed the gum for three months or more, 18 were abstinent at one year compared with only nine out of 34 who used it for less than three months. The equivalent figures for the placebo group were five out of eight and seven out of 50.

Side effects

Mild and transient symptoms were common with both the active and placebo gums (table IV). They were mainly non-specific effects of heavy chewing. Only in the case of hiccups, indigestion or stomach ache, and feeling sick was the incidence substantially higher and therefore interpretable as specific side effects of the active gum. In most cases these symptoms were mild and transient. In no cases were side effects cited as a cause for discontinuing the gum.

Acceptability of gum

Ten subjects in the active-treatment group and 13 in the placebo group did not attend the first meeting after the start of treatment. We do not know whether this was due to dislike of the gum, disappointment with its efficacy, or other reasons. Among the remainder the active group rated the gum as significantly stronger (p < 0·05) and more helpful (p < 0·05) than the placebo group. Both groups rated the gum as moderately satisfying and slightly unpleasant tasting, and these ratings did not differ significantly between the two groups when averaged over the first six weeks of treatment. In the first week, however, the active group rated their gum as tasting more unpleasant than did the placebo group (p < 0·05), a difference which disappeared by the second week. By the second week the active group found the gum more satisfying than did the placebo group (p < 0·05).

Withdrawal symptoms

Since the pattern of attendance at weekly treatment sessions did not differ between the active-treatment and placebo groups, each subject's

Table IV. *Incidence of unwanted symptoms reported at least once on check list administered weekly during first six weeks of treatment*

	Felt sick	Been sick	Dizziness	Sore throat	Headache	Sore mouth	Felt faint	Hiccups	Indigestion	Tiredness from chewing	Mouth ulcers
Active gum (n = 47)	18	2	10	19	14	28	5	14	24	25	1
Placebo gum (n = 44)	9	0	8	17	17	23	3	2*	12†	26	1

Note: Fewer than 58 subjects in each group owing to early drop-outs. Subjects asked to check whether they had "experienced any of the following this week."

*p < 0.05.
†p < 0.01.

ratings of withdrawal symptoms over the first six weeks of treatment were averaged. Subjects who received the active gum experienced less severe withdrawal symptoms than the placebo group. They felt less irritable ($p < 0.05$), less sleepy ($p < 0.01$), and less hungry ($p < 0.05$). Differences between the groups in ratings of tenseness, feeling miserable, and difficulty doing without cigarettes also favoured the active gum but did not reach statistical significance. The active group, however, also rated themselves as less alert but this difference was not significant.

Characteristics of subjects and outcome

The relation of the variables listed in table I to outcome at the one-year follow-up was similar in the active-treatment and placebo groups, so that the two groups were combined to provide 39 successes and 77 failures. The successes tended to be older (mean age 43 v 38 years; $p < 0.05$) and to have lower pretreatment carboxyhaemoglobin values (mean 6·0% v 7·6%; $p < 0.01$) and lower plasma nicotine concentrations (means 172.0 nmol/l (27·9 ng/ml) v 229·3 nmol/l (37·2 ng/ml); $p < 0.001$). Their mean pretreatment daily cigarette consumption was also lower (26·3 v 29·9) but this difference was not statistically significant. Social class and sex had no relation to outcome. The success rate among the men was 37% (19/52) compared with 31% (20/64) for the women ($\chi^2 = 0.36$; NS).

Discussion

Treatment with the active nicotine chewing-gum achieved results that were substantially better than with the placebo. Success rates, based on three different criteria, were more than double those obtained with placebo. By the conventional criterion of smoking status at follow-up 47% of the subjects in the active-treatment group were abstinent at one year compared with 21% of the subjects given placebo. By the criterion of abstinence at the end of treatment and at six months and one year the success rates were 38% and 16% respectively, and when based on lapse-free abstinence throughout the year from the first week of treatment to the one-year follow-up they were 31% and 14% respectively. The differences were statistically significant in all three cases and were of a similar order to our earlier study, which obtained a 38% success rate (conventionally defined) with nicotine chewing-gum compared with 14% for intensive psychological treatments.[9] In both studies the active gum alone gave results that were well above the range (about 15–25%) reported for all other methods.[2]

Our study was unusual in showing a better result at one year than at six months. This was because some subjects who relapsed returned for further treatment. This response contrasts with studies of other treatment methods, in which those who relapse tend to avoid returning even for follow-up. The tendency for those treated with nicotine gum to be more likely to return for a second course if they relapse may be a further reflection of its greater efficacy.

The rigorous design of our study with randomised allocation, double-blind placebo control, success rates based on all who started treatment, biochemical validation of reported abstinence, and the fact that the placebo provided nicotine to taste but with low biological availability all make it difficult to see how the gum could have achieved its effect other than by a specific action of the nicotine it provided. This further suggests an important role for nicotine in maintaining the habit of dependent smokers. That the active gum was significantly more effective in relieving withdrawal symptoms also supports the view that they may be caused partly be nicotine deprivation.

Another finding also has possible implications for the role of nicotine in smoking. This is that the extent of gum use was significantly related to pretreatment plasma nicotine values but not to cigarette consumption in those given the active gum, whereas the reverse was true for those using the placebo. This suggests that the active gum was fulfilling a pharmacological need while the placebo may have been acting more as an oral substitute. The pharmacological role of nicotine is also supported by the fact that 7% of those assigned to receive the active gum developed some degree of dependence on it, while there were no instances of dependence on the placebo.

On the practical side, the active gum was apparently more effective in helping smokers to stop smoking during the first four weeks of treatment than in reducing the tendency to relapse thereafter. Other studies have found higher rates of long-term success among those who continued using the gum for longer periods.[9] [13] While it was realised that this may have been attributable to self-selection with people continuing to chew while they were successfully keeping off cigarettes but giving up the gum as soon as they relapsed to smoking, this finding was nevertheless used as a reason for suggesting that longer-term use of the gum might improve outcome.[14] That our placebo group also showed a similar trend in this direction suggests that further study is needed to establish the optimal duration of gum use.

We emphasise that the high success rate achieved in this study was not necessarily due to the gum alone. The subjects had six group meetings with an experienced therapist. Above all they were given careful instructions on what they might realistically expect from the gum and how to use it correctly. This no doubt accounted for the lack of more than mild and transient side effects. That the active gum was initially more unpleasant to taste but subsequently became more satisfying points to the importance of encouraging subjects to persist with it for at least two weeks.

We conclude that after more than 20 years of unsuccessful research into all kinds of treatment methods for smokers, nicotine chewing-gum given to well-motivated smokers in a clinic setting is the first treatment to have been developed that has a specific effect over and above that attributable to an attention-placebo response. That it is also the first treatment to provide effective nicotine substitution has important implications for the role of nicotine in cigarette dependence.

Acknowledgements

We thank the Medical Research Council and Department of Health and Social Security for financial support, A B Leo for supplying the nicotine and placebo gum, and Vera Amato for secretarial help. Our colleagues Gill Devitt, John Stapleton, Steve Sutton, Colin Taylor, and Robert West gave helpful comments.

References

1 Ejrup B. Proposals for treatment of smokers with severe clinical symptoms brought about by their smoking habit. *British Columbia Medical Journal* 1960; 2:441–53.
2 Raw M. The treatment of cigarette dependence. In: Israel Y, Glaser FB, Kalant H, Popham RE, Schmidt W, Smart RG, eds. *Research advances in alcohol and drug problems*. Vol. 4. New York; Plenum, 1978:441–85.
3 Schwartz JL, Dubitsky M. Maximising success in smoking cessation methods. *Am J Public Health*, 1969;59:1392–9.
4 British Tuberculosis Association. Smoking deterrent study. *Br Med J* 1963;ii:486–7.
5 Russell MAH, Armstrong E, Patel UA. Temporal contiguity in electric aversion therapy for cigarette smoking. *Behav Res Ther* 1976;14:103–23.
6 Raw M, Russell MAH. Rapid smoking, cue exposure and support in the modification of smoking. *Behav Res Ther* 1980;18:363–72.
7 Berkowitz B, Ross-Townsend A, Kohberger R. Hypnotic treatment of smoking: the single-treatment method revisited. *Am J Psychiatry* 1979;136:83–5.
8 Lamontagne Y, Annable L, Gagnon MA. Acupuncture for smokers: lack of long-term therapeutic effect in a controlled study. *Can Med Assoc J* 1980;122:787–90.
9 Raw M, Jarvis MJ, Russell MAH. Comparison of nicotine chewing-gum and psychological treatments for dependent smokers. *Br Med J* 1980;281:481–2.
10 Feyerabend C, Russell MAH. Assay of nicotine in biological materials: sources of contamination and their elimination. *J Pharm Pharmacol* 1980;32:178–81.
11 Jarvis MJ, Russell MAH, Saloojee, Y. Expired air carbon monoxide: a simple breath test of tobacco smoke intake. *Br Med J* 1980;281:484–5.

12 Russell MAH, Cole PV, Brown E. Absorption by non-smokers of carbon monoxide from room-air polluted by tobacco smoke. *Lancet* 1973;i:576–9.

13 Wilhelmson L, Hjalmarson A. Smoking cessation experience in Sweden. *Canadian Family Physician* 1980;**26**:737–47.

14 Russell MAH, Raw M, Jarvis MJ. Clinical use of nicotine chewing-gum. *Br Med J* 1980;**280**:1599–1602.

Conditioned side effects induced by cancer chemotherapy: prevention through behavioral treatment

Thomas G. Burish, Michael P. Carey, Mary G. Krozely and
F. Anthony Greco

Vanderbilt University

Abstract

Cancer patients receiving chemotherapy often experience nausea and vomiting
that develop as a result of classical conditioning. In order to determine whether
this nausea and vomiting could be delayed or prevented, 24 cancer patients were
randomized either to a group that received progressive muscle relaxation training
(PMRT) plus guided imagery (GI), or to a no-treatment control group.
Relaxation training sessions were held before the initiation of chemotherapy and
during the first three chemotherapy treatments. Results indicated that patients
receiving PMRT and GI had significantly less nausea and vomiting and significantly lower blood pressures, pulse rates, and dysphoria, especially anxiety, than did
control patients. Nurse observations corroborated patient reports. These data
suggest that early training in PMRT and GI can reduce and perhaps prevent the
development of conditioned nausea and vomiting, and can alleviate high anxiety
levels, in cancer patients who receive emetogenic chemotherapy.

The side effects of cancer chemotherapy can be so aversive and
debilitating that some patients regard them as worse than the cancer
itself. Such patients often are noncompliant with their treatment, and a
few reject further treatment altogether (Wilcox, Fetting, Nettesheim, &
Abeloff, 1982). Among the most dreaded of the side effects are the
conditioned nausea and vomiting (CNV) experienced by approximately
25%–30% of all patients. Evidence suggests that CNV develop through a
classical conditioning process; that is, through their association with
pharmacologically induced side effects, various stimuli (e.g., smells,

Burish, T. G., Carey, M. P., Krozely, M. G. and Greco, F. A. Conditioned side
effects induced by cancer chemotherapy: prevention through behavioral treatment. *Journal of Consulting and Clinical Psychology*, 55, 42–8. Copyright (1987)
by the American Psychological Association. Reprinted by permission.

thoughts, tastes) become capable of eliciting nausea, vomiting, and intense emotional reactions (see Burish & Carey, 1986). Conditioned side effects can occur before the chemotherapy treatment begins, in which case they are referred to as *anticipatory side effects*, or they can occur during or after the treatment, in which case they appear with and are often indistinguishable from pharmacologically induced side effects. In all cases, once CNV have developed, they are highly resistant to antiemetic drugs.

The prevalence of CNV, as well as their resistance to pharmacological control, has produced considerable concern and research in recent years. Several investigators have studied the effectiveness of behavioral treatments such as progressive muscle relaxation training (e.g., Lyles, Burish, Krozely, & Oldham, 1982), systematic desensitization (e.g., Morrow & Morrell, 1982), biofeedback (e.g., Burish, Shartner, & Lyles, 1981), and hypnosis (e.g., Redd, Andresen, & Minagawa, 1982) in controlling conditioned side effects. In general, these interventions have been successful in producing decreases in the frequency and severity of conditioned responses. Of importance, however, is that there have been no reports of research in which an intervention has been used to *prevent* the development of conditioned side effects. However, because conditioned side effects are learned, one should be able to prevent or at least to retard their development. Obviously, the prevention of conditioned side effects could substantially reduce the aversiveness of cancer chemotherapy. On the basis of our prior research on the use of progressive muscle relaxation training (PMRT) plus guided relaxation imagery (GI) as a treatment intervention for CNV, we hypothesized that the introduction of a behavioral relaxation intervention before chemotherapy began could prevent or at least delay the development of conditioned responses. In addition, a behavioral relaxation procedure should reduce the emotional distress and psychological arousal generally experienced by cancer chemotherapy patients, thereby reducing the overall unpleasantness of the chemotherapy experience.

Therefore, in this study one group of cancer patients was taught PMRT and GI before beginning their first course of chemotherapy, whereas a second group received no training in PMRT or GI. All patients were then followed through their first five chemotherapy treatments. We hypothesized that conditioned side effects would develop in untreated patients by the fourth or fifth sessions (e.g., Nerenz, Leventhal, Easterling, & Love, 1986), but not in patients given PMRT and GI. Thus for the most part, differences between groups were expected primarily during these later sessions. We decided not to include a placebo- or attention-control group for ethical reasons; specifically, we chose not to ask new cancer patients to come to the oncology clinic at their own expense and on their own time exclusively for a "treatment" that was unlikely to be effective. Also, prior research has clearly and consistently demonstrated that patients receiving "placebo" or "nonspecific" treatments fare no better than do no-treatment control patients (e.g., Lyles et al., 1982; Morrow & Morell, 1982).

Method

Patients and design

Twenty-four patients with histologically confirmed cancer who had not previously received chemotherapy participated in the study. The specific types of cancer represented in the patient sample were as follows: 10 ovarian, 9 breast, 4 lung, and 1 Hodgkins. All patients received their chemotherapy on an outpatient basis. Only patients whose first treatment was scheduled at least 48 hr after the time they were referred to the study and who were scheduled to receive highly emetogenic chemotherapy regimens were invited to participate. Degree of emetogenicity was determined via the following procedure: The emetic potencies of various chemotherapy drugs and protocols were rated by each clinic physician and nurse on a scale from 1 (*no nausea and vomiting*) to 5 (*intense nausea and vomiting*). Only patients on protocols with an average rating of 3 or greater were considered for entry into the study.[1] This procedure was followed because previous data suggested that patients on emetogenic protocols are much more likely to develop CNV than are patients who are not on such protocols (e.g., Ingle, Burish, & Wallston, 1984; Morrow, 1984).

Patients were assigned either to a relaxation-training or to a no-relaxation-training (i.e., control) group according to a stratified random assignment procedure: Specific drug emetogenicity as well as antiemetic medications were equated for patients in the two conditions. The average length of time between treatments was approximately 15 days.

Evaluation technique

Physiological measures

Pulse rate and blood pressure levels were recorded immediately before and after each chemotherapy treatment. We monitored pulse rate by

---

[1] Mean nurse ($N = 5$) and physician ($N = 5$) ratings of emetogenicity were highly related, $r(8) = .87$, $p < .001$. Examples of protocols and their emetogenicity ratings are as follows: HCAP = 4.5; DTIC = 4.3; high-dose dioxorubicin = 4.1; MOPP = 3.7; CAV = 3.4; CMF = 3.0.

manually palpating the radial artery for 30 s; blood pressure was recorded from the brachial artery via the auscultatory method.

Multiple Affect Adjective Check List

A shortened version of the Multiple Affect Adjective Check List (MAACL; Zuckerman, Lubin, Vogel, & Valerius, 1964) was administered immediately after the physiological measures were obtained. The MAACL provided a self-report index of patients' anxiety (AACL), hostility (HACL), and depression (DACL).

Postchemotherapy rating scales

Immediately after the MAACL was completed, patients were asked to rate, on 7-point scales ranging from *not at all* (1) to *extremely* (7), the extent to which they felt anxious and nauseated during the chemotherapy treatment. Nurses who administered the chemotherapy were asked to rate the extent to which they perceived patients to be anxious and nauseated during the chemotherapy, and also to record the number of times that patients vomited while receiving the treatment. Although it was impossible for us to have the attending nurses unaware of whether patients received relaxation training, each nurse was unaware of the ratings made by patients and other nurses and of the physiological data.

Home records

After each chemotherapy treatment was completed and the other evaluation measures had been collected, patients were given the Home Record Form (HRF) with which they rated, on a 7-point scale ranging from *not at all* (1) to *extremely* (7), their level of anxiety and nausea as well as the number of times that they vomited during the 72 hr after chemotherapy. This time was divided into 12 consecutive periods (blocks) each lasting approximately 6 hr. The HRF thus provided a detailed self-report index of the anxiety, nausea, and vomiting that occurred during the hours and days that followed chemotherapy.

Procedure

Patients assigned to the relaxation-training condition were contacted before their first chemotherapy treatment, whereas patients in the control group were contacted on the day of their initial chemotherapy treatment. All patients were told that the general purpose of the study was to learn more about patients' responses to the chemotherapy process and how best to prevent the development of side effects. Patients were then given additional information specific to the group to which they had been assigned and were asked to read and sign an informed-consent form. The procedures then differed for patients in each group.

Relaxation training: Prechemotherapy sessions

Patients in the PMRT and GI group were given one to three relaxation-training sessions before their first chemotherapy treatment. The specific number of sessions depended on several factors, the most important being the amount of time available before the first treatment.[2] These sessions were held either in the clinic during nonclinic hours or in the patient's home if coming to the clinic was not possible. The patient's spouse and family members were invited to attend the sessions if they and the patient so desired. During the first training session, the therapist described in detail the purpose and nature of the relaxation-training procedure. The patient was told that relaxation training would enable him or her to recognize muscle tension in the body and would allow him or her to reduce unnecessary tension and become as calm as possible. Patients were told that being calm and relaxed before, during, and after chemotherapy would help to reduce the unpleasantness of the experience and the severity of some of the side effects. Patients were also told that relaxation is a general coping skill that can be used in a variety of unpleasant situations. The therapist then described and demonstrated a standard progressive muscle-relaxation-training procedure (Bernstein & Borkovec, 1973). The therapist explained that the patient would be asked to tense and then relax most of the major muscle groups in the body, focusing on the sensations of tension and relaxation that these exercises produced. The therapist explained that after this relaxing procedure was completed, the patient would be helped to relax even further by the use of relaxation imagery. The patient was then briefly interviewed to identify in some detail imagery that would be especially relaxing.

After this explanation, the patient and any family members were directed in PMRT, followed by GI. This procedure lasted approximately 30–45 min and was audiotaped. After the procedure was completed, the patient was interviewed in regard to the effectiveness of the relaxation procedure; if necessary, minor changes were made in the procedures in accordance with each patient's particular needs. The patient was given the tape of the session and encouraged to practice the procedure daily.

---

[2] Analyses indicated that the number of prechemotherapy relaxation training sessions was not related to treatment outcome.

One or two additional relaxation sessions were scheduled before the first chemotherapy treatment if time allowed. The patients were told that the therapist would guide them in PMRT and GI during chemotherapy and that they should call the therapist if they had any difficulties or question.

Relaxation training: Chemotherapy sessions

During the first five chemotherapy sessions, patients in the relaxation-training group were met in the clinic by the therapist approximately 45 min before the chemotherapy was scheduled. The patient was escorted to a private treatment room and seated in a comfortable recliner-type chair. The patient's pulse rate and blood pressure were recorded and the presession MAACL was administered. The therapist again explained briefly the purposes of the relaxation-training procedure and outlined what would happen during the remainder of the session.

The patient was then directed in PMRT and GI. Shortly after the imagery procedure started, the nurse entered the treatment room, administered the chemotherapy, and then left the room. The relaxation imagery was continued for 2–3 additional min, after which the therapist terminated the relaxation induction. The therapist recorded the patient's pulse rate and blood pressure, administered a postsession MAACL, and asked the patient and attending nurse to independently complete the postchemotherapy rating scales. Last, the patient was given the HRF and was encouraged to continue to practice the relaxation training procedure daily at home. On the day after the chemotherapy session, the therapist called the patient to remind him or her to complete the HRF and to encourage the continued practice of relaxation training.

The procedures during the patient's second and third chemotherapy treatments were similar to those of the first chemotherapy treatment with one major exception. During these subsequent treatments, the patient was taught progressively less time-consuming versions of relaxation training, and was given increasing responsibility in directing his or her own relaxation imagery. At the beginning of the fourth chemotherapy session, patients were told that they were ready to completely self-administer the relaxation training procedure. During this and subsequent chemotherapy sessions, patients were told to relax on their own as much as possible by applying the same relaxation techniques that they had used during previous chemotherapy sessions and had been practicing at home between chemotherapy sessions. Except for the fact that the patient self-administered the relaxation training, the procedures followed during the fourth and fifth sessions were virtually identical to those used during earlier sessions.

No relaxation training: Chemotherapy sessions

As described earlier, patients in the control condition were told about the nature of the study and signed the informed-consent form before their first chemotherapy treatment; they were also informed at this time that in order to help them relax before receiving chemotherapy, they would be taken to a private treatment room and would be allowed to rest comfortably in the reclining treatment chair. They were told that if a patient is relaxed and calm before and during chemotherapy, the experience of chemotherapy would be less unpleasant and the likelihood and severity of some side effects would be reduced. Presession dependent measures were then collected and patients were allowed to rest comfortably. At the scheduled time the nurse entered the room and administered the chemotherapy in the routine fashion. After the nurse left the room, the therapist entered and collected the postsession dependent measures, following the same procedures used with patients in the relaxation-training condition. Last, the patient was instructed in the use of the HRF. Patients in the no-relaxation-training condition were also called by the therapist on the day after their treatments and reminded to complete the HRF. These same procedures were followed during each of the subsequent chemotherapy sessions.

Results

Overview of Statistical Analyses

Data were analyzed as follows: Separate 2 (Group) × 5 (Session) mixed analyses of variance (ANOVAS) were carried out on the prechemotherapy and postchemotherapy physiological measures and MAACL data, and on the postchemotherapy rating scales and vomiting data. Separate 2 (Group) × 5 (Session) × 12 (6-hr Time Block) mixed ANOVAS were carried out on the HRF data. In appropriate cases, main effects and interactions that reached statistical significance were investigated further with Duncan multiple-range tests.

Nausea

The analyses of the patient ratings of nausea revealed main effects for group, $F(1, 22) = 6.60$, $p < .02$, and session, $F(4, 85) = 2.19$, $p < .05$, and a Group × Session interaction, $F(4, 85) = 3.08$, $p = .02$. The analyses of the nurse ratings of nausea revealed a similar pattern of results, corresponding $Fs(1, 22) = 12.06$ ($p = .002$), 6.23 ($p = .001$), and 4.26 ($p = .004$). Inspection of these data with Duncan multiple range tests

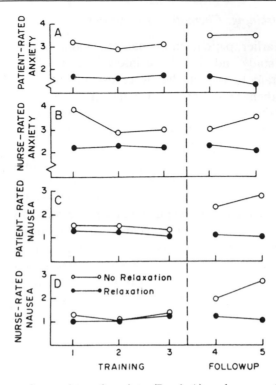

Figure 1. Mean patient ratings of anxiety (Panel A) and nausea (Panel C) during chemotherapy; and mean ratings by attending nurses of patients' anxiety (Panel B) and nausea (Panel D) during chemotherapy.

(see Figure 1) indicated that, as expected, there were no differences between groups during the first three chemotherapy treatments. However, most likely because of the initiation of conditioning, the nausea levels of the control patients increased during the fourth and fifth sessions, whereas the levels of patients who received relaxation training remained fairly constant. The difference between groups was significant, as rated both by patients ($p < .01$) and by nurses ($p < .02$).

The amount of nausea experienced at home during the 72 hr after chemotherapy was monitored with the HRF. Analysis of these data revealed main effects for group, $F(1, 22) = 7.52$, $p = .011$, and block, $F(11, 242) = 6.26$, $p < .001$, and a Group $\times$ Block interaction, $F(11, 242) = 2.00$, $p = .03$. Subsequent comparisons indicated that during the first 18 hr after chemotherapy (i.e., during the first three time blocks), both the relaxation-training patients and the control patients showed similar levels of nausea. However, whereas control patients still displayed elevated nausea levels 24 hr after chemotherapy, the nausea levels of

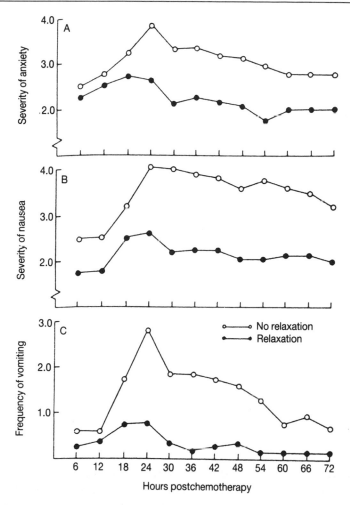

Figure 2. Mean patient ratings of anxiety (Panel A), nausea (Panel B), and vomiting (Panel C) during the 72 hr immediately after chemotherapy. (Scores are averaged across treatment sessions.)

relaxation-trained patients decreased significantly ($p < .05$) and remained significantly ($p < .05$) lower at each subsequent recording period until 60 hr postchemotherapy, at which time the nausea levels of patients in the control group finally decreased to a level that was statistically equivalent to that of the relaxation-training patients (see Figure 2). Overall, therefore, PMRT and GI were highly effective in minimizing the duration and severity of postchemotherapy nausea.

Last, in order to determine whether relaxation training actually prevented the development of conditioned nausea as opposed to simply

Table 1. *Fifth-session nausea intensity ratings by patients and nurse observers*

	Patient ratings		Nurse ratings	
Nausea intensity	RT	NRT	RT	NRT
None	90	46	80	27
Moderate	10	27	20	46
Severe	0	27	0	27

Note: RT = relaxation training; NRT = no relaxation training. On the 7-point nausea rating scale, intensity of nausea was determined as follows: 1 = *none*; 2–4 = *moderate*; 5–7 = *severe*. Data were unavailable for 4 patients on these measures during Session 5. Percentages reflect scores on the 20 remaining subjects.

reducing its severity, the percentage of patients experiencing no, mild, or severe nausea during the fifth chemotherapy session was calculated for each group (see Table 1). As inspection of these data shows, even by the last session the overwhelming majority of patients in the relaxation condition reported no nausea during chemotherapy; the nurse observations corroborated these ratings. These data suggest strongly that at least through the fifth treatment session, relaxation training prevented the development of conditioned nausea in most patients.

Vomiting

The frequency of vomiting during the short time in which chemotherapy was actually administered was very low in all patients (relaxation training: $M = 0.0$ per session; control: $M = 0.2$ per session); thus no significant differences emerged between groups. However, the frequency of vomiting reported by patients during the 72 hr after chemotherapy was affected by the PMRT procedure. Specifically, the analysis revealed main effects for group, $F(1, 22) = 7.54$, $p < .02$, session, $F(4, 84) = 3.72$, $p = .008$, and block $F(11, 242) = 4.13$, $p < .001$, and a Group × Block interaction, $F(11, 242) = 1.96$, $p < .04$. The session effect was attributable to the unusual and perhaps random finding that across both groups the frequency of vomiting was significantly lower after Session 2 ($M = 0.37$) than after any of the other sessions (overall $M = 0.98$). What is more important is that follow-up analysis of the Group × Block interaction revealed that, as with the nausea data, both groups showed similarly elevated frequencies of vomiting during the first 18 hr after chemotherapy. However, after this time the frequency of vomiting in relaxation-training patients began to stabilize and then returned to baseline levels. In contrast, the frequency of vomiting of control patients continued to rise at 24 hr and remained significantly higher ($p < .05$) than that of the PMRT patients until 54 hr after chemotherapy. After this point the control patients' vomiting frequency finally decreased to a level statistically equivalent to that of the relaxation-training patients (see Figure 2).

Emotional Distress

Patients ratings of how anxious (AACL), hostile (HACL), and depressed (DACL) they felt as they awaited their chemotherapy (i.e., at the pressession time) are displayed in Figure 3. Analyses on these data revealed significant Group × Session interactions for anxiety, $F(4, 83) = 4.95$, $p = .002$, and hostility, $F(4, 83) = 6.07$, $p < .001$. Patients in both groups showed similar presession scores on the AACL, HACL, and DACL during the first three chemotherapy sessions (see Figure 3). However, by Sessions 4 and 5, patients in the relaxation-training condition reported feeling significantly less anxious ($p < .01$) as they awaited chemotherapy, and by Session 5 they also reported feeling less hostile ($p < .01$). The postsession MAACL data were even stronger, and analyses revealed a group main effect for anxiety, $F(1, 22) = 4.58$, $p < .05$. amd a Group × Session interaction for hostility, $F(4, 830) = 19.53$, $p < .001$, and depression, $F(4, 830) = 3.83$, $p < .006$ (see Figure 4). As these data suggest, patients who received PMRT reported feeling significantly less anxious after each chemotherapy session than patients who did not receive relaxation training. Moreover, after Sessions 4 and 5, relaxation-training patients reported feeling significantly less depressed ($p < .05$) and, after Session 5, less hostile ($p < .05$) than patients in the control condition.

The analysis of the patients' ratings of anxiety during the actual chemotherapy infusion also revealed a significant difference: Patients who received PMRT and GI rated themselves as less anxious, main effect $F(1, 22) = 15.90$, $p < .001$, during all sessions than did the control patients. The nurses who administered the chemotherapy also rated the relaxation-training patients as being significantly less anxious, main effect $F(1, 22) = 12.52$, $p = .002$, than the control patients (see Figure 1).

Relaxation training also affected the anxiety levels that patients experienced at home after chemotherapy. Specifically, the data revealed a main effect for group, $F(1, 22) = 4.00$, $p = .055$, and a Group × Session interaction, $F(4, 84) = 5.40$, $p < .001$, and a Group × Block interaction, $F(11, 242) = 2.04$, $p = .025$. Further inspection of the Group × Block interaction (see Figure 2) indicated that, as with the nausea and vomiting data, there were no significant differences between groups during the first

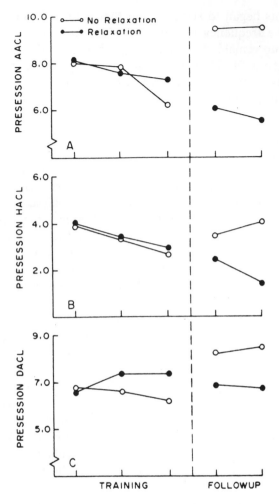

Figure 3. Mean anxiety (Panel A), hostility (Panel B), and depression (Panel C) scores before each chemotherapy session.

18 hr after chemotherapy. However, patients in the relaxation-training condition began to report significantly ($p < .05$) less anxiety by 24 hr, and continued to report significantly less anxiety throughout the remainder of the 72-hr home rating period. The Group × Session interaction suggested that if one collapses across time blocks, the significant ($p < .01$) posttreatment reduction in anxiety in the relaxation-training subjects began, not immediately, but rather during Session 3 and continued through the remaining sessions of the study.

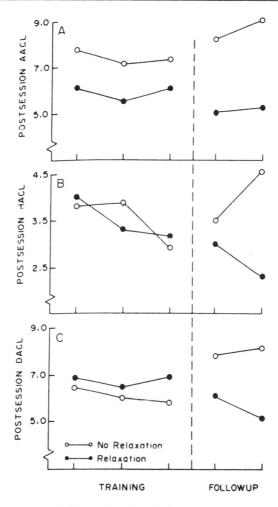

Figure 4. Mean anxiety (Panel A), hostility (Panel B), and depression (Panel C) scores after each chemotherapy session.

Physiological arousal

There were no significant differences between groups on any physiological measure at the beginning of the chemotherapy sessions, which indicates that the groups were comparable before the behavioral treatment. However, by the end of the chemotherapy treatments, the patients in the relaxation-training condition had significantly lower pulse rates, systolic blood pressures, and diastolic blood pressures than did patients in the control condition, main effect $Fs(1, 22) = 4.23$ ($p = .05$), 12.40 ($p = .002$), and 11.68 ($p = .003$), respectively (see Figure 5). Thus

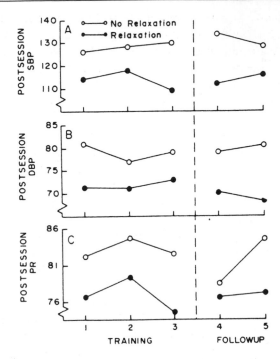

Figure 5. Mean systolic blood pressure (Panel A), diastolic blood pressure (Panel B), and pulse rate (Panel C) after each chemotherapy session.

relaxation training also proved to be effective in reducing patients' levels of autonomic arousal during the chemotherapy sessions.

Discussion

The results demonstrate that PMRT plus GI can be an effective procedure for reducing, and perhaps preventing, the CNV that frequently accompany cancer chemotherapy. Specifically, these data demonstrate that for many patients, relaxation procedures can prevent the development of anticipatory nausea and vomiting and can ameliorate the conditioned side effects that occur during the 72 hr that immediately follow chemotherapy. The study extended through five chemotherapy treatments, and it is possible that patients receiving additional treatments might develop CNV during later chemotherapy infusions. However, considerable prior research has documented that CNV usually develop by the third or fourth treatment (e.g., Nerenz et al., 1986). In accordance with that observation, the majority of control patients in this study appeared to develop conditioned side effects by the fourth treatment.

These data clearly suggest that the relaxation-training procedure protected patients through the time when conditioning usually emerges. During the fourth and fifth treatments, patients were actually relaxing themselves, demonstrating that they had learned the relaxation technique and could successfully use it on their own. The ability to self-administer relaxation should help to protect patients from developing conditioned symptoms during subsequent treatment.

An additional benefit of relaxation training is its effect on reducing dysphoria. Patients who received relaxation training reported feeling less anxious during and after chemotherapy than did patients who did not receive relaxation training. By the fourth treatment, relaxation-training patients were also reporting less anxiety as they sat in the treatment room and awaited their chemotherapy infusion—normally a very tense time for patients. This effect is probably attributable to patients' increased confidence in the effectiveness of the relaxation-training procedure. By the fourth and fifth treatments, relaxation-training patients also reported feeling less hostile or depressed, or both, than no-relaxation-training patients. Relaxation training also resulted in significant reductions in physiological arousal, namely, pulse rate, systolic blood pressure, and diastolic blood pressure. This finding is consistent with other studies that also have documented significant reductions in physiological arousal after the use of relaxation training (e.g., Paul, 1969). In summary, patients who used relaxation training were able to adopt a more positive emotional state and to decrease their physiological arousal, thereby reducing the general stressfulness of the chemotherapy session.

There are several possible mechanisms through which relaxation training may have exerted its effects. First, the results might be explained by the various "nonspecific" factors such as patient expectation of benefit and increased attention. However, this possibility has been previously investigated and ruled out in the chemotherapy context by Lyles *et al.* (1982) and by Morrow and Morrell (1982), and also has been studied and ruled out in a variety of other contexts (e.g., Jacob, Kraemer, & Agras, 1977). The results of these investigations have demonstrated that the effectiveness of relaxation training cannot be accounted for by patient expectancy (i.e., the placebo effect) or by the increased attention and support that these patients have received. Furthermore, research on the use of antiemetic treatments has shown that expectancy alone cannot produce a consistent reduction in nausea and vomiting (Laszlo, 1983). Overall, therefore, it is unlikely that the effectiveness of PMRT and GI can be accounted for by patient expectancy or other nonspecific factors.

A second and more likely mechanism contributing to the effectiveness of relaxation training is attentional diversion, that is, relaxation may exert its effect by diverting patients' attention away from the chemotherapy context and toward more pleasant and relaxing thoughts. Diverting attention is important in dealing with CNV because presumably attending to or even thinking about the chemotherapy situation has developed into a conditioned stimulus capable of eliciting CNV, intense anxiety, and so on. Thus to the extent that patients are able to divert their attention away from these conditioned stimuli, they should show a corresponding reduction in their conditioned responses. Several studies have documented the effectiveness of attentional diversion strategies for the reduction of stress and pain (McCaul & Malott, 1984), and it is likely that this aspect of relaxation training contributes to its efficacy with chemotherapy patients.

A third factor that may explain some of the effectiveness of PMRT and GI is the induction of a state of deep relaxation. Relaxation may reduce CNV through one or more of several mechanisms. First, relaxation may reduce muscular contractions in the gastrointestinal tract that are involved with vomiting. Second, relaxation may reduce CNV indirectly by reducing anxiety. Anxiety, because of its association with the side effects of chemotherapy, may become a conditioned stimulus for CNV and, of course, it also contributes directly to the stressfulness of overall chemotherapy experience. Therefore, by reducing anxiety, PMRT and GI may reduce the cues for CNV and relieve some of the distress that normally accompanies each treatment. Third, Borison and McCarthy (1983) suggested that physiological sedation may have antiemetic effects because of the biochemical changes that it produces. It is possible that behaviorally induced relaxation may have similar physiological sedation or relaxation effects. Unfortunately, few researchers have directly explored this possibility.

In summary, the data generated in this study provide the first evidence that behavioral changes may be effective in preventing, or at least retarding the development of, conditioned responses in cancer chemotherapy patients. Moreover, the data suggest that many patients are able to successfully induce self-relaxation after several therapist-directed sessions, thereby increasing the likelihood of relaxation's continued protective effects and its overall cost effectiveness. Taken together, these findings suggest that the early introduction of behavioral techniques, rather than their later introduction as is now commonly the practice, may have several clinical advantages in reducing the distress of chemotherapy.

Acknowledgements

This project was partly supported by Grant CA25516 from the National Cancer Institute.

We thank Dean Brenner and David Holmes for their helpful comments on the manuscript, Denise Matt for her help with the statistical analysis, and the entire staff of the Vanderbilt University Medical Center Oncology/Hematology Clinic for their contributions to this research.

References

Bernstein, D. A., & Borkovec, T. D. (1973). *Progressive relaxation training: A manual for the helping professions*. Champaign, IL: Research Press.

Borison, H. L., & McCarthy, L. E. (1983). Neuropharmacologic mechanisms of emesis. In J. Laszlo (Ed.), *Antiemetics and cancer chemotherapy* (pp. 6–20). Baltimore, MD: Williams & Wilkins.

Burish, T. G., & Carey, M. P. (1986). Conditioned aversive responses in cancer chemotherapy patients. Theoretical and developmental analysis. *Journal of Consulting and Clinical Psychology, 54*, 593–600.

Burish, T. G., Shartner, C. D., & Lyles, J. N. (1981). Effectiveness of multiple-site EMG biofeedback and relaxation in reducing the aversiveness of cancer chemotherapy. *Biofeedback and Self-Regulation, 6*, 523–535.

Ingle, R. J., Burish, T. G., & Wallston, K. A. (1984). Conditionability of cancer chemotherapy patients. *Oncology Nursing Forum, 11*, 97–102.

Jacob, R. G., Kraemer, H. C., & Agras, W. S. (1977). Relaxation therapy in the treatment of hypertension: A review. *Archives of General Psychiatry, 34*, 1417–1427.

Laszlo, J. (1983). Emesis as limiting toxicity in cancer chemotherapy. In J. Laszlo (Ed.), *Antiemetics and cancer chemotherapy* (pp. 1–5). Baltimore, MD: Williams & Wilkins.

Lyles, J. N., Burish, T. G., Krozely, M. G., & Oldham, R. K. (1982). Efficacy of relaxation training and guided imagery in reducing the adverseness of cancer chemotherapy. *Journal of Consulting and Clinical Psychology, 50*, 509–529.

McCaul, K. D. & Malott, J. M. (1984). Distraction and coping with pain. *Psychological Bulletin, 95*, 516–533.

Morrow, G. R. (1984). Clinical characteristics associated with the development of anticipatory nausea and vomiting in cancer patients undergoing chemotherapy treatment. *Journal of Clinical Oncology, 2*, 1170–1176.

Morrow, G. R., & Morrell, C. (1982). Behavioral treatment for anticipatory nausea and vomiting induced by cancer chemotherapy. *New England Journal of Medicine, 307*, 1476–1480.

Nerenz, D. R., Leventhal, H., Easterling, D. V., & Love, R. R. (1986). Anxiety and drug taste as predictors of anticipatory nausea in cancer chemotherapy. *Journal of Clinical Oncology, 4*, 224–233.

Paul, G. L. (1969). Physiological effects of relaxation training and hypnotic suggestion. *Journal of Abnormal Psychology, 74*, 425–437.

Redd, W. H., Andresen, G. V., & Minagawa, R. Y. (1982). Hypnotic control of anticipatory emesis in patients receiving cancer chemotherapy. *Journal of Consulting and Clinical Psychology, 50*, 14–19.

Wilcox, P. M., Fetting, J. H., Nettesheim, K. M., & Abeloff, M. D. (1982). Anticipatory vomiting in women receiving cyclophosphamide, methotrexate, and 5-FU (MF) adjuvant chemotherapy for breast carcinoma. *Cancer Treatment Reports, 66,* 1601–1604.

Zuckerman, M., Lubin, V., Vogel, L., & Valerius, E. (1964). Measurement of experimentally induced affects. *Journal of Consulting and Clinical Psychology, 28,* 418–425.

Improvement of medication compliance in uncontrolled hypertension

R. Brian Haynes, David L. Sackett, Edward S. Gibson, D. Wayne Taylor, Brenda C. Hackett, Robin S. Roberts and Arnold L. Johnson

Department of Clinical Epidemiology and Biostatistics, McMaster University Medical Centre, and Dominion Foundries and Steel Limited, Hamilton, Ontario, Canada

Summary

38 hypertensive Canadian steelworkers who were neither compliant with medications nor at goal diastolic blood-pressure six months after starting treatment were allocated either to a control group or to an experimental group who were taught how to measure their own blood-pressures, asked to chart their home blood-pressures and pill taking, and taught how to tailor pill taking to their daily habits and rituals; these men were also seen fortnightly by a high-school graduate with no formal health professional training who reinforced the experimental manœuvres and rewarded improvements in compliance and blood-pressure. Six months later, average compliance had fallen by 1·5% in the control group but rose 21·3% in the experimental group. Blood-pressures fell in 17 of 20 experimental patients (to goal in 6) and in 10 of 18 control patients (to goal in 2).

Introduction

The potential benefit of vigorous medical treatment for hypertension often remains out of reach, in part because the patient does not comply with treatment. We believe that this non-compliance is a major barrier to the effective control of hypertension[1] and that our understanding of this phenomenon is primitive.[2] In phase I of a trial of strategies for improving compliance we found[3] that neither the mastery of facts about hypertension nor receiving care and follow-up at work in "company time" led to any improvement. We describe here the second phase of this trial in

Reprinted from Haynes, R. B., Sackett, D. L., Gibson, E. S., Taylor, D. W., Hackett, B. C., Roberts, R. S. and Johnson, A. L. Improvement of medication compliance in uncontrolled hypertension. *Lancet*, i, 1265–8, 1976.

457

which the application of more behaviourally oriented strategies did lead to improvements in both compliance and blood-pressure control.

Methods

These have been described in detail elsewhere.[3] Briefly, the examination of 5400 men at Dominion Foundries and Steel Company (over 95% of a random two-thirds sample of male employees) yielded 245 who had high blood-pressures (when sitting quietly on three separate days, a standard series of fifth-phase diastolic blood-pressure were $\geqslant$95 mm Hg), were free of remediable forms of hypertension, were taking no daily medications (70 men were on treatment and were therefore excluded), and had not been treated for hypertension in the preceding six months.

In phase I of this trial,[3] men were randomly allocated into a factorial design in order to test strategies affecting either the convenience of their follow-up care or their knowledge about hypertension and its treatment. Phase II of this trial was designed to see whether a further set of strategies could salvage patients who, although put on recognised antihypertensive drugs in phase I, were neither compliant (pill-counts less than 80%) nor at goal diastolic blood-pressure (fifth phase $\geqslant$90 mm Hg) in the sixth month of treatment. Following stratification by diastolic blood-pressure and compliance level at six months, plus their phase I allocation, 39 such men were allocated by "minimisation" either to a control group or to an experimental group. Minimisation allows the simultaneous consideration of a large series of matching characteristics when allocating subjects to experimental and control groups, thereby minimising (using randomisation in the case of ties) between-group differences. The method is immune to experimenter bias and has been shown to substantially outperform simple randomisation in reducing the imbalance between treatment groups that has troubled several earlier randomised trials.[4] The experimental group received the following set of strategies:

Home self-measurement of blood-pressure

Each experimental patient was loaned an aneroid sphygmomanometer and stethoscope and instructed in its use. 18 men were loaned separate cuffs ('Nelkin' sphygmomanometer model 204M; Nelkin Medical Products, Inc., Kansas City, Missouri) and stethoscopes; two men with upper extremity impairments were loaned devices in which the stethoscope head was incorporated into the cuff ('Arden' sphygmomanometer-stethoscope model HRI 8104-705201; Taylor Consumer Products Division, Sybron Corporation, Arden, North Carolina).

Home blood-pressure and medication charting

Each experimental patient was issued with daily pill and blood-pressure charts and asked to record (by number and by a dot on the chart) his fifth-phase blood-pressure each day, along with both the number of pills taken and the number of pills missed during the previous day. The treatment goal of a fifth-phase blood-pressure below 90 mm Hg was clearly stated, and the background of the blood-pressure chart was red above, and blue below, this value.

Tailoring

Each experimental patient was interviewed to identify any daily habits or rituals. The resulting pattern was compared with the patient's anti-hypertensive regimen and when the two coincided, agreement was sought to take the pills immediately before executing the habit or ritual; it was also suggested that medications be placed at the sites of these rituals.

Increased supervision and reinforcement

Experimental patients were asked to report fortnightly for a review of their daily pill and blood-pressure charts and for a check of their blood-pressure. At each review, if the blood-pressure check was either <90 mm Hg or ⩾4 mm Hg below that observed at the sixth month, the patient was praised and received a $4 credit toward ownership of the home blood-pressure cuff and stethoscope. Praise was also received for periods of perfect compliance, and the reasons for every missed pill were sought in an effort to identify problems and solve them through further tailoring. If neither a blood-pressure fall nor perfect compliance had occurred, the patient was encouraged to do better over the next interval.

All phase-II interventions were executed by a 28-year-old female programme coordinator, a high-school graduate with no health professional training; after instruction in blood-pressure measurement and the phase-II strategies, she was given full responsibility for their implementation. Phase-II patients received follow-up care from the same source as in phase I, and the programme coordinator was not permitted to contact the treating physicians (a protocol for medical emergencies was devised but never had to be used).

At the end of phase II (in the twelfth month of treatment) patients were evaluated both at home and at the mill by examiners who were "blind" to their experimental group allocation. The home visitor verified each patient's drugs and doses and, while the patient was supplying a urine specimen (requested without prior warning), did an unobtrusive pill-count and compared it with a baseline established one month earlier. Within a few days of this home visit, the standardised blood-pressure measurement was repeated at the mill and a blood-sample was taken. In this paper, compliance-rates are reported as the proportion of pills prescribed for the twelfth month of therapy which were removed from their containers and, presumably, swallowed by the patients.

Criteria for success were set in advance. Intervention was to be considered clinically useful if the average twelfth-month compliance-rate among experimental patients met three conditions: first, it had to exceed the sixth-month baseline compliance among experimental patients by 20% or more; second, this difference had to be statistically significant; third, the twelfth-month mean compliance-rate among phase II experimental patients had to exceed that for controls by 20% or more.

Results

315 (6%) of the DOFASCO employees screened met our criteria for sustained primary hypertension. 70 were already on treatment and were thus ineligible. Of 245 eligible men, 230 (94%) agreed to take part in our trial. In phase I we tested the effects of "augmented convenience" by comparing outcomes in patients managed by industrial physicians' in company time with those handled by their general practitioners in the usual way, and we compared the effects of "mastery learning" (learning the facts about hypertension). Neither strategy led to the patient being more likely to take his pills or achieve goal blood-pressure.

The 20 experimental and 19 controls who, because they were neither compliant nor at goal blood-pressure in the sixth month were allocated to receive or not receive the phase-II strategies, were similar with respect to six month blood-pressures, previous compliance, and allocation to the phase-I interventions (these matching characteristics were used in their phase-II allocation by minimisation), and were also similar for age, height, weight, and complaints reported at their sixth-month evaluations.

1 control developed deep-vein thrombosis and his hypotensive drugs were stopped; this patient was removed from the study, leaving 20 experimental patients and 18 controls.

16 of the 20 experimental patients were cooperative throughout phase II and kept an average of just under ten appointments (mean duration = 30 min) with the programme coordinator. 1 refused the phase-II intervention entirely and 3 others repeatedly missed appointments completing an average of only 2.5 visits (mean duration = 40 min).

Phase-II outcomes are summarised in figs 1–3 and the table. Over the course of phase II, substantially more experimental than control patients exhibited increased compliance, decreased diastolic blood-pressure, or

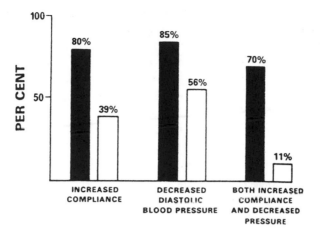

Fig. 1. Changes in patients between start and end of phase II. The closed bars represent experimental patients and the open bars, controls.

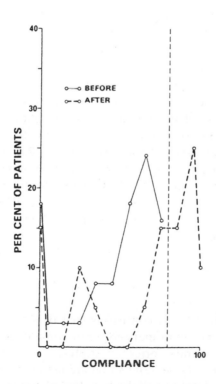

Fig. 2. Compliance distributions before and after phase II strategies among experimental patients.

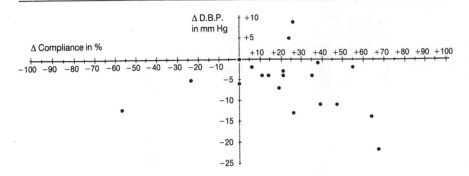

Fig. 3. Changes in diastolic blood-pressure and compliance between start and end of phase II among experimental patients.

both, and this is shown in fig. 1. Furthermore, as shown in the table, the changes in compliance among experimental patients met the previously established criteria for success: their twelfth-month compliance exceeded their sixth-month compliance by more than 20%, this difference was statistically significant, and the twelfth-month compliance among experimental patients exceeded that of control patients by 20% or more (this latter difference was also statistically significant). Fig. 2 illustrates the distribution of compliance levels among experimental patients at both the beginning and end of phase II.

These changes in compliance among experimental patients were paralleled by decreases in their diastolic blood-pressure (fig. 3). Although the average pressure fall was a modest 5.4 mm Hg it contributed to a total fall in diastolic blood-pressure of 11.6 mm Hg for the full twelve months of therapy, a drop which approaches the 13.2 mm Hg average fall observed among highly compliant patients at six months. Furthermore, this diastolic blood-pressure fall among experimental patients in phase II exceeded 10 mm Hg in 6 patients, and 4 of these (plus 2 other experimental patients with lesser falls) achieved the diastolic blood-pressure goal; 3 controls exhibited pressure falls of 10 mm Hg or more, and 1 of these (plus 1 other) achieved goal blood-pressure.

Discussion

The phase-II results of this controlled trial of strategies for improving medication compliance in primary hypertension are encouraging, for they suggest that behaviourally oriented strategies can salvage a clinically significant portion of hypertensives who are neither compliant nor at goal blood-pressure six months after the initiation of treatment. These results, if replicable in other settings, may also encourage clinicians who, because

Effects of phase-II strategies upon compliance and blood-pressure

Group	No. of patients	Sixth month	Twelfth month	Change	Probability of no real difference Within groups*	Probability of no real difference Between groups†
Effect upon mean compliance-rates (% ± S.E.):						
Experimental	20	44.5 (±5.6)	65.8 (±8.2)	+21.3 (±6.5)	0.001	⎱ 0.025
Control	18	44.7 (±7.1)	43.2 (±10.1)	−1.5 (±7.8)	N.S.	⎰
Effect upon diastolic blood-pressure (mm Hg ± S.E.):						
Experimental	20	98.5 (±1.3)	93.1 (±1.3)	−5.4 (±1.7)	0.001	⎱ 0.12
Control	18	98.3 (±1.5)	96.4 (±1.3)	−1.9 (±2.0)	N.S.	⎰

*Within group comparisons by paired t test, one-tailed.

†Between group comparisons by unpaired t test, one-tailed.

of prior disappointment over poor compliance, have been reluctant to label and treat hypertensives.

Although the combination of self-measurement, the recording of home blood-pressures and pill-taking, tailoring, and reinforcement seems responsible for the differences between experimental and control patients in the twelfth month, four alternative explanations must be considered. First, could these differences simply reflect a lack of comparability of experimental and control patients? This has been a major problem in interpreting other reports of new strategies for improving compliance and follow-up among hypertensives in which comparison groups have either been absent[5] or consisted of non-contemporaneous controls.[6] However, we compared outcomes between groups generated through the allocation of patients previously stratified for factors likely to affect subsequent compliance and blood-pressure, and the experimental and control groups in this trial were highly similar for prior compliance and blood-pressure levels, age, weight, height, complaints, and phase-I intervention strategy. Therefore, we are confident that this source of bias is absent.

Second, could the differences in blood-pressure we observed simply reflect a "training effect" in which experimental patients, more accustomed to having their blood-pressures measured, would exhibit lower, more "relaxed" readings, at the twelfth-month evaluation? This possibility has been tested, and the result is negative.[7] Carnahan and Nugent provided cuffs and stethoscopes to a random half of a group of 100 hypertensives and found no difference at six months between their diastolic blood-pressures and those of control patients who had not practised home blood-pressure measurement. It is therefore unlikely that the blood-pressure differences we observed were the result of a "training" bias.

Third, do the phase-II results simply reflect the "delayed action" of a phase-I strategy? More specifically, is a delayed effect of mastery learning, reinforced by the phase-II behavioural strategy, responsible for the differences observed in the twelfth month? Apparently not. Phase-I experiences were evenly divided between the phase-II groups (11 of 20 experimental patients and 10 of 18 controls had undergone mastery learning). Furthermore, although patients who had been through the mastery learning programme were slightly more responsive to the phase-II intervention, there was once again no correlation between knowledge about hypertension and compliance at twelve months.

We are not satisfied, however, that this investigation is free from a fourth potential source of bias, and this is the confounding of the compliance-improving strategies with the amount of attention shown to these patients. By design, phase-II experimental patients received more attention (five hours, spread over six months) than phase-II controls, and our review of the compliance literature suggests that simply spending more time with patients, regardless of the content of the interchange, is associated with increased compliance.[8] Is it possible that this increased attention all by itself, regardless of the precise compliance strategy, was responsible for some or all of the differences noted at the end of phase II? A review of the phase-I results is helpful here. Although patients who underwent mastery learning received more attention than their corresponding controls, they were no more compliant. On the other hand, this group was somewhat more responsive to the phase-II strategy, a result consistent with a cumulative "attention" effect. We have suggested elsewhere that future trials of compliance-improving strategies include "attention placebos",[9] and our subsequent randomised trial of home blood-pressures and home visits, now in progress, will determine the independent contribution of "attention" to the achievement of high compliance and goal blood-pressure.

We have done several other analyses of this controlled trial, and one deserves mention here. The effects of phase-II strategies were not limited to patients' compliance. Although the programme coordinator was not allowed to contact the treating physicians, these physicians were nonetheless more likely to increase the antihypertensive regimens of experimental patients than of controls. By the end of phase II the former were prescribed more vigorous therapy, on average, than the latter; this effect will be reported in detail elsewhere.

In adopting the strategy of the pharmacological trial to the testing of compliance-improving strategies we have searched for the counterpart of the untoward drug reaction. We have made serial measurements of these patients' social and emotional function and have monitored their absenteeism as well as their reports of side-effects. A preliminary analysis of these data shows no deleterious effect of the compliance-improving strategies on these indexes of function and self-image. (This portion of the investigation has been carried out in collaboration with Dr Jana Mossey, department of social and community medicine, University of Manitoba, and will be reported elsewhere).

This controlled trial, while not designed to describe the current state of hypertension at a community level, does provide an indication of the present situation in urban, industrial Canada. Among men working in a steel mill, 14% have diastolic (fifth phase) blood-pressure above 90 mm Hg and, of those with persistent pressures >95 mm Hg, 46% are aware of their condition and 22% are on drugs; these values are similar to those of earlier population surveys.[10] In view of this consistency, our subsequent discovery that only two-thirds of men with diastolic pressures consistently >95 mm Hg will be started on drugs, and that of those begun on medication only slightly more than half will be taking 80% or more of their prescribed doses, are sobering indeed. The inability of isolated screening programmes to solve these problems and the need for rigorous validation of strategies reputed to alter the behaviour of clinicians and patients are underscored.

Finally, the behaviourally oriented strategies we used in phase II, if confirmed in further trials, can be implemented in the existing system of clinical services. As we shall describe elsewhere, a simple interview can detect up to half of non-compliant hypertensive patients, obviating the need for pill-counts or body-fluid assays and rendering the identification of a substantial portion of non-compliers both quick and practicable. Second, virtually all patients can be taught home blood-pressure measurement, using equipment which is already in the clinician's office; neither automated nor integrated cuffs and stethoscopes are required. Third, this trial showed that effective compliance-improving strategies can be applied, maintained, and supervised by a layperson without demanding either more time from a busy clinician or more reorganisation from a beleaguered health service. In view of this potential, the need for further trials to confirm or refute the value of these and other compliance-improving strategies is great.

Acknowledgements

We thank Mrs Charmaine Turford who carried out the phase-II intervention programme, Dr Ian Cunningham and the nurses of the Hamilton Wentworth Health Unit who assisted with the twelve-month home visits, Dr Robert Martin, Mr Brian Austin, and the other members of the medical department at DOFASCO, and the physicians in Hamilton and the surrounding communities without whose encouragement and cooperation the trial could never have happened. This work was supported in part by grant no. MA-5159 from the Medical Research Council of Canada, National Health Grant 606-22-12 from Health and Welfare Canada, and a grant from Dominion Foundries and Steel Company of Canada. R. B. H. is a Physician's Services Inc. foundation fellow.

References

1. Sackett, D. L. *in* International Textbook on Hypertension (edited by J. Genest, E. Koiw, and O. Kuchel). New York (in the press).
2. Haynes, R. B. *in* Compliance with Therapeutic Regimens (edited by D. L. Sackett and R. B. Haynes). Baltimore (in the press).
3. Sackett, D. L., Haynes, R. B., Gibson, E. S., Hackett, B. C., Taylor, D. W., Roberts, R. S., Johnson, A. L. *Lancet*, 1975, **i**, 1205.
4. Taves, D. R. *Clin. Pharm. Ther.* 1974, **15**, 443.
5. Alderman, M. H., Schoebaum, E. E. *New Engl. J. Med.* 1975, **293**, 65.
6. Finnerty, F. A. Jr., Shaw, L. W., Himmelsbach, C. K. *Circulation*, 1973, **47**, 76.

7. Carnahan, J. E., Nugent, C. A. *Am. J. med. Sci.* 1975, **269**, 69.
8. Haynes, R. B. *in* Compliance with Therapeutic Regimens (edited by D. L. Sackett and R. B. Haynes). Baltimore (in the press).
9. Sackett, D. L. *ibid.*
10. Wilber, J. A., Barrow, J. G. *Am. J. Med.* 1972, **52**, 653.

Effect of psychosocial treatment on survival of patients with metastatic breast cancer

David Spiegel, Joan R. Bloom, Helena C. Kraemer and Ellen Gottheil

Department of Psychiatry and Behavioral Sciences, Stanford University School of Medicine, Stanford, California, USA;
Department of Social and Administrative Health Sciences, School of Public Health, University of California, Berkeley, California, USA

Summary

The effect of psychosocial intervention on time of survival of 86 patients with metastatic breast cancer was studied prospectively. The 1 year intervention consisted of weekly supportive group therapy with self-hypnosis for pain. Both the treatment (n = 50) and control groups (n = 36) had routine oncological care. At 10 year follow-up, only 3 of the patients were alive, and death records were obtained for the other 83. Survival from time of randomisation and onset of intervention was a mean 36.6 (SD 37.6) months in the intervention group compared with 18.9 (10.8) months in the control group, a significant difference. Survival plots indicated that divergence in survival began at 20 months after entry, or 8 months after intervention ended.

Introduction

Many studies have demonstrated positive psychosocial effects of group therapy in cancer patients, including improvements in mood, adjustment, and pain.[1-4] However, few studies have prospectively examined medical effects.[5-9] In general, patients who receive psychotherapy survived longer. Our objective was to assess whether group therapy in patients with metastatic breast cancer had any effect on survival. This group intervention has been reported[10] to improve the psychological well-being of such patients. We started with the belief that positive psychological and symptomatic effects could occur without affecting the course of the

Reprinted from Spiegel, D., Bloom, J. R., Kraemer, H. C. and Gottheil, E. Effect of psychosocial treatment on survival of patients with metastatic breast cancer. *Lancet*, **ii**, 888–91, 1989.

disease; we expected to improve the quality of life without affecting its quantity. Here we describe a 10 year follow-up of the effect of psychosocial intervention on disease progression and mortality.

Patients and methods

Patients

Only subjects with documented metastatic carcinoma of the breast were included. 109 women were referred by their oncologists. Those patients who agreed were called upon by our research interviewer, who told them about the study and invited them to participate. Of this group, 86 completed the first questionnaire, while 18 others refused to participate and 5 died before contact. After written informed consent was obtained (protocol approved by Stanford Human Subjects Committee), a battery of psychological tests was administered. The subjects were then randomly assigned to either the intervention or control groups, and initial follow-up was done every 4 months for a year. More subjects were randomly assigned to therapy (n = 50) than to control (n = 36) to ensure enough patients for group work. 14 subjects assigned to group therapy were too weak or ill at initial interview to participate; 6 died after entry but before the groups began and 2 others moved away. 12 subjects were lost from the controls; 4 were too ill to participate, 2 died, 4 refused to participate, and we were unable to contact 2. 30 of the 34 women in the intervention group and all 24 control women survived long enough to respond to at least one follow-up questionnaire during the year of study. During the first year there was no indication of improved survival in the treatment group; in fact, slightly more patients in this group died during this period (30 *vs* 22%, χ^2 not significant).

Survival time, obtained for all patients who entered the study, was based on state death records for 83 patients. All but 2 of these had breast cancer listed as the immediate or contributing cause of death. The 2 deaths not related to cancer occurred in the controls: 1 cerebrovascular accident and 1 suicide. We made phone contact with the 3 survivors. For other than the primary survival analysis, these 3 were treated as though their date of death was July 1, 1988, when all death records had been obtained. If there was any bias resulting from this decision, it would be in the direction of minimising the impact of intervention, since all 3 were in the treatment group.

The two groups were similar at study entry except for a nearly significant difference in staging at initial diagnosis (tables I and II). Staging information, based on medical records at study entry, was available for 70 of the 86 patients. Initial staging favoured the intervention

Table I. *Details of control and intervention patients*

	Control (n = 36)	Intervention (n = 50)
Age		
At initial diagnosis	49.3 (10.5)	49.9 (10.0)
At study entry	54.6 (10.2)	54.7 (9.9)
Married	25 *(69%)*	26 *(52%)*
Type of surgery		
Lumpectomy	6 *(17%)*	3 *(6%)*
Simple mastectomy	2 *(6%)*	2 *(4%)*
Modified radical mastectomy	11 *(31%)*	18 *(36%)*
Radical mastectomy	17 *(47%)*	26 *(52%)*
*Degree of metastatic spread**		
Soft tissue	0.3 (0.5)	0.5 (0.6)
Viscera	0.3 (0.5)	0.3 (0.5)
Bone	0.4 (0.7)	0.3 (0.7)
Initial stage†		
I	3 *(8%)*	8 *(16%)*
II	18 *(50%)*	16 *(32%)*
III	5 *(14%)*	11 *(22%)*
IV	7 *(19%)*	2 *(4%)*
No of mastectomies‡	1	1
Exercise		
Hours per week	1.7 (0.8)	1.6 (0.8)
Activity level§	1.8 (1.1)	1.8 (1.1)
No of treatment courses at entry‡		
Chemotherapy	1	1 (0, 1)
Oestrogen	0 (0, 1)	0
Androgen	0 (0, 1)	0
Steroid	0	0
Irradiation	1 (0, 1)	1 (0, 1)
Days of irradiation	41.7 (81.9)	18.8 (24.8)

Mean (SD) or no of cases.
*Spread of metastasis scaled as: 0 = no spread, 1 = one site, 2 = more than one site of a particular type, and 3 (bone only) = four or more sites.
†χ^2 for trend, $p < 0.07$.
‡Median (lower and upper quartiles = median except where indicated).
§Self-rating 1–5.

group. Initial staging took place, on average, 59.8 (SD 47.6) months before the beginning of the study. Patients were not referred to us until they had metastatic disease. Since some studies show that staging is a predictor of survival,[11–13] it could be that by chance the treatment sample had a better prognosis when initially diagnosed than the controls. We

Table II. *Disease course pre-entry (months)*

	Control	Intervention
Initial diagnosis to first metastasis	38.0 (44.9)	36.3 (35.6)
First metastasis to entry	24.4 (17.4)	21.9 (21.8)
Initial diagnosis to entry	62.3 (53.5)	58.0 (43.3)

Mean (SD).

found, however, that initial staging was unrelated to survival from the time of randomisation until death. Nonetheless, staging was a control variable during analysis.

Intervention

The intervention lasted for a year while both control and treatment groups received their routine oncological care. The three intervention groups met weekly for 90 min, led by a psychiatrist or social worker with a therapist who had breast cancer in remission. The groups were structured to encourage discussion of how to cope with cancer, but at no time were patients led to believe that participation would affect the course of disease. Group therapy patients were encouraged to come regularly and express their feelings about the illness and its effect on their lives. Physical problems, including side-effects of chemotherapy or radiotherapy, were discussed and a self-hypnosis strategy was taught for pain control.[14] Social isolation was countered by developing strong relations among members. Members encouraged one another to be more assertive with doctors. Patients focused on how to extract meaning from tragedy by using their experience to help other patients and their families. One major function of the leaders was to keep the groups directed toward facing and grieving losses.[10]

Analysis

The analysis used Cox's proportional hazards model to examine whether intervention affected survival. This model was chosen so that we could assess the influence of treatment assignment over and above the effect of pre-randomisation prognostic variables by O'Brien's logit-rank procedure.[15] The log-rank test was also used to ensure that main effect differences were significant although the hazards of survival differed. We also drew Kaplan–Meier plots, and used unpaired t, Wilcoxon's rank sum, and χ^2 tests where appropriate.

Table III. *Survival (months)*

	Control	Intervention
Survival from:		
Study entry to death*	18.9 (10.8)	36.6 (37.6)
Initial medical visit to death	81.2 (53.9)	94.6 (61.0)
First metastasis to death†	43.2 (20.5)	58.4 (45.4)

Mean (SD).
*$p < 0.0001$, Cox; $p < 0.005$, log-rank.
†$p < 0.01$, Cox; $p < 0.04$, log-rank.

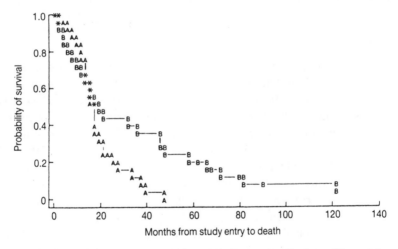

Kaplan-Meir survival plot. A = control (n = 36), B = treatment (n = 50), and * = overlapping control and treatment probabilities of survival. Some points represent more than 1 case.

Results

Most striking was the difference in survival from time of randomisation, when intervention began, until date of death. Survival time for the treatment group was significantly longer compared with controls (table III and figure). In addition the interval from first metastasis to death was significantly longer for the group randomised to treatment. Thus the intervention group lived on average twice as long as did controls.

Since initial staging differed, we examined whether the group randomised to treatment was not as ill and therefore survived longer. The following points make this unlikely: (1) all patients had metastatic disease at recruitment and randomisation, and therefore had a fairly uniform prognosis; (2) there were no differences in other important prognostic variables; and (3) although initial staging was, as expected, significantly correlated with time from initial medical visit to date of first metastasis (Spearman's r = −0.42, n = 70, p < 0.0003), this variable was not correlated with any survival variables, including the outcome variable that differentiated between treatment and control groups—ie, time from entry to date of death (r = 0.03, n = 70).

To address this potential problem directly, the between-group differences were examined controlling for initial staging. The difference in survival from randomisation to death between the treatment and control groups remained highly significant (n = 70, p < 0.0001). Staging had little influence on this survival variable (p < 0.86). Likewise the difference between the dates of metastasis and death remained significant (p < 0.02). In addition, examination of Kaplan-Meier curves for treatment versus control patients matched for initial staging revealed a pattern similar to that seen for the overall sample in the figure. Survival between intervention and control groups was different within each homogeneous staging group. This analysis indicated that initial staging differences do not account for the observed differences in survival between the groups.

Although there were no significant differences between treatment and control groups in chemotherapy and irradiation before randomisation, we tested the significance of the main effect for survival while controlling for each of these variables with the O'Brien procedure, entering the medical treatment variable first and then group status. In each case the treatment/control difference held. Of most interest was the significance of the treatment/control difference in survival after entering those variables that were close to being significantly different: days of irradiation (n = 69, p < 0.0005) and androgen (n = 86, p < 0.0004) and steroid treatment (n = 86, p < 0.0004). Differences in time from first metastasis to death also remained significant with this analysis. Thus these variables do not account for the enhanced survival.

There was variation in attendance among those randomised to group therapy. Illness accounted for some of this variation. Indeed, 15 patients in the treatment group and 8 controls died during the year. Some other patients moved away or were reluctant to attend their group. To examine between-group differences among those patients who where more actively involved, we did the same Cox regression analysis on the 54 patients who completed both a baseline and at least one of the three follow-up questionnaires during the year. The difference in survival time from randomisation to death between treatment and control groups again remained significant (p < 0.0001), even when staging was controlled (n = 42, p < 0.0001), and when log-ranks were used (p < 0.03).

Discussion

Patients with metastatic breast cancer randomised to weekly group therapy for a year lived significantly longer than did controls, by an average of nearly 18 months. This difference was statistically and clinically significant. Our results are consistent with but greater in magnitude than those of Grossarth-Maticek *et al.*,[6] and overcome the problem of differences in time from initial diagnosis to study entry which limited the findings of Morganstern *et al.*[7]

In agreement with Cassileth *et al.*[16] and Jamison *et al.*,[17] we found that a battery of extensive psychological assessments before intervention did not significantly predict survival. Indeed the only variable to affect survival time significantly was our complex psychosocial intervention. The effect of group interaction on longevity was not apparent in the year of intervention. Treatment and control groups did not diverge until about 8 months after the year was over (figure), which may be explained, as would the result of a somatic treatment, as a cumulative mild effect on time until death.

Our follow-up study was done to investigate whether psychosocial intervention, which significantly reduced anxiety, depression, and pain, would do so without having any effect on the course of the disease. We intended, in particular, to examine the often overstated claims made by those who teach cancer patients that the right mental attitude will help to conquer the disease. In these interventions patients often devote much time and energy to creating images of their immune cells defeating the cancer cells.[18] At no time did we take such an approach. The emphasis in our programme was on living as fully as possible, improving communication with family members and doctors, facing and mastering fears about death and dying, and controlling pain and other symptoms. To the extent that this intervention influenced the course of the disease, it did not do so because of any intention on the part of the therapists or the patients that their participation would affect survival time.

What could account for the differences observed? Social support may be an important factor in survival.[8,19] Even when matched for health habits, social relations affect survival.[20,21] The provision of social support for isolated individuals under stress can improve health outcome.[8] Social support is important in mediating how individuals cope with stress. For example, married cancer patients survive longer than unmarried patients.[22] In our study there was a higher proportion of married patients in the control group (70% *vs* 57%). The fact that treatment patients had longer survival may indicate the efficacy of psychosocial intervention. One role of the group might have been to provide a place to belong and to express feelings.[23] Clearly the patients in these groups felt an intense bonding with one another and a sense of acceptance through sharing a common dilemma. 1 patient with oesophageal strictures secondary to irradiation described her sense of estrangement from the world; while struggling to swallow soup at a restaurant, she thought: "These people don't realise how fortunate they are just to be able to eat". The therapy group patients visited each other in hospital, wrote poems, and even had a meeting at the home of a dying member. Thus the groups countered the social alienation that often divides cancer patients from their well-meaning but anxious family and friends.

Involvement in the group may have allowed patients to mobilise their resources better, perhaps by complying more vigorously with medical treatment or by improving appetite and diet through reduced depression. Treated patients learnt about hypnosis for pain control and therefore may have been more able to maintain exercise and other routine activities. Neuroendocrine and immune systems may be a major link between emotional processes and cancer course.[19,24] Future studies of the impact of psychosocial interventions on medical illness might profitably examine variables such as compliance, health habits, diet, and immune and neuroendocrine function.

Acknowledgements

This study was supported by grants from the National Cancer Institute (N01-CV-55313 [DHEW]), NIMH grant MH 16744, the American Cancer Research Fund, and the Alan and Laraine Fischer Foundation. We thank the other therapists, Dr Irvin D. Yalom, Dr Regina Kriss, and Susan Weissberg, Laiani Kuspa for data analysis, Arnold M. Rey for research assistance, and Helen Abrahamson for manuscript preparation. We also thank the following doctors for critiques of earlier drafts: Helen Blau, Kenneth Bowers, Barrie Cassileth, Hans Eysenck, Bernard Fox, James S. Goodwin, Jimmie Holland, Larry Kessler, Sandra M. Levy, Margaret Mattson, Rudolph Moos, Gary R. Morrow, Helen Pettinati, Frank Stockdale, Auke Tellegen, Lydia Temoshok, and Irvin D. Yalom.

References

1. Ferlic M, Goldman A, Kennedy BJ. Group counseling in adult patients with advanced cancer. *Cancer* 1979; **43**: 760.
2. Gustafson J, Whitman H. Towards a balanced social environment on the oncology service. *Soc Psychiatry* 1978; **13**: 147.
3. Wood PE, Milligan I, Christ D, Liff D. Group counseling for cancer patients in a community hospital. *Psychosomatics* 1978; **19**: 555.
4. Spiegel D, Bloom J. Group therapy and hypnosis reduce metastatic breast carcinoma pain. *Psychosom Med* 1983; **45**: 333.
5. Forester B, Kornfeld DS, Fleiss JL. Psychotherapy during radiotherapy: effects on emotional and physical distress. *Am J Psychiatry* 1985; **142**: 22.

6. Grossarth-Maticek R, Schmidt P, Veter H, Arndt S. Psychotherapy research in oncology. In: Steptoe A, Mathews A, eds. Health care and human behaviour. London: Academic Press, 1984: 325.
7. Morganstern H, Gellert GA, Walter SD, Ostfeld AM, Siegel BS. The impact of a psychosocial support program on survival with breast cancer: the importance of selection bias in program evaluation. *J Chron Dis* 1984; **37**: 273.
8. Rodin J. Managing the stress of aging: the role of control and coping. In: Levine S, Ursin R, eds. Coping and Health. London: Plenum, 1980: 171.
9. House JS, Landis KR, Umberson D. Social relationships and health. *Science* 1988; **241**: 540.
10. Spiegel D, Bloom J, Yalom ID. Group support for patients with metastatic breast cancer. *Arch Gen Psychiatry* 1981; **38**: 527.
11. Kamby C, Rose C, Ejlertsen B, Andersen J, Birkler NE, Rytter L. Stage and pattern of metastases in patients with breast cancer. *Eur J Cancer Clin Oncol* 1987; **23**: 1925.
12. Gaglia P, Bussone R, Caldarola B, Lai M, Jayme A, Caldarola L. The correlation between the spread of metastases by level in the axillary nodes and disease-free survival in breast cancer: a multifactorial analysis. *Eur J Cancer Clin Oncol* 1987; **23**: 849.
13. Schwartz GF, Feig SA, Pathefsky AS. Significance and staging of nonpalpable carcinomas of the breast. *Surg Gynecol Obstet* 1988; **166**: 6.
14. Spiegel D. The use of hypnosis in controlling cancer pain. *CA: Cancer J Clin* 1985; **35**: 221.
15. O'Brien PC. A non-parametric test for association with censored data. *Biometrics* 1978; **34**: 243.
16. Cassileth BR, Lusk EJ, Miller DS, Brown LL, Miller C. Psychosocial correlates of survival in advanced malignant disease? *N Engl J Med* 1985; **312**: 1551.
17. Jamison RN, Burish TG, Walston KA. Psychogenic factors in predicting survival of breast cancer patients. *J Clin Oncol* 1987; **5**: 768.
18. Achterberg J, Matthews-Simonton S, Simonton C. Psychology of the exceptional cancer patient: a description of patients who outlive predictive life expectancies. *Psychother Theory Res Practice* 1977; **14**: 416.
19. Kennedy S, Kiecolt-Glaser JK, Glaser R. Immunological consequences of acute and chronic stressors: mediating role of interpersonal relationships. *Br J Med Psychol* 1988; **61**: 77.
20. Berkman LF, Syme SL. Social networks, host resistance, and mortality: a nine-year follow-up study of Alameda County residents. *Am J Epidemiol* 1979; **109**: 186.
21. House JS, Robbins C, Metzner HL. The association of social relationships and activities with mortality: prospective evidence from the Tecumseh community health study. *Am J Epidemiol* 1982; **116**: 123.
22. Goodwin JS, Hunt WC, Key CR, Samet JM. The effect of marital status on stage, treatment and survival of cancer patients. *JAMA* 1987; **258**: 3125.
23. Friedman LC, Baer PE, Nelson DV, Lane M, Smith FE, Dworkin RJ. Women with breast cancer: perception of family functioning and adjustment to illness. *Psychosom Med* 1988; **50**: 529.

24. Pennebaker JW, Kiecolt-Glaser JK, Glaser R. Disclosure of traumas and immune function: health implications for psychotherapy. *J Consult Clin Psychol* 1988; **56**: 239.

Alteration of type A behavior and its effect on cardiac recurrences in post myocardial infarction patients: summary results of the recurrent coronary prevention project

Meyer Friedman, MD, Carl E. Thoresen, PhD, James J. Gill, MD, Diane Ulmer, RN, MS, Lynda H. Powell, PhD, Virginia A. Price, PhD, Byron Brown, PhD, Leonti Thompson, MD, David D. Rabin, MD, William S. Breall, MD, Edward Bourg, PhD, Richard Levy, MD, and Theodore Dixon, PhD

From Harold Brunn Institute, Mount Zion Hospital and Medical Center, San Francisco, USA; the Center for Advanced Study in Behavioral Sciences, Stanford, USA; the Division of Biostatistics, Stanford Medical Center, USA; Harvard University Health Services, Cambridge, USA; and the Department of Epidemiology, Yale University, New Haven, USA

Abstract

One thousand thirteen post myocardial infarction patients were observed for 4.5 years to determine whether their type A (coronary-prone) behavior could be altered and the effect such alteration might have on the subsequent cardiac morbidity and mortality rates of these individuals. Eight hundred sixty-two of these individuals were randomly assigned either to a control section of 270 participants who received group cardiac counseling or an experimental section of 592 participants who received both group cardiac counseling and type A behavioral counseling. The remaining 151 patients, serving as a "comparison group," did not receive group counseling of any kind. Using the "Intention-to-Treat" principle, we observed markedly reduced type A behavior at the end of 4.5 years in 35.1% of participants given cardiac and type A behavior counseling compared with 9.8% of participants given only cardiac counseling. The cumulative 4.5-year cardiac recurrence rate was 12.9% in the 592 participants in the

Reproduced from Friedman M, Thoresen CE, Gill JJ. Alteration of type A behavior and its effect on cardiac recurrences in post myocardial infarction patients: Summary results of the recurrent coronary prevention project. AM HEART J 1986; 112: 653–65 with permission from Mosby-Year Book, Inc.

experimental group that received type A counseling. This recurrence rate was significantly less ($p < 0.005$) than either the recurrence rate (21.2%) observed in the 270 participants in the control group or the recurrence rate (28.2%) in those of the comparison group not receiving any special treatment. After the first year, a significant difference in number of cardiac deaths between the experimental and control participants was observed during the remaining 3.5 years of the study. Overall, the results of this study demonstrate for the first time, within a controlled experimental design, that altering type A behavior reduces cardiac morbidity and mortality in post infarction patients. (AM HEART J 1986; 112:653).

Persons who exhibited an emotional syndrome characterized by a continuously harrying sense of time urgency and easily aroused free-floating hostility (i.e. type A behavior pattern) were observed in 1959 to have a sevenfold greater prevalence[1] and in 1975 a significantly greater incidence[2] of clinical coronary heart disease (CHD) than persons not exhibiting these two emotional components (i.e., type B persons).

Ever since this observed associational relationship between the presence of type A behavior and the prevalence and incidence of clinical CHD, hundreds of studies have been designed to investigate further the nature of this association. After various laboratory,[3] clinical,[4-8] pathologic,[9,10] and epidemiologic[11-15] studies further suggested the possible involvement of this behavior pattern in the pathogenesis of clinical CHD, a Review Panel of investigators was convened at the request of the National Heart, Lung, and Blood Institute to review these studies and come to some conclusion about the possible role of type A behavior in the development of clinical CHD.

This Review Panel concluded[16] that type A behavior was an independent coronary risk factor and of the same order of pathogenetic magnitude as that of previously accepted risk factors (e.g., hypertension, hypercholesterolemia, excess cigarette smoking). This same panel, however, pointed out that no available data suggested that type A behavior could be modified. Moreover, the panel pointed out that just as in the case of all other commonly accepted coronary risk factors, although the data suggested that an *associational* relationship existed between type A behavior and the increased prevalence and incidence of clinical CHD, proof was still lacking that a *causative* relationship existed between this emotional disorder and the pathogenesis of clinical CHD.

In view of these last two uncertainties, we initiated and carried out the Recurrent Coronary Prevention Project (RCPP)[17-19] to see whether answers could be found to two fundamental questions: (1) can the type A behavior pattern be substantially altered in a reasonably large cohort of persons who had survived one or more myocardial infarctions, and (2) if reductions in the intensity of type A behavior can be accomplished, can such reduction be directly related to documented decreases in coronary morbidity and mortality? The final results of this 4.5-year project reported herein clearly indicate that the intensity of type A behavior can be decreased and that such diminution appears to effect a significant decrease in both the morbidity and the mortality of CHD in post infarction patients.

Methods

Enrollment of participants

The methods used have been described.[17,19] In summary, over a period of 12 months we recruited 1013 participants who had had one or more documented myocardial infarctions 6 months or more earlier, were 64 years of age or younger, either had never smoked or had quit for 6 months or longer, and had never been treated for or exhibited signs of diabetes mellitus. As already described,[17] 90% of the participants were men. There were 13 blacks and three Asians; the remainder were white.

Eight hundred sixty-two of these participants volunteered to be randomized into either a control group of 270 participants (section 1) who received only group cardiac counseling or an experimental group of 592 participants (section 2) who received both group cardiac and type A behavioral counseling.* The remaining 151 participants were not counseled but were examined yearly and thus served as a nonrandom "comparison group" (section 3) to inform us of the cardiac recurrence rate of post infarction nonvolunteer participants who received no group counseling of any kind. Sixty-seven of these 151 comparison-group participants lived in a city approximately 100 miles from the San Francisco Bay area. They had not volunteered spontaneously to enter the study but had been asked by the two cardiologists attending them to agree to allow themselves to be examined and subsequently reexamined, as did the San Francisco Bay area volunteers. These participants were especially chosen because only several of them were cognizant of the possible relationship of type A behavior to the pathogenesis of CHD.

As reported previously,[17] the baseline sociodemographic and medical findings in both the randomized sections 1 and 2 and the nonrandomized comparison group were essentially the same. Thus the mean age was approximately 53 years, approximately 90% were men, the Peel Index[20] was 8.8, 74% had smoked cigarettes, 39% had a history of hypertension,

---

* Twice as many patients were randomly enrolled in the cardiac and type A behavioral-counseled section because we initially feared that twice as many of such patients might drop out of the program because of the demands that would be made on them by type A counseling.

39% had angina, and 25% had undergone bypass surgery. *More than 95% were found to exhibit type A behavior.*

Any section 1 or 2 participant was designated a "treatment failure" if he missed three successive meetings without a valid excuse or if he was in section 2 and refused to practice the assigned drills. All these treatment failures, however, continued to be reexamined yearly and behaviorally reassessed throughout the entire study period.

Initial and repeat examinations

As previously described,[17,19] all participants on entry received a cardiovascular examination that included an ECG, a serum cholesterol determination, and a urinalysis. The hospital records of approximately 93% of sections 1 and 2 participants were reviewed to provide the data for the calculation of the prognostically important Peel Index[20] based as it is on the number of previous infarctions and the possible occurrence of shock, complex arrhythmias, congestive heart failure, cardiomegaly, and the appearance of new Q waves, during the last acute infarction.† An interval medical history, physical examination, and ECG were repeated at 1.5, 3, and 4.5 years after entry. Repeat blood samples for serum cholesterol analysis were obtained biannually.

The criteria used for the determination of cardiac recurrences (i.e., nonfatal infarction or cardiac death) have been described in earlier reports.[17,19] In brief, the initial diagnosis of infarction was made by the participants' own cardiologists, who were independent of the study and not aware of their patients' status therein. This diagnosis, however, was accepted by us only if there was documentary evidence of the appearance of new and abnormal Q waves,[21] elevation of the MB isoenzyme fraction >5% of the total serum creatine kinase concentration or both. The diagnosis of the occurrence of a silent infarction sometime between the participant's enrollment in the study and his subsequent examinations was made by an independent cardiologist, blind to the treatment status of the participant, if new and diagnostic Q waves were observed in his last ECG. Only two such silent infarctions were detected during the entire study.

The diagnosis of cardiac death was made if a participant died during the course of an acute infarction or congestive heart failure, was witnessed to have died instantaneously without a history or signs of any other illness except his known CHD, or was found dead under circumstances suggesting to the participant's own physician or coroner that the

† It has been found[20] that whereas 66% of post infarction participants exhibiting a Peel Index of 8 or below were alive 5 years after their last infarction, only 37% were alive if their Index was 9 or above.

death was cardiac. An autopsy was performed in 16 of the 28 participants who were witnessed to have died instantaneously without premonitory symptoms or signs or who were found dead (four participants).

Diagnosis and assessment of intensity of type A behavior

The initial diagnosis and assessment of the intensity of type A behavior was determined by a videotaped clinical interview (VCI)* administered by an independent consultant who was blind to the treatment status of the participants at entry and at subsequent interviews, which were obtained at 3 and 4.5 years in both the active and the treatment failure participants. This interview consisted primarily of observation for the *clinical signs and symptoms* indicative of the presence of type A behavior. Details concerning the method of scoring, the validity, and the reliability of the VCI are described in previous reports.[17,18]

As an additional method to determine possible changes in the intensity of type A behavior, all participants at entry filled out a self-report (Participant Questionnaire) and repeated this procedure yearly. In addition, section 2 participants were asked to have similar questionnaires filled out by their spouse (Spouse Questionnaire) and by an associate at work (Monitor Questionnaire). These latter two questionnaires also were filled out yearly. Section 1 and 3 participants were not asked to have their spouse or a business associate fill out questionnaires because we believed that doing so could increase their cognizance and possible self-correction of their type A behavior.

Treatment

The 270 control section 1 participants given cardiac counseling only were enrolled in 22 groups and invited to attend a total of 33 group counseling sessions of 90 minutes duration over a period of 4.5 years. The average section 1 participant attended 25 counseling sessions (76% of total sessions). The cardiac treatment administered by cardiologists as previously described[17,19] consisted of advice and information concerning diet, exercise, drugs, possible surgical regimens, and cardiovascular pathophysiology.

The 592 section 2 participants were enrolled in 60 groups. Because they were scheduled to receive the same amount of cardiac counseling as

---

* In our earlier reports,[17–19] we referred to this type of interview as a videotaped *structured* interview (VSI), but we believe now that because this diagnostic method is primarily a *clinical* procedure (in that it allows the detection of specific physical signs and symptoms characteristic of type A behavior), it should be designated as a videotape *clinical* interview (VCI).

section 1 participants in addition to receiving type A behavioral counseling, they were invited to attend a total of 62 group cardiac and type A behavioral counseling sessions in their 4.5-year period of involvement in the study. However, the average section 2 participants actually attended only 38 counseling sessions (61% of total sessions). The components of type A behavioral counseling (instruction in progressive muscle relaxation, behavior alteration techniques, changes in certain belief systems, restructuring of various environmental situations, cognitive-affective learning, and involvement in specific drills) have been described fully in earlier publications.[17,19]

Statistical analysis

Change in type A behavior

Possible change in the intensity of type A behavior was determined in section 1 and 2 participants at the end of 1, 2, 3, and 4.5 years. At the end of the first year a participant was considered to have *reduced* type A behavior if his self-report questionnaire score was at least 1 SD or more lower than that at his entry. At the end of 4.5 years, a participant was considered to have *markedly reduced* type A behavior if both the VCI and Participant Questionnaire scores declined by 1 SD or more.

Cardiac recurrence rates over 4.5-year period

Total cardiac recurrence rates. The *total* cardiac recurrence rates (i.e., both nonfatal infarctions and cardiac deaths) of randomized section 1 and 2 participants were analyzed in two ways. First, the *cumulative annualized* cardiac recurrence rate was determined at 3-month intervals throughout the 4.5 years. This rate was calculated by using the "Intention-to-Treat" principle,[22] by which all participants originally allocated to sections 1 and 2 were included in the calculations up to the time of censoring.* Participants were censored before 4.5 years only in the case of cardiac recurrence or loss to follow-up (30 section 1 and 52 section 2 participants).

---

* The general formula used for calculation of the cumulative annualized cardiac recurrence rate was as follows: $R = (E/\Sigma Mi) \times 12 \times 100$, where R = the average annual recurrence rate per 100 participants at risk, recalculated at 3-month intervals; E = the total number of participants at risk suffering a cardiac recurrence (nonfatal or fatal); and ΣM_i = the total number of months at risk for participant (i), summed over all participants. The contribution of patients who are lost to follow-up terminates in the previous interval. Multiplying the rate by 12 converts it from a monthly to an annual rate, and multiplying it by 100 produces an annual rate per 100 persons at risk. Confidence intervals around the annual mean differences were computed for the $\alpha = 0.05$ level of significance.

Second, we computed and compared the *total 4.5-year cumulative* cardiac recurrence rate in section 1, 2, and 3 participants, again using the "Intention-to-Treat" principle.

All univariate comparisons were conducted by means of standardized tests: Student's *t* tests in the case of continuous variables and chi square tests of association in the case of categoric variables.[23]

Effect of modification of type A behavior at end of first year on subsequent 3.5-year cumulative cardiac recurrence rates in section 1 and 2 participants

To test more directly the possible relationship between documented reduction in type A behavior and cardiac recurrence, we computed and compared the cardiac recurrence rates for the last 3.5 years of the 4.5-year follow-up of (1) those section 2 participants who at the end of their first year reported a significant behavior reduction (i.e., decline of 1 SD or more in their first year self-report) with (2) those section 1 participants who failed to show such improvement.

Effectiveness of type A counseling in combination with other cardiac treatments on 4.5-year cumulative recurrence rate in section 1 and 2 participants

To determine whether type A counseling could offer protection against a cardiac recurrence over that provided by the standard cardiac treatments of beta-blocking drugs and coronary bypass surgery, we compared the cardiac recurrence rate in sections 1 and 2 for two subgroups of participants: (1) those who were taking beta-blocking drugs at entry and continuing, and (2) those who had undergone coronary bypass surgery at the time of entry into the study.

Cardiac death rates

Cumulative cardiac death rates.   The cumulative cardiac death rate was calculated in all sections, by use of the "Intention-to-Treat" principle. There may be a delay between the initiation of type A counseling and significant behavior modification.[18,19] There also may be a similar delay between behavior change and reduction in cardiac death rate. Therefore we computed the cumulative cardiac death rate separately for the first year and then for the subsequent 3.5 years.

Cumulative cardiac death rate in low and high peel index section 1 and 2 participants.   The occurrence of an earlier infarction, or severe left ventricular impairment or a dangerous arrhythmia arising in the course of an acute infarction are well-recognized ominous prognostic signs.[20]

Because such pathophysiologic risk factors might obscure the otherwise possible protective effect of type A behavior modification in our post infarction participants, we separately analyzed the 4.5-year cumulative cardiac death rate of the 415 section 1 and 2 participants who had not incurred these prognostically ominous catastrophes (as indicated by a Peel Index below 8) and those 303 section 1 and 2 participants who had incurred one or more of these serious defects (as indicated by a Peel Index above 8).

Results

Number of participants remaining in study after 4.5 years

One hundred sixty-one (59.6%) section 1 and 335 (56.6%) section 2 participants remains in group counseling for 4.5 years. One hundred four (38.6%) section 1 and 253 (42.7%) section 2 participants* withdrew from the study during the 4.5-year period. Five participants in section 1 and four participants in section 2 died a noncardiac death. Two hundred seventy-five (74 section 1 and 201 section 2 participants) of these treatment failures continued to be reexamined for cardiac recurrences and the intensity of their type A behavior reassessed at yearly intervals up to their death or for a minimum of 4.5 years after entry. Eighty-two (30 section 1 and 52 section 2 participants) were unable to be traced. Thus we were able to follow 88.9% of section 1 and 91.3% of section 2 participants for 4.5 years with regard to cardiac recurrences (nonfatal and fatal) and to possible changes in the intensity of their type A behavior as determined by self-reports and repeat VCIs.

Entry findings of section 1 and 2 participants who did and did not suffer cardiac recurrences

As found in our initial report,[17] no significant differences (see Table I) were found between the entry medical data of section 1 and 2 participants. However, as might be expected,[16,17] those section 1 and 2 participants who had a recurrence possessed (see Table I) at entry a higher Peel Index, had more often two or more infarctions, hypertension, and in the case of section 2 participants a greater prevalence of complex arrhythmias. Also section 1 participants who had undergone bypass

---

* All these participants voluntarily withdrew from their sections except for 40 section 2 (6.8% of initially enrolled) participants who were considered treatment failures and encouraged to drop out of the program by their respective group counselors because of their outright failure or refusal to practice the drills ordered for section 2 participants. None of these latter participants had suffered a cardiac recurrence before their withdrawal. It should be emphasized that none of the participants who withdrew from the study did so because they were too ill to attend group sessions.

Table I. *Findings at entry in section 1 and 2 participants who did and did not have cardiac recurrences (4.5 years)*

		Section 1			Section 2	
		Participants having recurrences (n = 50)	Participants not having recurrences (n = 185)	Level of significance (p value)	Participants having recurrences (n = 69)	Participants not having recurrences (n = 467)	Level of significance (p value)
Sociodemographic characteristics							
Age (yr)	$\bar{X}$	53.1	53.7	NS	53.2	53.2	NS
	SD	±6.6	±6.1		±5.9	±6.5	
Height (in)	$\bar{X}$	69.4	69.4	NS	69.8	70.2	NS
	SD	±2.9	±2.7		±2.6	±2.7	
Weight (lb)	$\bar{X}$	175.0	173.0	NS	175.5	169.9	NS
	SD	±24.5	±25.9		±23.8	±22.5	
CHD risk factors							
Peel index	$\bar{X}$	10.4	8.3	0.01	10.2	8.5	0.02
	SD	±5.7	±4.8		±5.7	±5.2	
Serum cholesterol (mg/dl)	$\bar{X}$	266.0	258.0	NS	268.0	262.0	NS
	SD	±42.0	±42.3		±47.5	±47.2	
Familial history of CHD		32 (64.0%)	112 (58.9%)	NS	43 (62.3%)	258 (54.8%)	NS
Two or more infarctions		13 (26.0%)	32 (17.0%)	NS	22 (31.9%)	84 (17.8%)	0.01
History of past smoking		34 (68.0%)	141 (74.4%)	NS	49 (71.0%)	340 (72.1%)	NS

Symptoms of cardiovascular disease			p		p			p
History of								
Hypertension		28 (56.0%)	0.02	70 (37.1%)		30 (43.5%)	166 (35.2%)	NS
Angina		21 (42.0%)	NS	70 (36.8%)		28 (40.6%)	166 (35.2%)	NS
Complex arrhythmia		0 (0.0%)	NS	3 (1.6%)		3 (4.3%)	5 (1.1%)	0.04
Congestive heart failure		7 (14.0%)	NS	17 (9.1%)		10 (14.5%)	46 (9.8%)	NS
CHD treatment								
History of bypass surgery		19 (38.0%)	0.03	42 (22.1%)		19 (27.5%)	113 (24.0%)	NS
Beta blockers		17 (34.0%)	NS	48 (25.3%)		18 (26.1%)	99 (21.0%)	NS
Videotaped interview score	$\bar{X}$	29.3	NS	29.3		31.4	29.0	NS
	SD	±14.2		±11.4		±12.2	±11.4	
Participant interview score	$\bar{X}$	2.63	NS	2.66		2.73	2.74	NS
	SD	±0.43		±0.39		±0.45	±0.41	

NS = not significant.

surgery before entry appeared to have a greater incidence of cardiac recurrence.

Although a history of congestive heart failure was obtained more frequently in both section 1 and 2 participants who subsequently had a recurrence than in those who escaped a recurrence, this difference was not statistically significant.

As previously reported,[17,19] here again more than 96% of the section 1 and 2 participants at entry exhibited type A behavior as diagnosed by the VCI test. Moreover, 97% of the 67 comparison group participants, who lived elsewhere than the San Francisco Bay area, had not spontaneously volunteered but had been requested to join the study, and were essentially unaware of the possible relevance of type A behavior to CHD, also exhibited a VCI score that was positive for the presence of type A behavior. The average VCI scores of section 1 and 2 participants (see Table I) also were not significantly different from the average VCI score (27.0 [SD $\pm$ 9.0]) of the above 67 comparison group members living away from the San Francisco Bay area. These findings suggest that the very high frequency of type A behavior detected in all post infarction patients of this study was not a result of a self-selection process in which only patients aware of the possible cardiac importance of type A behavior had volunteered for this study.

Although the entry VCI scores of more than 95% of all post infarction participants were positive for the presence of type A behavior, the average VCI score of either section 1 or 2 participants who suffered recurrences was not significantly different from the average VCI score of those section 1 and 2 participants who did not encounter a recurrence.

Reduction in type A behavior

As determined by participant's questionnaire

As Fig. 1 shows, a significant reduction occurred in the initial intensity of the type A behavior of the section 2 participants given both type A behavior and cardiac counseling throughout the 4.5-year period. The most significant decremental change occurred at the end of the first year, at which time the mean entry score of 2.74 ($\pm$0.42) dropped to 2.34 ($\pm$0.40), a reduction of approximately 1 SD. The average score continued to fall (see Fig. 1) so that at the end of 4.5 years, the mean score was 2.11 ($\pm$0.40), a significant ($p < 0.00001$) decline of 1.5 SD.

A reduction in the intensity of type A behavior also occurred in section 1 participants. However, as Fig. 1 illustrates, the decline was far less dramatic. Thus the initial mean entry score of 2.69 ($\pm$0.42) fell at the end

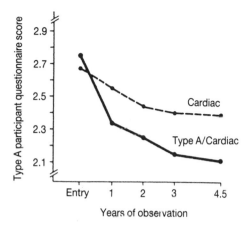

Fig. 1. Decremental change in type A behavior observed each year for 4.5 years in average type A behavior questionnaire scores of section 1 (cardiac-counseled) and section 2 (type A and cardiac-counseled) participants. Questionnaires were obtained at entry and 1, 2, 3 and 4.5 years from 225 (83.3%), 145 (61.7%), 188 (71.6%), 177 (75.3%), and 207 (88%) of section 1 active and treatment-failure participants, respectively. Similar questionnaires were obtained at entry and 1, 2, 3, and 4.5 years from 570 (96.3%), 387 (72.2%), 424 (79.1%), 432 (80.6%), and 450 (84.0%) section 2 active and treatment-failure participants, respectively.

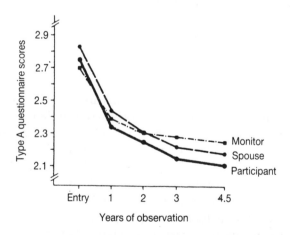

Fig. 2. Decremental changes in type A behavior observed each year for 4.5 years in average type A behavior questionnaire scores of spouses and monitors of section 2 active and treatment-failure participants. Spouse Questionnaires were obtained at entry and 1, 2, 3, and 4.5 years from spouses of 495 (83.6%), 245 (45.7%), 345 (64.4%), 312 (58.2%), and 259 (48.1%) section 2 active and treatment-failure participants, respectively. Monitor Questionnaires were obtained at entry and 1, 2, 3, and 4.5 years from monitors of 527 (89.0%), 256 (47.8%), 356 (66.4%), 315 (58.8%), and 265 (49.4%) section 2 active and treatment-failure participants, respectively. Note that degree of behavior change observed by participants, spouses, and monitors was essentially the same.

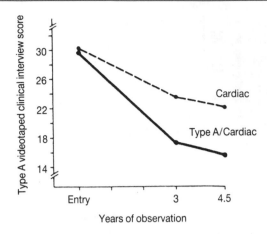

Fig. 3. Decremental changes in type A behavior as estimated by VCI scores in section 1 (cardiac-counseled) and section 2 (type A and cardiac-counseled) active and treatment-failure participants.

of 4.5 years to 2.39 ($\pm$0.41), a decline of 0.71 SD, and significantly less ($p < 0.001$) than those observed in the Section 2 participants.

As we previously reported,[19] the self-reports of section 1 and 2 participants appeared to be relatively accurate because a comparison of both entry and subsequent questionnaire scores of section 2 participants with those of their spouses and monitors (see Fig. 2) showed no statistically significant differences.

As determined by VCI

The VCI scores of the section 2 participants also declined during their 4.5 years in the study, from their mean entry score of 28.0 ($\pm$11.9). At the end of 3 years the mean VCI score was 17.3 ($\pm$8.5), a decline almost equal to 1 SD. At the end of 4.5 years, the mean VCI had dropped even further to 15.5 ($\pm$8.9). This total decremental change from entry to 4.5 years was highly significant ($p < 0.0001$). A significant reduction ($p < 0.05$) also was observed at the end of 3 and 4.5 years in section 1 participants, but the extent of the decline (30.2 $\pm$ 12.3 at entry to 22.1 $\pm$ 9.7) was significantly less ($p < 0.001$) than that (see Fig. 3) in Section 2 participants.

As determined by both questionnaire and VCI

Using the "Intention-to-Treat" principle, we observed at the end of 4.5 years a markedly reduced type A behavior (as manifested by a decline of 1 SD in *both* the participant questionnaire and VCI scores) in 188

Table II. *Cumulative cardiac recurrence rates in sections 1, 2, and 3*

Section	Total number at risk (4.5 years)*	Total recurrence (nonfatal infarctions and cardiac deaths)	Nonfatal infarctions			Cardiac deaths		
			First year†	Remaining 3.5 years	Total 4.5 years	First year	Remaining 3.5 years	Total 4.5 years
1	235	50 (21.2%)	7 (2.7%)	26 (11.1%)	33 (14.0%)	2 (0.8%)	15 (6.4)	17 (7.2%)
2	536	69 (12.9%)‡	6 (1.0%)§	35 (6.5%)‖	41 (7.6%)¶	10 (1.7%)	18 (3.4%)#	28 (5.2%)**
3	109	22 (20.2%)	5 (4.0%)	5 (4.0%)	10 (9.2%)	2 (1.8%)	10 (9.2%)	12 (11.0%)

*These recurrence rates are calculated on entire initial cohort, censoring those who died of a noncardiac death (five, four, and three in sections 1, 2, and 3, respectively) and those who were unable to be traced (30 section 1, 52 section 2, and 43 section 3 participants).

†At end of first year, 262 section 1, 579 section 2, and 124 section 3 participants were at risk.

‡$p < 0.005$ vs section 1; $p < 0.05$ vs section 3.

§$p < 0.07$ vs section 1; $p < 0.02$ vs section 3.

‖$p < 0.05$ vs section 1.

¶$p < 0.02$ vs section 1.

#$p < 0.05$ vs sections 1 and 3.

**$p < 0.05$ vs section 3.

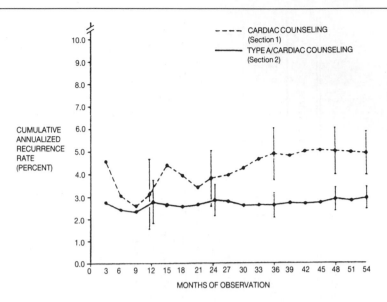

Fig. 4. Cumulative annualized recurrence rate in section 1 (cardiac-counseled) and section 2 (type A and cardiac-counseled) participants calculated quarterly for 4.5 years. Note that 95% confidence limits of quarterly calculated cardiac recurrence rates of two sections no longer intersect at end of 36 months.

(35.1%) of the 536 section 2 participants at risk.* We observed a similar decline in only 23 of the 235 (9.8%) section 1 participants at risk.* This difference in behavior change was highly significant ($p < 0.0001$).

Total cardiac recurrence rate

Cumulative annualized cardiac recurrence rate in randomized section 1 and 2 participants

The respective cumulative annualized total cardiac recurrent rates during the 4.5 years of follow-up of section 1 and 2 participants are depicted in Fig. 4. As can be seen from the graph, the average recurrence rate of section 2 participants from the outset was less than that of section 1 participants, but it was not until shortly after the second year of follow-up that this difference became and remained statistically significant. With use of the "Intention-to-Treat" principle, the average annual recurrence rate

---

* Number of initially enrolled participants *minus* participants who had a noncardiac death or who could not be traced (see Table II for details).

(for the entire 4.5 years of follow-up) was 4.97% in section 1 and 2.96% in section 2. This difference was statistically significant ($p < 0.01$). This analysis is based on 50 events for section 1 and 69 events for section 2 participants with 11.1% and 8.7% losses to follow-up, respectively.

The cumulative annualized total cardiac recurrence rate of those participants who remained active in group counseling throughout the 4.5 years was 5.49% in section 1 and 2.55% in section 2 ($p < 0.01$).

Cumulative total cardiac recurrence rate for 4.5 years in all participants

Again with use of the "Intention-to-Treat" principle, of the 536 section 2 participants* still at risk at the end of 4.5 years, 69 (12.9%) had either a recurrent nonfatal infarction or cardiac death (see Table II) during their 4.5 years at risk. This 4.5-year cumulative recurrence rate was significantly less than the rates observed (see Table II) in section 1 and 3 participants.

Cumulative recurrent nonfatal infarction rate for 4.5 years

As Table II demonstrates, the mean 4.5-year cumulative recurrent nonfatal infarction rate (7.6%) of the section 2 participants was significantly less than that of section 1 participants.

Cumulative cardiac death rate for 4.5 years

Table II indicates, the total 4.5-year cardiac death rate in section 2 participants was less than that observed in the participants of the other two sections, but significantly less than that of section 3 participants only.

The decreased death rate in section 2 participants, as Table II illustrates, was not achieved during the first year of the study. In this connection, nine of the 10 section 2 participants (90%) who succumbed to a cardiac death during the first year at entry had had attacks of angina, four (40%) congestive heart failure, four (40%) episodes of serious arrhythmias, and six (60%) two or more infarctions before entry. Just as ominous, nine of these participants (90%) had a very high Peel Index (average 16.2).

The cumulative cardiac death rate (3.4%) in the section 2 participants, however, during the last 3.5 years of the study (see Table II) was significantly less than the rate in section 1 (6.4%) and section 3 (9.2%) participants.

---

* This number represents the initially enrolled participants minus the 56 participants who (1) died a noncardiac death (four), or (2) were unable to be traced (52).

Cardiac death rate for 4.5 years in low and high Peel Index section 1 and 2 participants

At entry there were 415 participants (119 section 1 and 296 section 2 participants) who exhibited a low and 303 participants (102 section 1 and 201 section 2 participants) who exhibited a high Peel Index. The number of cardiac deaths occurring in the low Peel Index participants was 16 (3.9%), a number significantly ($p < 0.001$) less than the 30 (9.9%) cardiac deaths that occurred in the high Peel Index participants.

The observed 4.5-year cumulative cardiac death rate (2.7%) in the low Peel Index section 2 participants was significantly less ($p < 0.05$) than that (6.7%) observed in the low Peel Index section 1 participants during the same period. However, the cardiac death rate (9.9%) of the high Peel Index section 2 participants was not significantly different from that (9.8%) of the high Peel Index section 1 participants. A detailed analysis of these findings will be reported in the future.

Cumulative recurrence rate for 4.5 years in section 1 and 2 treatment failures

The 4.5-year total cumulative cardiac recurrence rate in the 28 section 1 treatment failures was 32.1% (four nonfatal infarctions and five cardiac deaths). This recurrence rate was not significantly greater than that (21.4%) observed in the 192 section 1 participants who continued to receive counseling for the 4.5-year period. However, this recurrence rate in the section 1 treatment failures was significantly greater ($p < 0.001$) than that (13.0%) observed in the section 2 participants who continued to receive type A counseling.

Similarly, the 4.5-year total cumulative cardiac recurrence rate in the 63 section 2 treatment failures was 33.3% (12 nonfatal infarctions and nine cardiac deaths), which was not significantly different from the recurrence rate observed in the *active* 192 section 1 participants but again significantly greater ($p < 0.001$) than that (13.0%) observed in the *active* section 2 participants.

Cardiac recurrence rate in section 2 participants who exhibited significant type A behavioral reduction at the end of their first year

The first year self-reports of 167 section 2 participants exhibited significant reduction in their type A behavior (i.e., a decrease of 1 SD or more at the end of the first year from the entry score). On the other hand, the first-year questionnaires of 116 section 1 participants failed to indicate significant improvement.

As Table III shows, the cumulative cardiac recurrence rate in the behaviorally improved participants (8.3%) during the last 3.5 years of the total 4.5 years of follow-up was less than half that (21.5%) occurring in the behaviorally unimproved section 1 participants. The difference in recurrence rates was significant.

The entry date of these two groups (see Table III) indicate that they were essentially the same except for a significantly higher entry participant questionnaire score in the section 2 group.

Cumulative rate for 4.5 years of two cardiac recurrences in randomized section 1 and 2 participants

Again when the "Intention-to-Treat" principle was used, eight of the 235 initially enrolled section 1 participants (3.4%) had two cardiac recurrences during the 4.5 years of follow-up. Four of these second cardiac recurrences were fatal. During the same time period only two of the 536 section 2 participants (0.4%) had two recurrences (one of which was fatal). This difference in the rate of two recurrences between section 1 and 2 participants was significant ($p < 0.001$).

Perusal of the entry characteristics of the 10 section 1 and 2 participants having two recurrences indicates that, like participants having one recurrence (see Table I), at entry these participants also exhibited a higher Peel Index (mean 13.3) and more often had experienced at entry two infarcts (50%), congestive heart failure (40%), complex arrhythmias (20%), and angina (50%) than the section 1 and 2 participants who did not have a single recurrence during the 4.5-year study period.

Cardiac recurrence rate for 4.5 years in participants with prior coronary bypass surgery and participants taking beta-blocking drugs at entry

Using the "Intention-to-Treat" principle we found that 38 cardiac recurrences (14 of which were fatal) occurred during the 4.5-year period of follow-up in the 208 section 1 and 2 participants (18.3%) who had had coronary bypass surgery before entry. Eighty-one cardiac recurrences (31 of which were fatal) occurred in the 563 section 1 and 2 participants (14.4%) who had not undergone such surgery before entry. Thus, no significant difference was found in either the total cardiac recurrence or the cardiac death rates between these two groups of participants. However, a significantly greater percentage of the participants entering with prior bypass surgery had had two or more infarcts and also showed a significantly higher Peel Index (10.75) than the participants who had not undergone bypass surgery.

Table III. Entry characteristics and cardiac recurrence rate of section 1 and 2 participants who exhibited reduced or unchanged type A behavior at end of first year of follow-up

		Section 2 participants with reduced type A behavior (n = 167)	Section 1 participants with unchanged type A behavior (n = 116)	Level significance (p value)
Sociodemographic characteristics				
Age (yr)	$\bar{X}$	53.7	54.6	NS
	SD	±6.4	±5.4	
Height (in)	$\bar{X}$	69.3	69.5	NS
	SD	±3.2	±2.8	
Weight (lb)	$\bar{X}$	168.1	172.1	NS
	SD	±22.0	±25.6	
CHD risk factors				
Peel Index	$\bar{X}$	9.2	8.8	NS
	SD	±5.5	±4.5	
Serum cholesterol (mg/dl)	$\bar{X}$	257.7	259.3	NS
	SD	±45.5	±39.3	
Familial history of CHD		93 (55.7%)	65 (56.0%)	NS
More than one prior infarction		42 (25.1%)	25 (21.6%)	NS
History of past smoking		120 (71.9%)	89 (76.9%)	NS

Videotaped clinical interview score	$\bar{X}$ SD	30.1 ±11.6	30.3 ±13.1	NS
Participant questionnaire score	$\bar{X}$ SD	2.9 ±0.36	2.63 ±0.39	0.001
CHD therapy				
History of bypass surgery		42 (25.0%)	32 (27.6%)	NS
Drugs taken at entry				
Beta blocking		32 (19.2%)	26 (22.4%)	NS
Vasodilating		65 (38.9%)	38 (32.8%)	NS
Digitalis glycosides		16 (9.6%)	17 (14.7%)	NS
Antiarrhythmic		13 (7.8%)	13 (11.2%)	NS
Symptoms of cardiovascular disease				
History of				
Hypertension		55 (32.9%)	49 (42.2%)	NS
Angina		63 (37.7%)	40 (34.5%)	NS
Complex arrhythmia		2 (1.2%)	1 (0.9%)	NS
Congestive heart failure		20 (12.0%)	9 (7.8%)	NS
Cumulative recurrence rate (years 2 through 4.5)		14 (8.3%)	25 (21.5%)	0.002
Nonfatal infarctions		11 (6.6%)	20 (17.2%)	0.01
Cardiac deaths		3 (1.8%)	5 (4.3%)	NS

NS = not significant.

Table IV. *Cumulative cardiac recurrence rates in section 1 and 2 participants with prior coronary bypass surgery or taking beta-blocking drugs*

	Section 1		Section 2		
	Number at risk	Cardiac recurrences	Number at risk	Cardiac recurrences	Level of significance (*p* value)*
Participants with prior coronary bypass surgery at entry	67	23 (30.3%)	141	21 (14.0%)	0.01
Participants taking beta-blocking drugs before and during study	62	17 (27.4%)	120	18 (15.0%)	0.05

*Comparison of recurrence rates in sections 1 and 2.

It was of interest, however, that the 4.5-year cumulative cardiac recurrence rate (28.4%) in bypass participants enrolled in section 1 (see Table IV) was significantly higher than the cardiac recurrence rate (13.5%) observed in the section 2 bypass participants who received type A behavior counseling.

Thirty-five cardiac recurrences (14 of which were fatal) occurred in the 4.5-year period in the 178 section 1 and 2 participants (19.7%) who were taking beta-blocking drugs at entry. Eighty-five recurrences (33 of which were fatal) occurred in the 593 section 1 and 2 participants (14.3%) who had not taken beta-blocking drugs at entry. Thus no significant difference was found in either the total cardiac recurrence or the fatal cardiac rates between these two groups.

However, as noted above in the bypass and nonbypass participants, the 4.5-year cumulative cardiac recurrence rate (27.4%) in section 1 participants taking beta-blocking drugs (see Table IV) was significantly greater than the recurrence rate (15.0%) observed in section 2 participants taking beta-blocking drugs.

Changes in medical and surgical treatment, symptoms, and signs of coronary heart disease after 4.5 years

Table V indicates that section 1 and 2 participants received after entry essentially the same surgical and medical treatment during the 4.5 years of follow-up. Thus the percentages of section 1 participants undergoing coronary bypass surgery, or taking beta-blocking drugs, vasodilators, digitalis glycosides, or antiarrhythmic drugs were essentially the same as those of section 2 participants. Moreover, the incidence of arrhythmia, congestive heart failure, and hypertension (see Table V) was not significantly different in the two sections. The mean serum cholesterol levels of both section 1 and 2 participants, which had dropped significantly from their entry levels at the end of the third year of the study,[19] dropped even more at the end of 4.5 years (see Table V). Thus the decline from entry was 16.3% in the section 1 and 18.6% in the section 2 participants.

Discussion

The present report summarizes the final results obtained in the RCPP study, whose initially designed 5 years of type A behavioral counseling of

Table V. Incidence of coronary bypass surgery, cardiovascular manifestations, ingestion of drugs, and serum cholesterol levels in section 1 and 2 participants (4.5 years)

Section	Number of living, active participants (4.5 years)	Number of coronary bypass operations (4.5 years)	Number of participants currently having			
			Angina	Arrhythmia	Congestive heart failure	Hypertension
1	161	34 (21.1%)	94 (58.4%)	34 (21.1%)	12 (7.5%)	69 (42.9%)
2	335	65 (19.3%)	167 (49.7%)	62 (18.5%)	23 (6.8%)	118 (35.1%)

Section	Number of participants current taking				Mean ± SD serum cholesterol (mg/dl)	
	Beta blockers	Vasodilators	Digitalis glycosides	Antiarrhythmics	At entry	4.5 years
1	74 (46.0%)	72 (44.7%)	25 (15.5%)	32 (19.9%)	258 ± 41.2	216 ± 46.2*
2	139 (41.4%)	142 (42.3%)	59 (17.6%)	58 (17.3%)	264 ± 51.6	215.2 ± 46.3

*p < 0.001 vs entry value.

post infarction participants was shortened to 4.5 years because the protective influence against a cardiac recurrence of such behavioral counseling became statistically obvious as early as the third year of the study.[19] *

We believe that one of the most important findings of this study is the observation that more than 95% of the 1013 successively admitted and examined post-infarction participants exhibited type A behavior, varying from moderate to very severe intensity. Moreover, the almost ubiquitous presence of this behavior pattern was not a result of any voluntary self-selection, because the same prevalence rate was detected in the 67 participants who had not volunteered initially, almost all of whom were not aware of the possible relationship of type A behavior to the pathogenesis of CHD.

This finding of course is at variance with the observations of Shekelle *et al.*,[24] Ruberman *et al.*,[25] Case *et al.*,[26] and even the earlier results obtained in the Western Collaborative Group Study.[2] We believe that there are two probable reasons for this significant difference between the prevalence rate of type A behavior observed in the present study and that of these other studies.

First, the diagnosis of type A behavior in these earlier studies was attempted by presenting the patients with a list of stereotyped questions that were either printed (i.e., a questionnaire) or verbally administered by nonmedical personnel who previously had no experience at all in the diagnosis of any kind of medical disorder but received only a few hours of training concerning how to ask the predetermined set of questions. Also in most cases, these ad hoc interviewers were trained by nonmedical personnel.

The diagnosis of type A behavior in the present study was accomplished, as all diagnoses of all medical disorders, by the *clinical examination* of each participant in which the various clinical signs and symptoms characteristic of type A behavior were noted by a technician who possessed 26 years' experience in diagnosing the presence of type A behavior.

The second probable reason is that these earlier investigations used questions that were formulated by one of us (M.F.) more than a quarter of a century ago.[1] Since that time, as we previously pointed out,[27,28] more than a dozen new physical signs and symptoms suggestive of the presence

---

* This reduction of the initially planned 5 years of type A counseling to 4.5 years was advised by a special committee of the National Heart, Lung, and Blood Institute after its perusal of all the data accumulated at the end of the third year of the study.

of type A behavior have been uncovered. Although these diagnostics formed a key component of the VCI,[18,28] none of them was used in the studies of Shekelle *et al.*,[24] Ruberman *et al.*,[25] and Case *et al.*[26] Indeed, these investigators used questionnaires that contained no questions concerning the presence of free-floating hostility, one of the two core components of type A behavior.[1-3] How can the presence of type A behavior be detected or diagnosed by a questionnaire if such a questionnaire contains no questions concerning the possible presence of one of the characteristic components of this behavior?

As previously reported,[19] although almost all post infarction patients were observed to exhibit varying degrees of severity of type A behavior, the degree of this severity did not appear to carry prognostic relevance. This may well result from the probability, as Halperin and Littman,[29] Pickering,[30] and Ketterer[31] have pointed out in their criticism of results of the study of Case *et al.*,[26] that the physical status of the left ventricle after an infarction plays a far greater role in determining subsequent mortality than even severe type A behavior. If, then, the possible prognostic importance of a severe degree of type A behavior is to be determined accurately, the presence of such ominous risk factors as post infarction congestive heart failure, reduced left ventricular ejection fraction, and serious arrhythmias must be controlled.

It is of interest that although the cumulative annualized cardiac recurrence rate (4.97%) observed in our control section 1 participants receiving only group cardiac counseling was not significantly different from the recurrence rates of 5.7%, 4.9%, and 4.4% observed respectively in the 2789 control post infarction patients of the Coronary Drug Project,[32] the 2257 control subjects of the Aspirin Myocardial Study,[33] and the 80 control post infarction patients of the Coronary Artery Surgery Study,[34] the recurrence rate (2.96%) in our experimental section 2, type A-counseled participants was significantly lower than each of the recurrence rates observed in these three other studies.

Thus there appears to be little doubt that when group type A behavioral counseling together with cardiac counseling was given to the RCPP post infarction participants, a significant decrease in both cardiac morbidity and mortality was achieved *after the first year of such combined counseling*. Moreover, this decrease appears to be greater than that achieved in previously reported studies in which post infarction patients were administered various drugs or underwent various surgical procedures.

The relative protection against recurrent infarction or cardiac death afforded to section 2 participants seemed to be a result of the type A behavioral counseling for two reasons: first, the treatment of section 2 participants essentially differed from that given the control section 1

participants only in that they were exposed to type A counseling.*
Second, those section 2 participants who were found to exhibit significant
behavioral change at the end of the first year of the study subsequently
had significantly fewer cardiac recurrences in the remaining 3.5 years than
those section 1 participants who failed to exhibit any significant behavioral change at the end of the first year.

The final results of the RCPP study also suggest that besides the
already demonstrated associational relationship between type A behavior
and the prevalance[1,11] as well as the incidence[2,15,16] of CHD, this
behavioral syndrome also has a causal relationship to the continued
progress of clinical CHD. Such relationship appears probable because
when type A behavior and no other possible risk factor was modified in
one of two sections of post infarction patients this section exhibited
significantly fewer cardiac recurrences.

We believe that the results of the present study will be replicated when
other post infarction patients are counseled by *adequately trained and
dedicated* professional personnel. If such confirmation does occur, we
believe that it will be an immediate and urgent necessity to begin
administering type A behavioral counseling to all post infarction patients
for the following reasons: first, unlike other putative risk factors (e.g.,
hypertension, excess smoking of cigarettes, hypercholesterolemia, and
positive family history of CHD), which are not found in all post infarction
patients (see Table I), type A behavior was observed in 97.5% of the
1013 initially enrolled post infarction participants of this study.[17] Second,
type A counseling appears to provide the post infarction participants of
this study powerful protection against subsequent recurrent myocardial
infarction or cardiac death (including those participants who have
undergone coronary artery bypass surgery or who are taking beta-
blocking drugs). Third, unlike various other medical or surgical procedures used in treating coronary patients, modification of the type A

---

* It might be argued that section 2 participants spent approximately 27 hours more in group
sessions than section 1 participants during the 4.5 years and therefore some nonspecific
psychologic factor might have been responsible for the approximate halving of their
cardiac recurrence rate. However, if mere attendance at group sessions played a critical
role in preventing cardiac recurrences, then section 1 participants who attended many
group sessions in turn should have had a significantly lower recurrence rate than (1)
section 3 participants who received no group counseling and (2) those section 1 and 2
participants who very early dropped out of the study. However, as already indicated, no
such difference in cardiac recurrence rates was observed. Also, the cardiac recurrence
rate in the control post infarction patients of the Coronary Drug,[32] Aspirin,[33] and
Coronary Artery Surgery[34] studies who did not receive group counseling of any kind was
essentially the same as that of our section 1 participants who did receive cardiac
counseling.

behavior of a person frequently appears *to enhance the quality of that person's familial and vocational relationships.*[35]

Acknowledgements

Supported by grants from the National Heart, Lung, and Blood Institute (21427), Bank of America, Chevron Oil Company, the Kaiser Hospital Foundation, and the Mary Potishman Lard Trust, Fort Worth, Texas.

We thank Nancy Fleischmann and Drs. Gary S. Gelber, Raphael B. Reider, Bernard DeHovitz, Paul Loftus, Michael Grossman, Peter J. Wolk, and Rene Bine, Jr., who served as group counselors, independent referees, or consultants. We also thank Drs. Berton Kaplan, Michael A. Ibrahim, and David G. Kleinbaum for statistical assistance. We acknowledge the advice of Professor Byron W. Brown, Jr., Ph.D., Head of Division of Biostatistics, Stanford University, School of Medicine, in the analysis of the data for this study, and the preparation of this report.

References

1. Friedman M, Rosenman RH. Association of specific overt behavior pattern with blood and cardiovascular findings. JAMA 1959;169:1286.
2. Rosenman RH, Brand RJ, Jenkins CD, Friedman M, Straus R, Wurm M. Coronary heart disease in the Western Collaborative Group Study: final follow-up experience of 8½ years. JAMA 1975;23:872.
3. Friedman M. Pathogenesis of coronary artery disease. New York: McGraw-Hill, 1949.
4. Friedman M, St. George S, Byers SO, Rosenman RH. Excretion of catecholamines, 17 ketosteroids, 17-hydroxycorticoids and 5-hydroxindole in men exhibiting a particular behavior pattern (A) associated with a high incidence of clinical coronary artery disease. J. Clin Invest 1960;39:735.
5. Carruthers ME. Aggression and atheroma. Lancet 1969;2:1170.
6. Friedman M, Byers SO, Rosenman RH. Coronary prone individuals (type A behavior pattern): some biochemical characteristics. JAMA 1970;212:1030.
7. Friedman M, Byers SO, Rosenman RH. Plasma ACTH and cortisol concentration of coronary prone subjects. Proc Soc Exp Biol Med 1972;140:681.
8. Williams RB Jr, Lane JD, Kuhn CM, Meosh W, White AD, Schanberg SM. Type A behavior and elevated physiological and neuroendocrine responses to cognitive tasks. Science 1976;136:1234.
9. Blumenthal JA, Williams RB Jr, Kong Y, Schanberg SM, Thompson LW. Type A behavior pattern and coronary atherosclerosis. Circulation 1978;58:634.
10. Zyzanski SJ, Jenkins CD, Ryan TJ, Flessas A, Everist M. Psychological correlates of coronary angiographic findings. Arch Intern Med 1976;136:1234.
11. Caffrey B. Behavior patterns and personality characteristics related to prevalence rates of coronary heart disease in American monks. J Chronic Dis 1969;22:93.

12. Jenkins CD. Recent evidence supporting psychological and social risk factors for coronary disease. Part II. N Engl J Med 1976;294:1033.

13. Dembroski TM, Weiss SM, Shields JL, Haynes SG, Feinleib M. Coronary prone behavior. New York: Springer-Verlag, 1978.

14. Matthews KA, Glass DC, Rosenman RH, Bortner RW. Competitive drive, pattern A and coronary heart disease: a further analysis of some data from the Western Collaborative Group Study. J Chronic Dis 1977;30:489.

15. Haynes SG, Feinleib M, Levine S, Scotch N, Kannel WB. The relationship of psychosocial factors to coronary heart disease in the Framingham Study. III. Eight year incidence of coronary heart disease. Am J Epidemiol 1980;111:37.

16. The Review Panel on Coronary-Prone Behavior and Coronary Heart Disease. A critical review. Circulation 1981;63:1199.

17. Friedman M, Thoresen CE, Gill JJ, Ulmer D, Thompson L, Powell LH, Price V, Elek SR, Rabin DD, Breall WS, Piaget G, Dixon T, Bourg E, Levy RA, Tasto DL. Feasibility of altering Type A behavior pattern. Recurrent Coronary Prevention Project Study. Methods, baseline results and preliminary findings. Circulation 1982;66:83.

18. Powell LH, Friedman M, Thoresen CE, Gill JJ, Ulmer D. Can the Type A behavior pattern be altered after myocardial infarction? A second year report from the Recurrent Coronary Prevention Project. Psychosom Med 1984;46:293.

19. Friedman M, Thoresen CE, Gill JJ, Powell LH, Ulmer D, Thompson L, Price VA, Rabin DD, Breall WS, Dixon T, Levy R, Bourg E. Alteration of type A behavior and reduction in cardiac recurrences in postmyocardial infarction patients. Am Heart J 1984;108:237.

20. Peel A, Semple T, Wong I, Lancaster WM, Dahl JLG. A coronary prognostic index for grading the severity of infarction. Br Heart J 1962;24:745.

21. Blackburn H. Electrocardiographic classification for population comparisons. The Minnesota Code. J. Electrocardiol 1969;2:5.

22. Peto R, Pike M, Armitage P, Breslow NE, Cox DR, Howard SV, Mantel N, McPhersen K, Peto J, Smith PG. Design and analysis of randomized clinical trials requiring prolonged observation of each patient. Introduction and design. Br J Cancer 1976;34:585.

23. Hays WL. Statistics. 3rd ed. New York: Holt, Rinehart & Winston, 1981.

24. Shekelle R, Hully SB, Neaton, J. Et al. The MRFIT behavior pattern study. II. Type A behavior and incidence of coronary heart disease. Am J Epidemiol 1985;122:555.

25. Ruberman W, Weinblatt E, Goldblatt JD, Chaudharry BS. Psychosocial influences on mortality after myocardial infarction. N Engl J Med 1984;311:552.

26. Case RB, Heller SS, Case NB, Moss AJ, and The Multicenter Post-Infarction Research Group. Type A behavior and survival after acute myocardial infarction. N Engl J Med 1985;312:737.

27. Friedman M, Thoresen CE, Gill JJ. Type A behavior, its possible role, detection and alteration in patients with ischemic heart disease. In: Hurst JW, ed. The heart update V. New York: McGraw-Hill, 1981:81.

28. Friedman M, Powell LH. The diagnosis and quantitative assessment of Type

A behavior: introduction and description of the videotaped structured interview. Integrative Psychiatry 1984;2:121.

29. Halperin PJ, Littman AB. Type A behavior and survival after myocardial infarction. N Engl J Med 1985;313:448.

30. Pickering TG. Type A behavior and survival after myocardial infarction. N Engl J Med 1985;313:450.

31. Ketterer MK. Type A behavior and survival after myocardial infarction. N Engl J Med 1985;313:449.

32. The Coronary Drug Project. Clofibrate and niacin in coronary heart disease. JAMA 1975;231:360.

33. Aspirin Myocardial Infarction Study Research Group. A randomized control trial of aspirin in persons recovered from myocardial infarction. JAMA 1980;243:661.

34. Coronary Artery Surgery Study Principal Investigators and Their Associates. Myocardial infarction and mortality in the coronary artery surgery study (CASS) randomized trial. N Engl J Med 1984;310:750.

35. Gill JJ, Price VA, Friedman M, Thoresen CE, Powell LH, Ulmer D, Brown B, Drews FR. Reduction in type A behavior in healthy middle-aged American military officers. Am Heart J 1985;110:503.

Can lifestyle changes reverse coronary heart disease? The Lifestyle Heart Trial

Dean Ornish, Shirley E. Brown, Larry W. Scherwitz, James H. Billings, William T. Armstrong, Thomas A. Ports, Sandra M. McLanahan, Richard L. Kirkeeide, Richard J. Brand and K. Lance Gould

Pacific Presbyterian Medical Center, Preventive Medicine Research Institute, and Departments of Medicine and Psychology, University of California San Francisco School of Medicine, USA (D. Ornish, MD, S. E. Brown, MD, J. H. Billings, PhD); UCSF School of Dental Public Health and Hygiene, USA (L. W. Scherwitz, PhD); Cardiac Catheterisation Laboratories, Pacific Presbyterian Medical Center, USA (W. T. Armstrong, MD); Cardiovascular Research Institute, UCSF School of Medicine, USA (T. A. Ports, MD); Integral Health Services, Inc, Richmond, Virginia, USA (S. M. McLanahan, MD); Center for Cardiovascular and Imaging Research, University of Texas Medical School, USA (R. L. Kirkeeide, PhD, Prof K. L. Gould, MD); and Department of Biomedical and Environmental Health Science, University of California School of Public Health, Berkeley, California, USA (Prof R. J. Brand, PhD)

Abstract

In a prospective, randomised, controlled trial to determine whether comprehensive lifestyle changes affect coronary atherosclerosis after 1 year, 28 patients were assigned to an experimental group (low-fat vegetarian diet, stopping smoking, stress management training, and moderate exercise) and 20 to a usual-care control group. 195 coronary artery lesions were analysed by quantitative coronary angiography. The average percentage diameter stenosis regressed from 40·0 (SD 16·9)% to 37·8 (16·5)% in the experimental group yet progressed from 42·7 (15·5)% to 46·1 (18·5)% in the control group. When only lesions greater than 50% stenosed were analysed, the average percentage diameter stenosis regressed from 61·1 (8·8)% to 55·8 (11·0)% in the experimental group and progressed from

Reprinted from Ornish, D., Brown, S. E., Scherwitz, L. W., Billings, J. H., Armstrong, W. T., Ports, T. A., McLanahan, S. M., Kirkeeide, R. L., Brand, R. J. and Gould, K. L. Can lifestyle changes reverse coronary heart disease? *Lancet*, **336**. 129–33, 1990.

61·7 (9·5)% to 64·4 (16·3)% in the control group. Overall, 82% of experimental-group patients had an average change towards regression. Comprehensive lifestyle changes may be able to bring about regression of even severe coronary atherosclerosis after only 1 year, without use of lipid-lowering drugs. *Lancet* 1990; **336**: 129–33.

Introduction

The Lifestyle Heart Trial is the first randomised, controlled clinical trial to determine whether patients outside hospital can be motivated to make and sustain comprehensive lifestyle changes and, if so, whether regression of coronary atherosclerosis can occur as a result of lifestyle changes alone. Over twenty clinical trials are being carried out to determine whether the progression of coronary atherosclerosis can be modified; in all of these, cholesterol-lowering drugs, plasmapheresis, or partial ileal bypass surgery are the primary interventions.[1]

We carried out trials in 1977 and 1980 to assess the short-term effects of lifestyle changes on coronary heart disease with non-invasive endpoint measures (improvements in cardiac risk factors, functional status, myocardial perfusion,[2] and left ventricular function[3]). However, the subjects of those studies were not living in the community during the trial, and we did not use angiography to assess changes in coronary atherosclerosis.

Patients and methods

Patients with angiographically documented coronary artery disease were randomly assigned to an experimental group or to a usual-care control group. Experimental-group patients were prescribed a lifestyle pro-gramme that included a low-fat vegetarian diet, moderate aerobic exercise, stress management training, stopping smoking, and group support. Control-group patients were not asked to make lifestyle changes, although they were free to do so. Progression or regression of coronary artery lesions was assessed in both groups by quantitative coronary angiography at baseline and after about a year.

Patients were recruited from Pacific Presbyterian Medical Center (PPMC) and from Moffitt Hospital of the UCSF School of Medicine according to the following criteria: age 35–75 years, male or female; residence in the greater San Francisco area; no other life-threatening illnesses; no myocardial infarction during the preceding 6 weeks, and no history of receiving streptokinase or alteplase; not currently receiving lipid-lowering drugs; one, two, or three vessel coronary artery disease (defined as any measurable coronary atherosclerosis in a non-dilated or non-bypassed coronary artery); left ventricular ejection fraction greater than 25%; not scheduled to have coronary artery bypass grafting; and permission granted by patient's cardiologist and primary care physician. We screened and recruited only patients who were having angiograms for clinical reasons unrelated to this study so that only one additional angiogram was needed for research purposes.

A total of 193 patients who met the first five entry criteria underwent quantitative coronary arteriography at UCSF and PPMC. 94 of these patients (49%) met the remaining entry criteria. Of the 94 eligible patients, 53 were randomly assigned to the experimental group and 43 to the control group; 28 (53%) and 20 (42%), respectively, agreed to take part. All patients who were eligible and volunteered were accepted into the study. These patients represented a cross-section of age, gender, race, ethnic group, socioeconomic status, and educational level. Each gave fully informed written consent and the study was approved by the relevant ethical committees.

Follow-up angiographic data were not available for 7 patients: 1 control-group patient underwent emergency, non-quantitative angiography in another hospital; and of the 6 experimental-group patients, 1 died while greatly exceeding exercise recommendations in an unsupervised gym, 1 could not be tested owing to a large unpaid hospital bill, 1 was a previously undiagnosed alcoholic who dropped out, 1 patient's preintervention angiogram was lost in transit to Houston for quantitative analysis, and 2 patients' angiographic views before and after intervention did not match adequately owing to technical difficulties.

Selective coronary angiography was done by the percutaneous femoral technique. The two laboratories were calibrated at baseline and every 6 months thereafter. Orthogonal views were obtained, and the angle, skew, rotation, table height, and type of catheter were recorded during the baseline angiogram to allow these measurements to be reproduced during angiography about a year (15 [SD 3] months) later. Baseline and follow-up measures were identical in the view angles, their sequence, type of contrast dye, the angiographer, and the cine arteriographic equipment. Catheter tips were saved and used as reference measures for quantitative analyses of films. Cine arteriograms made in San Francisco were sent to the University of Texas Medical School at Houston for quantitative analyses by a protocol described elsewhere in detail.[4]

Blood samples for measurement of serum lipids were drawn (after a 14 h fast) at baseline, after 6 months, and after a year. Total cholesterol, HDL-cholesterol, and triglyceride concentrations were measured by 'Astra' enzymic assays (Beckman Instruments, Brea, California).[5] LDL was calculated as total cholesterol minus HDL-cholesterol plus

0·16 × triglycerides. Apolipoproteins A-I and B were measured by disc gel electrophoresis and by isoelectric focusing.[6]

To check adherence to the programme patients completed a 3-day diet diary at baseline and after a year to assess nutrient intake and dietary adherence.[7] These diaries were analysed by means of the CBORD diet analyser based upon the USDA database (CBORD Group Inc, Ithaca, New York, USA). Patients were asked to complete a questionnaire describing the type, frequency, and duration of exercise and of each stress management technique. Patients who said they had stopped smoking underwent random tests of plasma cotinine.[8] Information from the adherence questionnaires was quantified by a formula determined before the study. A total score of 1 indicated 100% adherence to the recommended lifestyle change programme, and 0 indicated no adherence. Patients who did more than we recommended achieved a score greater than 1.

To reduce the possibility that knowledge of group assignment might bias the outcome measurements, the investigators carrying out all medical tests remained unaware of both patient group assignment and the order of the tests. Different people provided the lifestyle intervention, carried out the tests, analysed the results, and carried out statistical analyses. Coronary arteriograms were analysed without knowledge of sequence or of group assignment.

The intervention began with a week-long residential retreat at a hotel to teach the lifestyle intervention to the experimental-group patients. Patients then attended regular group support meetings (4 h twice a week).

Experimental-group patients were asked to eat a low-fat vegetarian diet for at least a year. The diet included fruits, vegetables, grains, legumes, and soybean products without caloric restriction. Some take-home meals were provided for those who wanted them. No animal products were allowed except egg white and one cup per day of non-fat milk or yoghurt. The diet contained approximately 10% of calories as fat (polyunsatured/ saturated ratio greater than 1), 15–20% protein, and 70–75% predominantly complex carbohydrates. Cholesterol intake was limited to 5 mg/day or less. Salt was restricted only for hypertensive patients. Caffeine was eliminated, and alcohol was limited to no more than 2 units per day (alcohol was excluded for anyone with a history of alcoholism, and no one was encouraged to drink). The diet was nutritionally adequate and met the recommended daily allowances for all nutrients except vitamin B_{12}, which was supplemented.

The stress management techniques included stretching exercises, breathing techniques, meditation, progressive relaxation, and imagery.[3,9–12] The purpose of each technique was to increase the patient's sense of relaxation, concentration, and awareness. Patients were asked to practise these stress management techniques for at least 1 h per day and were given a 1 h audiocassette tape to assist them.

Only 1 patient in the experimental group was smoking at baseline, and she agreed to stop on entry.

Patients were individually prescribed exercise levels (typically walking) according to their baseline treadmill test results. Patients were asked to reach a target training heart rate of 50–80% of the heart rate at which 1 mm ST depression occurred during baseline treadmill testing or, if not ischaemic, to 50–80% of their age-adjusted maximum heart rate based on level of conditioning. Patients were also trained to identify exertional levels by means of the Borg rate of perceived exertion scale.[13] Patients were asked to exercise for a minimum of 3 h per week and to spend a minimum of 30 min per session exercising within these target heart rates. A defibrillator and emergency drugs were available at all times.

The twice-weekly group discussions provided social support to help patients adhere to the lifestyle change programme.[14] The sessions were led by a clinical psychologist who facilitated discussions of strategies for maintaining adherence to the programme, communication skills, and expression of feelings about relationships at work and at home.

Differences in baseline characteristics of the two groups were tested for statistical significance by conventional *t* tests. Comparisons of the two study groups' baseline coronary artery lesion characteristics (measured by quantitative coronary angiography) and changes in lesion characteristics after intervention were examined by a mixed-model analysis of variance.[15] These analyses used lesion-specific data but allowed for the possibility that lesion data in a given subject could be statistically dependent. Mean changes in other endpoint measures were analysed for statistical significance by repeated-measures analysis of variance.

Results

At baseline, there were no significant differences between the experimental and control groups in demographic characteristics (table I), diet and lifestyle characteristics, functional status, cardiac history, or risk factors in the 41 subjects who completed angiography before and after the intervention. The control group had significantly higher levels of HDL-cholesterol (1·33 [SD 0·52] *vs* 1·02 [0·31] mmol/l; p = 0·029) and apolipoprotein A-I (156 (36) *vs* 133 (21)mg/dl; p = 0·0155) than the experimental group, but the ratios of total/HDL cholesterol and LDL/HDL cholesterol did not differ significantly between the groups at baseline. The experimental and control groups did not differ significantly in disease severity at baseline. The mean values in table II do not fully reflect the severity of coronary atherosclerosis in these patients for the following

Table I. *Baseline characteristics of experimental and control groups*

	Mean (SD)	
	Experimental group (n = 22)	Control group (n = 19)
Male/Female	21/1	15/4
Age (yr)	56.1 (7.5)	59.8 (9.1)
Weight (kg)	91.1 (15.5)	80.4 (22.8)
Body mass index (kg/m²)	28.4 (4.1)	26.5 (5.3)
Education (yr)	15.9 (2.9)	14.2 (3.0)

Table II. *Mean lesion characteristics at baseline*

	Mean (SEM)	
	Experimental group (n = 22)	Control group (n = 19)
% diameter reduction	40.0 (1.78)	42.7 (1.95)
Stenosis flow reserve	3.96 (0.12)	3.88 (0.13)
Minimum diameter (mm)	1.67 (0.10)	1.73 (0.10)
Normal diameter (mm)	2.76 (0.14)	2.96 (0.15)

195 lesions: 105 experimental, 90 control.

reasons: quantitative analyses of coronary arteriograms tend to assess stenoses as being less severe than do qualitative assessments; we analysed all detectable lesions, including minor ones; and we excluded from analysis 33 lesions that were 100% occluded at baseline.

Adherence to the diet, exercise, and stress management components of the lifestyle programme in the experimental group was excellent (table III). Patients in the control group made more moderate changes in lifestyle consistent with more conventional recommendations.

Table IV summarises changes in risk factors during the intervention period. In the experimental group, total cholesterol fell by 24·3% and LDL-cholesterol by 37·4%. These falls occurred even though patients had already reduced fat consumption to 31·5% of calories and cholesterol intake to 213 mg/day on average before baseline testing. HDL-cholesterol did not change significantly in either group. Apolipoprotein B fell substantially in the experimental group but it did not change in the

Table III. *Compliance with exercise, stress management, and dietary changes*

| | Mean (SD) at baseline | | Mean (SD) at 122 mo | | p (two-sided) |
	Experimental (n = 20–22)	Control (n = 17–19)	Experimental (n = 20–22)	Control (n = 17–19)	
Exercise					
Times/day	0.26 (0.37)	0.35 (0.39)	0.69 (0.20)	0.39 (0.37)	0.0008
Min/day	11.0 (17.7)	18.4 (27.7)	38.1 (17.4)	20.6 (27.7)	0.0004
Stress reduction					
Times/day	0.50 (1.21)	0.16 (0.34)	5.94 (2.62)	0.42 (0.74)	<0.0001
Min/day	5.09 (12.7)	1.76 (4.34)	82.1 (36.6)	4.50 (10.2)	<0.0001
Fat intake					
g/day	67.4 (18.6)	58.2 (25.9)	14.0 (8.6)	55.2 (21.1)	<0.0001
% of energy intake	31.5 (7.6)	30.1 (10.7)	6.8 (3.5)	29.5 (8.6)	<0.0001
Dietary cholesterol (mg/day)	213 (111)	205 (127)	12.4 (45.8)	190 (99)	<0.0001
Energy intake (MJ/day)	8.2 (1.8)	7.2 (2.2)	7.6 (2.1)	7.1 (1.9)	0.5082
Total adherence score*	0.55 (0.22)	0.56 (0.30)	1.22 (0.22)	0.62 (0.30)	<0.0001

*Percentage of minimum recommended level of combined lifestyle change; includes all the above plus smoking cessation.

Table IV. *Changes in risk factors*

	Mean (SD) at baseline		Mean (SD) at 12 mo		p
	Experimental group (n = 20–22)	Control group (N = 17–19)	Experimental group (n = 20–22)	Control group (n = 17–19)	p (two-sided)
Serum lipids (mmol/l)					
Total cholesterol	5.88 (1.29)	6.34 (1.02)	4.45 (1.15)	6.00 (1.55)	0.0192
LDL cholesterol	3.92 (1.25)	4.32 (0.77)	2.46 (1.55)	4.07 (1.17)	0.0072
HDL cholesterol	1.00 (0.26)	1.35 (0.52)	0.97 (0.40)	1.31 (0.38)	0.8316
Triglycerides	2.38 (1.26)	2.45 (2.47)	2.91 (1.47)	2.24 (1.79)	0.2472
Apolipoproteins (mg/dl)					
A-I	133 (21)	156 (36)	135 (26)	166 (47)	0.4612
B	104 (33)	104 (21)	79 (23)	105 (28)	0.0104
Lipid ratios					
Total/HDL cholesterol	6.33 (2.14)	5.32 (1.89)	5.15 (2.23)	4.93 (1.59)	0.1734
LDL/HDL cholesterol	4.18 (1.53)	3.59 (1.37)	2.89 (1.92)	3.33 (1.42)	0.0348
Blood pressure (mm Hg)					
Systolic	134 (13)	140 (26)	127 (13)	131 (20)	0.7550
Diastolic	83 (8)	82 (13)	79 (7)	77 (11)	0.8987
Weight (kg)	91.1 (15.5)	80.4 (22.8)	81.0 (11.4)	81.8 (25.0)	<0.0001

Table V. *Changes in angina symptoms*

	Mean (SD) at baseline		Mean (SD) at 12 mo		
	Experimental group (n = 20)	Control group (n = 17)	Experimental group (n = 20)	Control group (n = 17)	p (two-sided)
Chest pain frequency	5.10 (14.1)	2.35 (3.77)	0.45 (0.76)	6.24 (12.9)	0.0578
Chest pain duration (min)	2.73 (4.69)	3.47 (7.95)	1.58 (4.48)	6.97 (14.5)	0.1390
Chest pain severity	2.3 (1.6)	1.8 (1.1)	1.7 (1.2)	2.5 (1.2)	0.0006

*Scale of 1 to 7, 1 least severe.

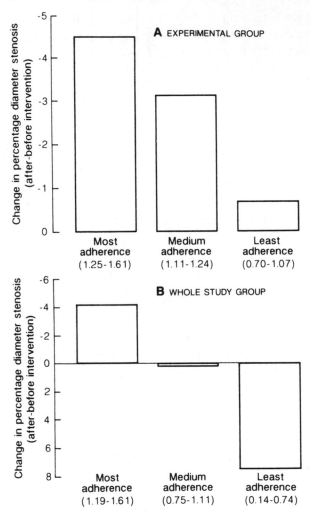

Correlation of overall adherence score and changes in percentage diameter stenosis in experimental group only (A) and in whole study group (B). A = 7 subjects in each tertile; B = 13, 14, 13.

control group. Neither group had significant changes in apolipoprotein A-I.

Patients in the experimental group reported a 91% reduction in the frequency of angina, a 42% reduction in duration of angina, and a 28% reduction in the severity of angina. In contrast, control-group patients reported a 165% rise in frequency, a 95% rise in duration, and a 39% rise in severity of angina (table V). In previous studies,[2,3] we found that similar improvements in functional status occurred in only 1 month, which suggests that improvements in angina may precede regression of coronary atherosclerosis, perhaps by changing platelet-endothelial interactions, vasomotor tone, or other dynamic characteristics of stenoses.

All 195 detectable lesions were included in the quantitative analysis. The average percentage diameter stenosis decreased from 40·0 (SD 16·9)% to 37·8 (16·5)% in the experimental group yet progressed from 42·7 (15·5)% to 46·1 (18·5)% in the control group (p = 0.001, two-tailed). When only lesions greater than 50% stenosed were analysed, the average percentage diameter stenosis regressed from 61·1 (8·8)% to 55·8 (11·0)% in the experimental group but progressed from 61·7 (9·5)% to 64·4 (16·3)% in the control group (p = 0.03, two-tailed).

The average lesion change scores (% diameter stenosis after intervention minus before intervention) in the experimental group were in the direction of regression of coronary atherosclerosis in 18 of the 22 patients (82%) including the 1 woman, in the direction of slight progression in 3 patients, and in the direction of substantial progression in 1 patient with poor adherence. In contrast, in the control group the average lesion change scores were in the direction of progression of coronary atherosclerosis in 10 of 19 (53%), in the direction of regression (including all 4 women) in 8, and 1 showed no change.

In the experimental group and in the whole study group, overall adherence to the lifestyle changes was strongly related to changes in lesions in a "dose-response" manner, suggesting that the relation was causal. The differences in overall adherence are sufficient to explain the observed differences in percentage diameter stenosis. To assess whether programme adherence was related to lesion changes, the experimental group and the combined study group were divided into tertiles based on overall adherence score. Degree of adherence was directly correlated with changes in percentage diameter stenosis (see accompanying figure).

Discussion

This clinical trial has shown that a heterogeneous group of patients with coronary heart disease can be motivated to make comprehensive changes in lifestyle for at least a year outside hospital. The changes in serum lipid levels are similar to those seen with cholesterol-lowering drugs. The lifestyle intervention seems safe and compatible with other treatments of coronary heart disease.

After a year, patients in the experimental group showed significant overall regression of coronary atherosclerosis as measured by quantitative coronary arteriography. Since coronary atherosclerosis occurs over a period of decades, one would not expect to find larger changes in only a year. Perfusion is a fourth-power function of coronary artery diameter, so even a small amount of regression in a critically stenosed artery has a large effect on myocardial perfusion and thus on functional status. In contrast, patients in the usual-care control group who were making less comprehensive changes in lifestyle showed significant overall progression of coronary atherosclerosis. This finding suggests that conventional recommendations for patients with coronary heart disease (such as a 30% fat diet) are not sufficient to bring about regression in many patients.

The strong relation between programme adherence and lesion changes showed that most patients needed to follow the lifestyle programme as prescribed to show regression. Those who made the greatest changes showed the biggest improvement. Since degree of stenosis change was correlated with extent of lifestyle change across its whole range, small changes in lifestyle may slow the progression of atherosclerosis, whereas substantial changes in lifestyle may be required to halt or reverse coronary atherosclerosis.

The 5 women in our study (1 experimental group, 4 control group) were the notable exceptions. All 5 made only moderate lifestyle changes, yet all showed overall regression. All 5 were postmenopausal, and none was taking exogenous oestrogens. The 4 women in the control group showed more regression than any of the men in that group, even though some men made greater lifestyle changes. Although the numbers are small, these findings suggest the possibility that gender may affect progression and regression of atherosclerosis. Further studies may determine whether women can reverse coronary atherosclerosis with more moderate lifestyle changes than men.

5 men in the control group showed very slight regression of atherosclerosis. These patients exercised more often, for longer periods, and consumed fewer calories and less cholesterol than the control-group patients who showed progression of atherosclerosis.

We found that the severely stenosed lesions showed the greatest improvement. Although the opposite of what we expected, the finding is important since more severely stenosed lesions are the most important clinically. More work is needed to determine the extent to which the relation between change and initial site of lesions is affected by the phenomenon of regression to the mean.

Increasing evidence supports the roles of diet, exercise, emotional stress, and smoking in the pathogenesis of coronary heart disease,[16–18] but until lately evidence for regression of coronary atherosclerosis was limited or anecdotal. There are case-reports of regression involving femoral[19] and renal arteries,[20] and one case-report of spontaneous regression in a coronary artery.[21] However, several studies have found that regression of coronary atherosclerosis can occur spontaneously in the absence of lifestyle changes or treatment with drugs,[22–24] thereby making it necessary for intervention trials to be controlled. Only two other randomised, controlled trials showing regression of coronary atherosclerosis have been reported,[22,23,25] and both used cholesterol-lowering drugs as the primary interventions.

Some important questions remain unanswered. Can these comprehensive lifestyle changes be sustained in larger populations of patients with coronary heart disease? The point of our study was to determine what is true, not what is practicable. The adherence measures and the angiographic findings suggest that adherence to this lifestyle programme needs to be very good for overall regression to occur, although more moderate changes have some beneficial effects. Further research will be necessary to determine the relative contribution of each component of the lifestyle programme and the mechanisms of changes in coronary atherosclerosis. It would be interesting to examine the effects of lifestyle changes in a larger sample of postmenopausal women with coronary atherosclerosis. Also, direct comparison of intensive lifestyle changes with pharmacological or surgical interventions would be interesting. Our trial suggests that comprehensive lifestyle changes may begin to reverse coronary atherosclerosis in only a year.

Acknowledgements

This study was supported by grants from the National Heart, Lung, and Blood Institute of the National Institutes of Health (RO1 HL42554), the Department of Health Services of the State of California (no 1256SC-01), Gerald D. Hines Interests, Houston Endowment Inc, the Henry J. Kaiser Family Foundation, the John E. Fetzer Institute, Continental Airlines, the Enron Foundation, the Nathan Cummings Foundation, the Pritzker Foundation, the First Boston Corporation, Quaker Oats Co., Texas Commerce Bank, Corrine and David Gould, Pacific Presbyterian Medical Center Foundation, General Growth Companies, Arthur Andersen and Co., and others.

Investigators who took part in the trial include: administrator, Myrna Melling; counsellors, Pamela Lea Byrne, Carol Naber; stress management instructor, Mary Dale Scheller; exercise instructors, Terri Merrit, Lawrence Spann, Sarah Spann; chefs, Celeste Burwell, Mary Carroll, Carol Connell, Jean-Marc Fullsack, Mark Hall, Jules Stenzel; quantitative angiography analysers, Dale Jones, Yvonne Stuart; head angiography nurses, LaVeta Luce, Geogie Hesse; angiographers, Craig Brandman, Bruce Brent, Ralph Clark, Keith Cohn, James Cullen, Richard Francoz, Gabriel Gregoratos, Lester Jacobsen, Roy Meyer, Gene Shafton, Brian Strunk, Anne Thorson; radiologists Robert Bernstein, Myron Marx, Gerald Needleman, John Wack; lipid laboratory directors, Washington Burns, John Kane, Steve Kunitake; medical liaison, Patricia McKenna; research assistants, Patricia Chung, Stephen Sparler; secretaries, Claire Finn, Kathy Rainbird.

References

1. Arntzenius AC. Regression of atherosclerosis. Presented at the Second International Conference on Preventive Cardiology, Washington, DC, June, 1989.
2. Ornish DM, Gotto AM, Miller RR, et al. Effects of a vegetarian diet and selected yoga techniques in the treatment of coronary heart disease. *Clin Res* 1979; **27**: 720A.
3. Ornish DM, Scherwitz LW, Doody RS, et al. Effects of stress management training and dietary changes in treating ischemic heart disease. *JAMA* 1983; **249**: 54–59.
4. Gould KL. Identifying and measuring severity of coronary artery stenosis. Quantitative coronary arteriography and positron emission tomography. *Circulation* 1988; **78**: 237–45.
5. Current status of blood cholesterol measurement in clinical laboratories in the US: a report from the Laboratory Standardization Panel of the National Cholesterol Education Program. *Clin Chem* 1988; **34**: 193.
6. Kane JP, Sata T, Hamilton RK, Havel RJ. Apoprotein composition of very low density lipoproteins of human serum. *J Clin Invest* 1975; **56**: 1622–34.
7. Stuff JE, Garza C, Smith EO, et al. A comparison of dietary methods in nutritional studies. *Am J Clin Nutr* 1983; **37**: 300–06.
8. Benowitz NL. Pharmacologic aspects of cigarette smoking and nicotine addiction. *N Engl J Med* 1988; **319**: 1318–30.
9. Ornish DM. Reversing heart disease. New York: Random House, 1990.
10. Patel C, North WR. Randomised controlled trial of yoga and biofeedback in management of hypertension. *Lancet* 1975; **ii**: 93–95.
11. Patel C, Marmot MG, Terry DJ, Carruthers M, Hunt B, Patel M. Trial of relaxation in reducing coronary risk: four year follow up. *Br Med J* 1985; **290**: 1103–06.
12. Benson H, Rosner BA, Marzetta BR, Klemchuk HM. Decreased blood pressure in pharmacologically treated hypertensive patients who regularly elicited the relaxation response. *Lancet* 1974; **i**: 289–91.
13. American College of Sports Medicine, Guidelines for exercise testing and prescription. Philadelphia: Lea & Febiger, 1986.
14. Orth-Gomer K, Unden AL, Edwards ME. Social isolation and mortality in ischemic heart disease. *Acta Med Scand* 1988; **224**: 205–15.
15. Dixon WS, ed, et al. BMDP3V statistical software, 1983 printing with additions. Berkeley: University of California Press, 1983.
16. Kornitzer M, DeBacker G, Dramaix M, et al. Belgian heart disease prevention project: incidence and mortality results. *Lancet* 1983; **i**: 1066–70.
17. Kaplan JR, Manuck SB, Clarkson TB, et al. Social stress and atherosclerosis in normocholesterolemic monkeys. *Science* 1983; **220**: 733–35.
18. US Department of Health and Human Services. Reducing the health consequences of smoking: 25 years of progress. A report of the Surgeon General. Washington DC: DHHS Publication # (CDC) 89-8411, 1989.
19. Barndt R, Blankenhorn DH, Crawford DW, et al. Regression and progression of early femoral atherosclerosis in treated hyperlipoproteinemic patients. *Ann Intern Med* 1977; **86**: 139–46.
20. Basta LL, Williams C, Kioschos JM. Regression of atherosclerotic stenosing

lesions of the renal arteries and spontaneous cure of systemic hypertension through control of hyperlipidemia. *Am J Med* 1976; **61**: 420–23.

21. Roth D, Kostuk WJ. Noninvasive and invasive demonstration of spontaneous regression of coronary artery disease. *Circulation* 1980; **62**: 888–96.

22. Blankenhorn DH, Nessim SA, Johnson RL, et al. Beneficial effects of combined colestipol-niacin therapy on coronary atherosclerosis and coronary venous bypass grafts. *JAMA* 1987; **257**: 3233–40.

23. Brown BG, Lin JT, Schaefer SM, et al. Niacin or lovastatin, combined with colestipol, regress coronary atherosclerosis and prevent clinical events in men with elevated apolipoprotein B. *Circulation* 1989; **80**: II–266.

24. Brown BG, Bolson EL, Dodge HT Arteriographic assessment of coronary atherosclerosis. Review of current methods, their limitations, and clinical applications. *Arteriosclerosis* 1982; **2**: 2–15.

25. Blankenhorn DH, Johnson RL, El Zein HA, et al. Dietary fat influences human coronary lesion formation. *Circulation* 1988; **78** (suppl II): 11.

Index